Vulvar Pain

Alessandra Graziottin • Filippo Murina

Vulvar Pain

From Childhood to Old Age

Springer

Alessandra Graziottin
Center of Gynecology and Medical Sexology
San Raffaele Resnati Hospital
Milan
Italy

Filippo Murina
Lower Genital Tract Disease Unit
V. Buzzi Hospital
University of Milan
Milan
Italy

ISBN 978-3-319-82635-6 ISBN 978-3-319-42677-8 (eBook)
DOI 10.1007/978-3-319-42677-8

Softcover reprint of the hardcover 1st edition 2017

Printed on acid-free paper

This Springer imprint is published by Springer Nature
The registered company is Springer International Publishing AG
The registered company address is Gewerbestrasse 11, 6330 Cham, Switzerland

Preface

Why a Book About Vulvar Pain?

The vulva has been a most neglected organ, from the medical point of view, until recently. Symptoms related to it have been largely underreported by women ("too intimate to be spoken of"), underinvestigated, and undertreated by physicians. In the last two decades, the problem of a "mysterious" pain referred to the vestibulum of the vagina or the entire vulva has been increasingly investigated. The currently defined "provoked vestibulodynia" (formerly called "vulvar vestibulitis") and "vulvodynia" are now undergoing intense scrutiny: their characteristics of chronic up to neuropathic vulvar pain are now familiar to an increasing number of gynecologists and healthcare providers (HCPs).

Unfortunately, today every vulvar pain is labeled as "vestibulodynia" and "vulvodynia," i.e., as neuropathic, which is not the case.

Women may have different types of pain perceived from or referred to the vulvar organ: acute, chronic, and pathologic/neuropathic. Time is not the only defining criteria. The second criterion implies a (partly) different pathophysiology of pain and the progressive involvement of the brain in the pain-generating and pain-perceiving dynamics. A solid neuropathological process underlies and determines its psychological and relational correlates. Acute vulvar pain may become chronic, but not necessarily neuropathic. Location of pain within the vulvar organ is the third defining criterion: it can be located at the entrance of the vagina (vestibular pain), with a focus around the urethra (urethral pain), in the clitoris (clitoral pain), or perceived in a part of or the entire vulva (vulvar pain). Only when the neuropathic component is there, the suffix "dynia" is appropriate: the pertinent name then becomes vestibulodynia, clitorodynia, vulvodynia, and urethrodynia, when the "burning" pain is perceived in and around the urethra as well. Immediate and appropriate diagnosis, cure, and care of acute vulvar pain would prevent its becoming chronic and, even worse, neuropathic.

Is vulvar pain a marginal, rare, "niche" symptom? No, many women have this intimate problem, acute vulvar pain, chronic vulvar pain, and neuropathic vulvar pain, defined as vulvodynia, as it is termed in medical words. Vulvodynia alone may affect 12–15 % of women: it is therefore a common disorder that every family doctor and every gynecologist see every day, in his/her routine work.

The first good reason to write – and read – this book is that vulvar pain *is frequent*, much more frequent than ever considered, and yet it remains *unaddressed* for years. Indeed, this genital pain specifically affecting the vulva is *neglected* by the majority of physicians, because it is perceived as difficult to address or as being "psychogenic" in nature and therefore more of an issue for psychologists than medical doctors. Contrary to this obsolete view, *vulvar pain* is a disorder with *solid biological etiologies* that are absolutely in the domain of a medical diagnosis and treatment. Psychosexual contributors and consequences are certainly relevant and should be accurately considered from the diagnostic and therapeutic point of view. However, pain and the underlying inflammation are first of all powerful biological signals that must be investigated, respected in their physical relevance, and appropriately addressed as first and absolute priority.

Yes, like all types of pain, vulvar pain can be *multifactorial*. As it is appropriate in every medical field, the diagnosis requires careful listening to the woman's *symptoms*, an accurate reading of vulvar pain's *pathophysiology*, a competent *physical examination* focused on detecting all the clinical signs, and a renewed attention to the frequent *comorbidities* (medical and sexual) with which vulvar pain can be associated.

There are *medical* comorbidities, as vulvar pain may be associated with *bladder symptoms* (postcoital cystitis, urethralgia/urethrodynia, painful bladder syndrome), *endometriosis*, *irritable bowel syndrome*, *fibromyalgia*, and *headache*, to quote the most frequent, and *sexual comorbidities*: *coital pain, or painful intercourse*, at the entrance of the vagina ("introital dyspareunia") is the leading symptom, with its cohort of secondary loss of desire, vaginal dryness, orgasmic difficulties, postcoital cystitis, and sexual dissatisfaction that can deeply affect a couple's relationship. In the current passion for renaming symptoms and comorbidities, genito-pelvic pain penetration disorder (GPPPD) is the definition of choice. However, in the dialogue with patients, a more simple "pain during or after intercourse" is to be preferred.

The clinical method for addressing pain of any kind is familiar to every physician: it simply requires a specific focus on the vulvar area, with a specially sensitive and gentle approach. Why? Because *vulvar pain involves the most secret part of the body*: the vulva and the introitus of the vagina. Sometimes it may be difficult to disclose the problem even to the most intimate friends.

The most exciting goal of this book is to increase the awareness of women and healthcare providers on this undisputable fact: *vulvar pain is real*, *is frequent*, *and has very solid biological contributors*. For some specialists, like pediatricians, it is so unknown that even the word "vulvar pain" is not used. Only a most generic and imprecise "genital pain" is reported in the medical records. And this is the same for the female genital mutilation/cutting. FGM/C causes excruciating vulvar pain for obvious reasons – the extremely rich nerve network of the vulva – and yet is (almost) never mentioned as such in the huge existing literature.

On the positive side, *curing vulvar pain may be extremely rewarding*, as it can offer to affected women the real chance to get back to their full well-being, with an intimate satisfying life and the possibility to make love again with passion and joy.

This is a practical book: its primary goal is to ease the way to a proper diagnosis and treatment for every physician motivated to really help women presenting with genital/vulvar pain. Yes, a physician's life is professionally too busy. We all have too little time to stay up to date, and we all need concise, distilled information, in order to get rapidly to the essence of a true clinical picture. Even more importantly, we need *practical suggestions* to be used in our *daily practice*: *a practice-based-evidence perspective*, supported, when appropriate, by a distilled, concise evidence-based medicine. The practical vision that inspired this book is based on the huge clinical experience of the two authors, distilled over decades of daily clinical commitment to help women desperate because of vulvar pain, sexual pain disorders, and associated comorbidities, with hundreds of women successfully treated, getting back to a painless, more fulfilling life.

In conclusion, this book is first of all *a call for awareness* on the many types and characteristics of vulvar pain in the lifespan, from childhood (when even the wording is nonexistent) to the late postmenopausal years. Areas of unbelievable neglect include vulvar pain after childbirth and the dramatic situation of female genital mutilation/cutting (FGM/C), where every genital symptom is reported except vulvar pain, in spite of the fact that it is exactly the vulva that is mutilated.

Physicians are therefore required *to open their mind to the existence of vulvar pain*, to its different time and site-related characteristics, etiology, pathophysiology, and diagnostic and treatment perspectives.

In short, we have a dream: *to empower physicians' competence in rapidly addressing vulvar pain and its associated comorbidities*. The sooner, the better. Women would be most grateful. And their families too. A healthier and happier woman is a gift to herself, her family, and our society.

Milan, Italy

Alessandra Graziottin, MD
Filippo Murina, MD

Acknowledgments

To our families, for their love, patience, and proud support.

To our patients, for their encouragement for this book, their endless source of inspiration through smart and challenging questions, and their empowering gratitude when vulvar pain fades away and they are back to enjoy a healthier and more fulfilling life.

To our colleagues, who welcomed the former book on vulvodynia and stimulate the rethinking of a broader teaching and learning project on *vulvar pain in the lifespan*.

To the publisher, for the encouraging trust in a writing project more demanding than originally thought.

To the beauty of life, when the happy smile of a woman finally rid of pain gives motivation and meaning to the daily work of every committed healthcare provider. A real blessing that is a deep pleasure to share with our readers.

Contents

Vulvar Pain: What's Behind a Name

1

"Vulvar pain" is a comprehensive term. Its main characteristics are described in Box 1.1.

Box 1.1. Vulvar Pain: Key Descriptors

Acute Vulvar Pain

- Is referred to the *vulvar organ*, or part of it:
  - The vulvar vestibule (*vestibular pain*)
  - The clitoris (*clitoral pain*)
  - Localized vulvar pain in parts other than the vestibule or the clitoris (*localized vulvar pain*), i.e., affecting the left labia majora or right labia minora, or the Bartholin gland (Bartolinitis)
  - The entire vulva (*vulvar pain*)
- Has a *precise*, *objective etiology*, *easy to be visualized*, *described*, and *recorded*
- *Acute tissue inflammation* is the *common denominator*, resulting, among others, from:
  - *A trauma*:
    - *Unintentional*, such as blunt lesions during sport or accidental falls, cutting, and burning, among others
    - *Intentional*, including sexual abuse and female genital mutilations/modifications (FGM/M)
  - *Infections*, such as in *Candida* vulvitis, in herpes virus, and in pyogenic abscesses or parasitic infections
  - *Acute nerve traumas*, such as mechanical traumas
  - *An iatrogenic damage*:
    - *Chemical*, during topical treatment with immunomodulants, or chemotherapy
    - *Physical*, such as after laser therapy, diathermocoagulation, and radiotherapy

A. Graziottin, F. Murina, *Vulvar Pain*, DOI 10.1007/978-3-319-42677-8_1

    - *Surgical, during episiotomy/episiorrhaphy, vulvar surgery* (excisional or not), and "*cosmetic*" vulvar interventions
  - A *painful acute skin disease*
- *It is a defensive, alerting response* to an acute damage, unintentional or intentional, to the vulvar region and organ:
  - *Nociceptive*, i.e., a sign of an ongoing acute damage
  - *A* "friend signal," in some ways, indicating the urgent need to withdraw from the cause of pain, understanding, and treating it
- It can be *continuous or remitting, constant,* or have *a circadian rhythm.*
- Acute vulvar nociceptive pain is usually *worse at night.*
- *Objective findings* include:
  - *Vulvar skin and mucosa turning red*
  - *Vulvar edema/swelling*
  - *Vulvar increase in temperature*
  - *Vulvar pain, spontaneous or provoked at gentle touching*
  - *Impaired functions*, including sexual symptoms (Graziottin 2009), cosmetic functions, and impossibility to behaviors such as stay seated or wearing tight trousers
- *Response to treatment*:
  - In acute vulvar pain, *removal of the damaging agent* and treatment of the lesions should *resolve/restore normal vulvar cytoarchitecture and function, with or without scars.*

Key Point

The *acute inflammation* underlying *acute vulvar pain* has three main characteristics. It is:

- *Resolving*, i.e., finalized to restore the return to normality in terms of vulvar cytoarchitecture, anatomy, and function
- *Limited in time*, usually within 3 months from the onset of traumatic agent
- *Limited in intensity*, adequate and proportionate to cope with the ongoing tissue insult

Chronic Vulvar Pain

- *Time* is the leading differentiating criteria: vulvar pain is defined as *chronic* when it persists more than 3–6 *months*, still maintaining most of the abovementioned characteristics.
- *Inflammation* shifts progressively from physiologic to pathologic and tends to become "anarchic," non-resolving, and of increasing and disproportionate severity (Graziottin et al. 2013, 2014, 2015; Graziottin and Gambini 2016).

Pathologic/Neuropathic Vulvar Pain

- *Pain progressively becomes a* "disease per se": symptoms of vulvar pain are included within the "dynia" *group*:
  - *Vestibulodynia*, when pain is referred to the vestibule
  - *Clitorodynia*, where pain is referred to the clitoris
  - *Vulvodynia*, where pain can be referred to part of it (*localized vulvodynia*) or to the entire organ (*generalized vulvodynia*)
- *The vulvar skin and mucosal damage are no more objectively identifiable*:
  - *Peripheral inflammatory signs gradually disappear.*
  - *Central involvement of the CNS* (*neuroinflammation*) *becomes prominent*, the common denominator of all types of pain becoming neuropathic (Haanpää et al. 2011; Hampson et al. 2013; Regauer et al. 2015; Schaible 2015).
- *Vestibulodynia, clitoridynia, or vulvodynia* can be spontaneous or provoked, with a remitting or persisting course.
- Neuropathic vulvar pain usually *disappears during night sleep.*
- *Inflammation becomes pathologic and self-maintained* by the upregulation of the immunitary system (with mast cells and microglia leading the pathophysiologic immunitary response) and the pain system (Graziottin et al. 2013, 2014, 2015; Graziottin and Gambini 2016). It is:
  - *Not finalized, i.e., non-resolving.*
  - *Persistent, chronic.*
  - *Of variable intensity.*
  - *Highly sensible to stressors*, physical and emotional. They can upregulate the central inflammatory process with further worsening of the vulvar pain perception.
- *Treatment* of *neuropathic vulvar pain/vulvodynia* and its subtypes is therefore oriented at *modulating the CNS components of vulvar pain*, while keeping attention to persistent vulvar trigger of pain, when present:
  - *Relaxation of the tightened, hyperactive pelvic floor*, either primarily or in response to the persisting pain, is a critical part of an effective treatment.
  - *Avoidance of penetrative vaginal intercourse is essential*, to avoid further microtraumas of the vulnerable introital mucosa, until vulvar pain is adequately addressed.
  - *Antalgic peripheral treatment* with temporary, periodic block of the Walter ganglion can be reserved to cases resisting to the standard treatment.

The goal of this chapter is to alert clinicians to devote more attention to this (still) neglected organ, the vulva, and to the leading symptom affecting it: pain, in the lifespan.

The rich innervation of the "vulvar organ" makes the vulvar pain particularly troublesome and invalidating. Its localization and multiple functions have complex implications on different aspects of the woman's daily living. Its peculiar emotional significance further potentiates the meaning and impact of vulvar pain. The vulva's leading role in intimate seduction and erotic pleasure makes even more challenging and troubling the shift from pleasure to invalidating pain (Graziottin 2006; Graziottin et al. 2015; Graziottin and Gambini 2016).

Its leading role in the woman's and couple's sexuality gives to vulvar pain a (still) unappreciated potential for disrupting and devastating women's and couple' lives. Healthcare providers (HCPs) should therefore consider the vulva, related sexual and nonsexual symptoms, and associated comorbidities, with the highest clinical diagnostic and therapeutic attention and care.

1.1 How to Diagnose Vulvar Pain in the Clinical Setting

The field of vulvar pain is pervaded by a dramatic nosographic and diagnostic confusion. Vulvar pain is credited to be either a "nonexistent," just a psychogenic invention, all created "in the woman's head," or a *mysterious symptom*, included *tout court* under the modern umbrella of "vulvodynia/vestibulodynia." The first goal of this section is to summarize in a structured and hopefully clear-cut nosography the different characteristics of vulvar pain (Box 1.1).

Different characteristics of vulvar pain have been "polarized" under three major headings:

- *Acute vulvar pain*, essentially *nociceptive*, with:
  - Prominent *vulvar-focused inflammation*
  - *Finalized to resolve the inflammation and the tissue damage*
  - *Duration* less than 3 months
  - *Intensity* appropriate to restore the normal tissue cytoarchitecture
- *Chronic vulvar pain*, where inflammation tends to:
  - Progressively involve neighbor organs ("pelvic comorbidity").
  - Be not finalized to resolve and heal the wound.
  - *Last more than 3–6 months.*
  - *Have an intensity disproportionate with respect to the damaging factor.*
  - Progress to the *central nervous system* (CNS), with *neuroinflammation*, involving as well *neurons and microglia*. This latter's role shifts gradually from a neuroplastic, protective role toward neurons to a neurotoxic, damaging activity (Haanpää et al. 2011; Hampson et al. 2013; Regauer et al. 2015; Schaible 2015).
- *Pathologic/neuropathic vulvar pain*:
  - Where pain progressively becomes a disease per se. Conditions where the etiology of pain is "invisible" to the clinical examining eyes are included within the "dynia" group:
    - *Vestibulodynia*, when pain is referred to the vulvar vestibule
    - *Clitorodynia*, where pain is referred to the clitoris

- *Vulvodynia*, where pain can be referred to part of it (*localized vulvodynia*) or to the entire organ (*generalized vulvodynia*) (*spontaneous or provoked*) (Bornstein et al. 2016)

Vulvodynia was first described by Thomas in 1880 as hyperesthesia of the vulva, that is, "excessive sensibility of the nerves supplying the mucous membrane of some portion of the vulva."

In 2015, the International Society for the Study of Vulvovaginal Disease, the International Society for the Study of Women's Sexual Health, and the International Pelvic Pain Society revised the current terminology of vulvar pain, on the basis of the significant increase in high-quality etiologic studies published in the last decade (Bornstein et al. 2016).

A section called "Vulvar pain caused by a specific disorder" was introduced. This section contains vulvar pain conditions for which a cause can be clearly identified:

- Infectious (e.g., recurrent candidiasis, herpes)
- Inflammatory (e.g., lichen sclerosus, lichen planus)
- Neoplastic (e.g., Paget disease, squamous cell carcinoma)
- Neurologic (e.g., postherpetic neuralgia, nerve compression or injury, neuroma)
- Trauma (e.g., female genital cutting, obstetrical)
- Iatrogenic (e.g., postoperative, chemotherapy, radiation)
- Hormonal deficiencies (e.g., genitourinary syndrome of menopause)

Other factors, however, may not be as clearly associated with the pain; hence, the second section of the definition is "Vulvodynia: vulvar pain of at least 3 months' duration, without clear identifiable cause, which may have potential associated factors."

The consensus development process identified several important factors potentially associated with vulvodynia. They may be clinically prominent and may help in choosing further evaluation methods or a treatment path:

- Comorbidities and other pain syndromes (e.g., painful bladder syndrome)
- Genetics
- Hormonal factors (e.g., pharmacologically induced)
- Inflammation (level of evidence 2)
- Musculoskeletal (e.g., pelvic muscle overactivity, myofascial, biomechanical)
- Central neurologic mechanisms (spine, brain)
- Peripheral: neuroproliferation
- Psychosocial factors (e.g., mood, interpersonal, coping, role, sexual function)

Key Point

The critical pathophysiologic change from acute vulvar pain to chronic to pathologic/neuropathic is that neuroinflammation, within the CNS, takes the leadership of the pain process that gradually becomes "a disease per se."

Gradual *attenuation/disappearance of the peripheral vulvar objective signs of inflammation* ("You have nothing") is substituted by a progressively challenging *inflammatory involvement of the brain*, with two major consequences:

- *A neurogenic inflammation in the peripheral organ*, the vulva in this case.
- *A neurogenic inflammation within the brain*. It further maintains and worsens the pain scenario and symptomatology (Graziottin et al. 2013, 2014; Xanthos et al. 2011; Xanthos and Sandkühler 2014; Walker et al. 2013; Graziottin and Gambini 2016; Watson and Sandroni 2016).

The differences highlighted in the box have been "polarized" for the sake of clarity, to ease the clinician to have in mind a clear-cut scenario. In real life, the shifting from acute to chronic to neuropathic, in more unfortunate challenging cases, can be more gradual and insidious.

Understanding and describing the *precise characteristics of pain in the individual consulting woman* is essential for a number of reasons:

- A precise diagnosis is essential to plan a successful treatment.
- The pessimistic labeling of every type of vulvar pain within the "dynia," neuropathic group, gives the woman, and her family, the sense of having an "untreatable" disease. This may have three very *negative emotional consequences*:
  - *Trigger reactive depression and potentiate anxiety*, both powerful potentiators of pain perception
  - *Predispose the woman to accept any type of* "solution," including surgery ("vestibulectomy"), which is not the appropriate answer in the vast majority of cases
  - *Induce or worsen catastrophism*, the most negative coping attitude a patient can have toward pain

Conclusion

The description of different types of vulvar pain is kept very "dry" on purpose, to maintain the core message. Details of vulvar pain will be discussed in every chapter, where more appropriate.

References

Bornstein J, Goldstein AT, Stockdale CK, Bergeron S, Pukall C, Zolnoun D, Coady D. 2015 ISSVD, ISSWSH, and IPPS consensus terminology and classification of persistent vulvar pain and vulvodynia. J Sex Med. 2016;13:607–12.

Graziottin A. Sexual pain disorders: dyspareunia and vaginismus. In: Porst H, Buvat J, editors. ISSM (International Society of Sexual Medicine) standard committee book, standard practice in sexual medicine. Oxford, UK: Blackwell; 2006. p. 342–50.

Graziottin A. Mast cells and their role in sexual pain disorders. In: Goldstein A, Pukall C, Goldstein I, editors. Female sexual pain disorders: evaluation and management. Chichester: Blackwell Publishing; 2009. p. 176–9.

Graziottin A, Gambini D. Evaluation of genito-pelvic pain penetration disorder. In: Waguih WI, editor. The textbook of sexual medicine. Philadelphia: Springer Verlag; 2016.

Graziottin A, Skaper S, Fusco M. Inflammation and chronic pelvic pain: a biological trigger for depression in women? J Depress Anxiety. 2013;3:142–50.

Graziottin A, Skaper S, Fusco M. Mast cells in chronic inflammation, pelvic pain and depression in women. Gynecol Endocrinol. 2014;30(7):472–7.

Graziottin A, Gambini D, Bertolasi L. Genital and sexual pain in women In: Vodusek D. Boller F, editors. Neurology of sexual and bladder disorders. Handbook of clinical neurology, vol. 130, 3rd Series, Edinburgh: Elsevier, 2015, p. 395–412

Haanpää M, Attal N, Backonja M, Baron R, Bennett M, Bouhassira D, Cruccu G, Hansson P, Haythornthwaite JA, Iannetti GD, Jensen TS, Kauppila T, Nurmikko TJ, Rice AS, Rowbotham M, Serra J, Sommer C, Smith BH, Treede RD. NeuPSIG guidelines on neuropathic pain assessment. Pain. 2011;152(1):14–27. doi:10.1016/j.pain.2010.07.031. Epub 2010 Sep 19.

Hampson JP, Reed BD, Clauw DJ, et al. Augmented central pain processing in vulvodynia. J Pain. 2013;14:579–89.

Regauer S, Eberz B, Beham-Schmid C. Mast cell infiltrates in vulvodynia represent secondary and idiopathic mast cell hyperplasias. APMIS. 2015;123:452–6.

Schaible HG. Emerging concepts of pain therapy based on neuronal mechanisms. Handb Exp Pharmacol. 2015;227:1–14.

Walker AK, Kavelaars A, Heijnen CJ, Dantzer R. Neuroinflammation and comorbidity of pain and depression. Pharmacol Rev. 2013;66(1):80–101.

Watson JC, Sandroni P. Central neuropathic pain syndromes. Mayo Clin Proc. 2016;91(3):372–85.

Xanthos DN, Sandkühler J. Neurogenic neuroinflammation: inflammatory CNS reactions in response to neuronal activity. Nat Rev Neurosci. 2014;15(1):43–53. doi:10.1038/nrn3617. Epub 2013 Nov 27.

Xanthos DN, Gaderer S, Drdla R, Nuro E, Abramova A, Ellmeier W, Sandkühler J. Central nervous system mast cells in peripheral inflammatory nociception. Mol Pain. 2011;7:42. doi:10.1186/1744-8069-7-42.

2 Epidemiology of Vulvar Pain

Vulvar pain is a very common problem that affects women of all age groups. Too often, women endure pain and sexual dysfunction for years without an adequate definitive diagnosis. They are desperate for help, looking for every type of medical and alternative treatment and regularly self-treat, wasting a lot of money a year in disappointing/frustrating consultations, anti-yeast creams, and other over-the-counter treatments.

The incidence of vulvar pain has increased over the past three decades. The reason is twofold: on one hand, there is certainly *greater awareness* about vulvar pain, which is increasingly reported to healthcare providers (HCPs), and on the other hand, there is a *real increase of etiologic factors* (please see the Chaps. 3 and 6).

Among the most frequent, physicians should consider the *Candida vaginitis epidemic*, secondary to the *antibiotic abuse* and to the increase in *dismetabolic diseases*, *diabetes* first. Diabetes can triple Candida vaginitis and other infections, such as recurrent cystitis from the uropathogenic *Escherichia coli* (UPEC), so frequently comorbid with provoked vestibulodynia, up to 60 % in the Salonia et al. series (2013).

Nevertheless, vulvar pain is not a recent diagnosis.

As early as 1874, T. Galliard Thomas wrote: "This disorder, although fortunately not very frequent, is by no means very rare" (Thomas 1874). He went on to express "surprise" that it had not been "more generally and fully described." Despite the focus Thomas directed to the issue, vulvar pain did not get much attention until the twenty-first century, when a number of studies began to gauge its prevalence. With the foundation of the International Society for the Study of Vulvovaginal Disease in the 1970s, interest and research in vulvar pain and other vulvar conditions increased.

The prevalence of isolated pain syndromes causing vulvar pain is difficult to estimate because of the private nature of this symptom, the lack of widespread knowledge among healthcare providers about vulvar pain disorders, and the belief, by some women, that vulvar or sexual pain of some extent is normal.

A. Graziottin, F. Murina, *Vulvar Pain*, DOI 10.1007/978-3-319-42677-8_2

2.1 Dyspareunia: A Red Alert to Vestibular Pain

Coital pain at the entrance of the vagina ("introital dyspareunia") has been relatively more investigated in comparison to vulvar pain. It can be considered the sexual correlate of vestibular pain. Its prevalence can therefore indirectly suggest the likely prevalence of vestibular pain, at least to some extent.

Latthe et al. (2006) identified 54 studies that specifically assessed dyspareunia. The reported prevalence rates of dyspareunia ranged widely, from 1 % in Sweden to 46 % in one US study. By restricting the review to the 18 well-designed studies with representative samples, prevalence rates ranged from 8 to 22 % (Latthe et al. 2006).

In the Study on Women's Health Across the Nation (SWAN) (Avis et al. 2005), 17 % percent of premenopausal women complain of constant or occasional coital pain, compared with 24 % of postmenopausal women.

In the classic epidemiological study of Laumann et al. (1999) in the USA, carried out among women aged 18–55, 21 % report dyspareunia. In an older cohort of sexually active women, aged 57–85, dyspareunia was reported in 10.5 % (Laumann et al. 2008).

A European survey, carried out on 2467 women aged 18–70 in UK, France, Germany, and Italy, through validated questionnaires, found that the prevalence of dyspareunia was 14 % (Graziottin 2007).

Overall the most frequent prevalence figures range between 10 and 20 %.

2.2 Vulvar Pain in the Lifespan

2.2.1 Vulvar Pain in Childhood

Different etiologies may contribute to vulvar pain in prepubertal girls (please see the Chap. 4).

- *Traumatic* unintentional *accidental lesions of the vulva* in childhood usually cause acute, intense, excruciating vulvar pain, given the extremely rich innervation of the area.
- Pediatric genital injuries represented 0.6 % of all pediatric injuries. The mean age at injury was 7.1 years old and was distributed 56.6 % girls and 43.4 % boys. A total of 43.3 % had lacerations and 42.2 % had contusions/abrasions. The majority of injuries occurred at home (65.9 %), and the majority of patients (94.7 %) were treated and released from the hospital. The most common consumer products associated with pediatric genital trauma were bicycles (14.7 % of all pediatric genital injuries), bathtubs (5.8 %), daywear (5.6 %), monkey bars (5.4 %), and toilets (4.0 %) (Casey et al. 2013).
- Traumatic *intentional* vulvar lesions
  - *Sexual abuse*. Every year, about 4–16 % of children are physically abused, and one in ten is neglected or psychologically abused. During childhood,

between 5 and 10 % of girls and up to 5 % of boys are exposed to penetrative sexual abuse, causing severe genital (and vulvar!) pain. Up to three times this number are exposed to any type of sexual abuse. However, official rates for substantiated child maltreatment indicate less than a tenth of this burden (Gilbert et al. 2009; Bailhache et al. 2013).

 - *Female genital mutilation/cutting* (*FGM/C*) is defined by the World Health Organization (WHO) as "all procedures that involve partial or total removal of the external female genitalia or other injury to the female genital organs for non-medical reasons" (WHO 2008) (please see the Chap. 5). Worldwide, an estimated 125–140 million girls and women live with FGM/C. The long-term gynecologic and obstetric outcomes of FGM/C include significantly increased risks of urinary tract infections (unadjusted RR = 3.01), bacterial vaginosis (adjusted OR (AOR) = 1.68), dyspareunia (RR = 1.53), prolonged labor (AOR = 1.49), caesarean section (AOR = 1.60), and difficult delivery (AOR = 1.88). Unfortunately *vulvar pain is not mentioned* in spite of the fact that the violent cutting trauma on the vulvar tissue causes excruciating acute pain and potential long-lasting consequences.
   Only a few recently published clinical cases report vulvar epidermoid inclusion cysts, with inguinal (Birge et al. 2015) and/or acute vulvar pain (Gudu 2014), and the first case of neuropathic pain with sensory neuropathy has been published in June 2015 (Hadid and Dahan 2015).

- *Lichen sclerosus* (LS), the most relevant vulvar dermatosis, is an inflammatory dermatologic condition of autoimmune etiology, usually affecting the anogenital area in both sexes. Less than 10 % occurrence is reported elsewhere on the skin (Murphy 2010).
- LS has been reported in *all age groups* and *both sexes*. Most often it occurs in postmenopausal females, but:
  - Approximately *7–15 %* of all cases are found in *prepubertal females*, with a prevalence that has been reported to be 1 in 900–1100 (Lagerstedt et al. 2013).
  - A study on 44 Finnish girls diagnosed under the age of 19 with LS found a *mean age of onset of symptoms of 7 years*, and 86 % were prepubertal at the time of presentation (Lagerstedt et al. 2013).
  - *Recurrence rates* of prepubertal LS after medical therapy have been reported to range from *44 to 82 %* (Smith and Fischer 2009; Focseneanu et al. 2013).
  - Recent studies have shown that the symptoms and signs of the disease persist after puberty in the majority (75 %) of patients (Smith and Fischer 2009; Powell and Wojnarowska 2002).

Key Point
LS should be considered as a chronic autoimmune condition with intermittent symptoms (vulvar itching and pain first). Symptoms may recur in the lifespan even after appropriate treatment.

2.2.2 Vulvar Pain in Adolescents and Young Women

Prevalence studies focusing on adolescents under 20 years of age have not yet been carried out. Available studies include larger age cohorts, usually from 18 to 40 years of age. Reported prevalence varies across studies.

A self-administered questionnaires from 5440 women in Boston Metropolitan area (BMA) and 13,681 in Minneapolis/Saint Paul Metropolitan area (MSP), 18–40 years of age, described their history of vulvar burning or pain on contact that persisted >3 months and that limited/prevented intercourse (Harlow et al. 2014). The study indicates that by age of 40 years, *7–8 %* in BMA and MSP *reported vulvar pain consistent with vulvodynia*. Women of Hispanic origin compared to whites were 1.4 times more likely to develop vulvar pain symptoms (95 % confidence interval, 1.1–1.8). Many women in MSP (48 %) and BMA (30 %) never sought treatment, and *>50 % who sought care with known healthcare access received no diagnosis* (Harlow et al. 2014)!

The diagnostic neglect is even more likely in adolescents who have less access to medical facilities, less probability of being listened to with a caring diagnostic attention, less assertiveness toward healthcare providers (HCPs). Access to healthcare does not increase the likelihood of seeking (and finding!) care for chronic vulvar pain.

In a study on 1795 women participating in the Woman to Woman Health Study, a multiethnic population-based study, women who screened positive for depression had a 53 % higher prevalence of having vulvodynia (PR = 1.53; 95 % CI: 1.12, 2.10) compared with women who screened negative for depression. Women who screened positive for post-traumatic stress disorder (PTSD) had more than a twofold increase in the prevalence of having vulvodynia (PR = 2.37; 95 % CI: 1.07, 5.25) compared with women who screened negative for PTSD (Iglesias-Rios et al. 2015).

The increased prevalence of vulvodynia among those screening positive for depression or PTSD suggests that these disorders may contribute to the likelihood of reporting vulvodynia. Alternatively, vulvodynia, depression, and PTSD may have a common pathophysiologic and risk profile (Iglesias-Rios et al. 2015). The most pertinent hypothesis is that neuroinflammation associated with chronic vulvar pain and vulvodynia contributes to depression. Prospective studies are needed to improve our understanding of the temporal relation between mental health conditions and vulvar pain.

2.2.3 Vulvar Pain After Childbirth

The prevalence of vulvar pain and sexual dysfunction is high after childbirth and in the postpartum and puerperium periods, and data indicate that up to 86 % of women report one or more vulvar complain soon after delivery (Leeman and Rogers 2012) (please see the Chap. 7).

Dyspareunia and vaginal dryness frequently occur after childbirth and may independently contribute to a reduction in sexual drive, because of the negative feedback from the genitals.

The reported prevalence rates of perineal pain at 12–24 months postpartum range from 5 to 33 % (Williams et al. 2007).

In a prospective cohort study of 484 women, vaginal dryness, vaginal tightness, vaginal looseness, bleeding or irritation after sex, and loss of sexual desire were all reported as having significantly increased from 38 % before delivery to 64 % at 3 months postpartum. Within 6 months from delivery, 89 % of participants had resumed sexual activity. While significant improvements were noted in all of these parameters, they had not returned to predelivery levels (Barrett et al. 2000).

Postpartum genital and pelvic pain has also been shown to persist for longer than a year, particularly for women with a history of no genital chronic pain before childbirth (Paterson et al. 2009).

A recent Australian prospective study on 1507 nulliparous women indicates that prevalence of dyspareunia at 3, 6, 13, and 18 month is of 44, 45, 28, and 23 % respectively (McDonald et al. 2015). Lack of professional recognition and treatment of postpartum dyspareunia, and associated vestibular and/or vulvar pain, persists all over the world.

2.2.4 Vulvar Pain After Menopause

During menopause, women experience many physical changes caused by a decrease in estrogen and other hormones and the effects of aging.

In addition to vasomotor symptoms, sleep disturbances, and mood alterations, menopausal women experience an increase in vulvovaginal symptoms, like vulvar pain, burning, fissuring, irritation, dyspareunia, and urogenital symptoms (please see the Chap. 8).

The new term "genitourinary syndrome of menopause" (GSM), that combines the conditions of vulvovaginal atrophy (VVA) and urinary tract dysfunction, is now considered more appropriate.

It is important to note that most menopausal women remain sexually active after the menopause:

- In one study on 94,000 postmenopausal women 50–79 years of age, 52 % reported that they had been sexually active (McCall-Hosenfeld et al. 2008).
- A review of published literature revealed that 22 % of married women, 70–79 years of age, report that they still have sexual intercourse (Schneidewind-Skibbe et al. 2008).

Menopause-related genitourinary symptoms affect up to 50 % of midlife and older women. Their severity ranges from mild to debilitating. They are not limited to sexually active women (NAMS 2013; Parish et al. 2013).

The prevalence of vulvovaginal discomfort increased with the menopausal stage: in early perimenopause the prevalence is about 4 %, rising to 25 % one year after menopause and to 47 % three years after menopause (Dennerstein et al. 2000).

VVA remains underreported, underdiagnosed, and undertreated (please see the Chap. 8). General lack of communication about female sexual health issues has been noted in the clinical setting. It was found that postmenopausal women reported that only 19 % of healthcare professionals addressed their sexual lives, and only 13 % specifically raised the issue of genitourinary symptoms, despite the fact that 40 % of women expected their healthcare professional to initiate discussions related to menopausal symptoms (Kingsberg et al. 2013).

In a relevant online survey, less than half of US respondents were aware of available treatments (nonhormonal or hormonal) to improve vaginal discomfort (Gott and Hinchliff 2003).

These findings are important because they highlight the lack of communication and discussion, the underdiagnosis, and the undertreatment of vulvar, vaginal, sexual, and urinary symptoms associated with the menopause.

2.3 Vulvodynia

Vulvodynia is a vulvar pain disorder that is typically chronic and occurs in women of all ages and ethnic groups. Once believed to be rare, vulvodynia has been shown to be very common. A large epidemiologic study showing an incidence of 17 % with a prevalence of 7 % has been confirmed by subsequent researchers from several countries (Reed et al. 2012a) (Box 2.1).

Box 2.1. The Vulvodynia Numbers

- 14,000,000 women in the United States have experienced chronic vulvar pain.
- Lifetime prevalence of unexplained vulvar pain ranges from 16 to 28 %. These estimates may be low given that 40 % of women who suffer from vulvar pain fail to seek treatment.
- Women who present symptoms of vulvodynia vary in age from 16 to 80 years, but the majority is between 20 and 60 years of age.
- White women and women of 77 African genetic background have an equivalent risk for vulvodynia, whereas Latina women have a higher risk

Harlow and Stewart (2003), Arnold et al. (2007), Reed et al. (2004, 2006).

Embarrassment and resulting silence of patients, dismissal of vulvar pain as a "psychological disorder" by clinicians ("pain is all in your head" or "your vulvar pain is psychogenic") and provider discomfort with management of these women have resulted in widespread ignorance about this destructive condition. Delayed diagnosis increases the women's risk for sexual dysfunction and diminished quality of life.

One leading factor influencing this diagnostic delay is the *lack of training of the specialists* who see these patients. Studies in the USA have estimated a high financial burden for vulvodynia, with an increased individual and social financial burden and impaired quality of life (Xie et al. 2012).

Vulvodynia may be associated with other chronic comorbid pain conditions such as fibromyalgia, interstitial cystitis, irritable bowel syndrome, endometriosis, and headache, individually and in combination. The presence of vulvodynia or any of the other comorbid pain conditions increases the likelihood that a woman will have one or more of the other chronic pain conditions (Reed et al. 2012b).

The presence of vulvodynia was associated with the presence of each of the other comorbid pain conditions ($P<.001$, odds ratio 2.3–3.3). Furthermore, these comorbid conditions may be premorbid identifiers of vulvodynia risk. The recognition of this risk may help identify pathophysiologically similar phenotypic subgroups. This may contribute to a better pathophysiologically based understanding of the multifactorial etiology of vulvodynia. It could improve the therapeutic strategies for this population (Reed et al. 2014).

2.4 Pudendal Neuralgia

Pudendal neuralgia is a painful, neuropathic condition involving the dermatome of the pudendal nerve and triggering vulvar pain. This condition is not widely known and often unrecognized by many practitioners. The International Pudendal Neuropathy Association (www.tipna.org) estimates the incidence of this condition to be 1/100,000 of the general population.

Spinosa et al. document the incidence at 1 % in the general population, affecting women more than men. Orphanet (www.orpha.net), a European website providing information about orphan drugs and rare diseases, states that pudendal neuralgia affects 4 % of patients undergoing consultation for pain and affects 7 women for every 3 men. These results exemplify the inability to derive the precise incidence of pudendal neuralgia (Spinosa et al. 2006).

Conclusions

Vulvar pain is still an underreported, underdignosed, and undertreated condition in the lifespan. Terminology further complicates the difficulties in finding reliable prevalence data. "Vulvar pain" is not even mentioned during childhood and after female genital mutilation, with the exception of a few case reports.

In postpubertal women, prevalence of vulvar pain is reported around 7–8 %, in a US study. Lifetime prevalence of unexplained vulvar pain ranges from 16 to 28 %. These estimates may be low, given that 40 % of women who suffer from vulvar pain fail to seek treatment ("a disorder too intimate to be spoken of"). Sad to say, more than 50 % of those women who dare to disclose about their vulvar pain and ask for help do not find an adequate diagnostic and therapeutic answer by their physician.

Coital pain at the entrance of the vagina ("introital dyspareunia") has been relatively more investigated in comparison to vulvar pain. It can be considered the sexual correlate of vestibular pain. Its prevalence varies between 10 and 20 % across studies. Prevalence of introital dyspareunia can indirectly suggest the likely prevalence of vestibular pain, at least to some extent.

Appropriate training of HCPs on vulvar pain, sexual pain, and associated comorbidities should be empowered during the medical school and in the specialties more afferent to the area (gynecolgists, urologists, pediatricians, physiatrists/physiotherapists, sexologists, neurologists, psychiatrists, oncologists, and, certainly, family physicians).

To increase a pathophysiologically based knowledge of vulvar pain in HCPs is the prerequisite to offer women an earlier, more competent diagnosis and treatment. This is why this book has been written, with a practical perspective hopefully useful for clinicians in their daily activity.

References

Arnold LD, Bachmann GA, Rosen R, Rhoads GG. Assessment of vulvodynia symptoms in a sample of US women: a prevalence survey with a nested case control study. Am J Obstet Gynecol. 2007;196:128.e1–6.

Avis NE, Zhao X, Johannes CB, Ory M, Brockwell S, Greendale GA. Correlates of sexual function among multi-ethnic middle-aged women: results from the Study of Women's Health Across the Nation (SWAN). Menopause. 2005;12:385–98.

Bailhache M, Leroy V, Pillet P, Salmi LR. Is early detection of abused children possible?: a systematic review of the diagnostic accuracy of the identification of abused children. BMC Pediatr. 2013;13:202–2010.

Barrett G, Pendry E, Peacick J, Victor C, Thakar R, Manyonda I. Women's sexual health after childbirth. BJOG. 2000;107:186–95.

Birge O, Ozbey EG, Arslan D, Erkan MM, Demir F, Akgor U. Vulvar epidermoid cyst and type 2 radical genital mutilation. Case Rep Obstet Gynecol. 2015;2015:520190.

Casey JT, Bjurlin MA, Cheng EY. Pediatric genital injury: an analysis of the national electronic injury surveillance system. Urology. 2013;82(5):10.1016.

Dennerstein L, Dudley EC, Hopper JL, Guthrie JR, Burger HG. A prospective population-based study of menopausal symptoms. Obstet Gynecol. 2000;96(3):351–8.

Focseneanu MA, Gupta M, Squires KC, et al. The course of lichen sclerosus diagnosed prior to puberty. J Pediatr Adolesc Gynecol. 2013;26:153.

Gilbert R, Widom CS, Browne K, Fergusson D, Webb E, Janson S. Burden and consequences of child maltreatment in high-income countries. Lancet. 2009;13(9657):68–81.

Gott M, Hinchliff S. Barriers to seeking treatment for sexual problems in primary care: a qualitative study with older people. Fam Pract. 2003;20(6):690–5.

Graziottin A. Prevalence and evaluation of sexual health problems – HSDD in Europe. J Sex Med. 2007;4 suppl 3:211–9.

Gudu W. Acute vulvar pain in a lady with post circumcision inclusion cyst of the vulva containing stones: a case report. BMC Womens Health. 2014;14:2.

Hadid V, Dahan MH. A case of chronic abdominal neuropathic pain and burning after female genital cutting. Case Rep Obstet Gynecol. 2015;2015:906309.

Harlow BL, Stewart EG. A population-based assessment of chronic unexplained vulvar pain: have we underestimated the prevalence of vulvodynia? J Am Med Womens Assoc. 2003;58:82–8.

Harlow BL, Kunitz CG, Nguyen RH, Rydell SA, Turner RM, MacLehose RF. Prevalence of symptoms consistent with a diagnosis of vulvodynia: population-based estimates from 2 geographic regions. Am J Obstet Gynecol. 2014;210(1):40.e1–8.

Iglesias-Rios L, Harlow SD, Reed BD. Depression and posttraumatic stress disorder among women with vulvodynia: evidence from the population-based woman to woman health study. J Womens Health (Larchmt). 2015;24(7):557–62.

Kingsberg SA, Wysocki S, Magnus L, Krychman ML. Vulvar and vaginal atrophy in postmenopausal women: findings from the REVIVE (REal Women's VIews of Treatment Options for Menopausal Vaginal ChangEs) survey. J Sex Med. 2013;10(7):1790–9.

Lagerstedt M, Karvinen K, Joki-Erkkilä M, Huotari-Orava R, Snellman E, Laasanen SL. Childhood lichen sclerosus – a challenge for clinicians. Pediatr Dermatol. 2013;30(4):444–50. doi:10.1111/pde.12109. Epub 2013 Feb 26.

Latthe P, Latthe M, Say L, et al. WHO systematic review of prevalence of chronic pelvic pain: a neglected reproductive health morbidity. BMC Pub Health. 2006;6:177.

Laumann EO, Paik A, Rosen RC. Sexual dysfunction in the United States: prevalence and predictors. JAMA. 1999;281:537–44.

Laumann EO, Das A, Waite LJ. Sexual dysfunction among older adults: prevalence and risk factors from a nationally representative U.S. probability sample of Men and women 57–85 years of age. J Sex Med. 2008;5(10):2300–11.

Leeman LM, Rogers RG. Sex after childbirth: postpartum sexual function. Obstet Gynecol. 2012;119(3):647–55.

McCall-Hosenfeld JS, Jaramillo SA, Legault C, et al. Correlates of sexual satisfaction among sexually active postmenopausal women in the Women's Health Initiative Observational Study. J Gen Intern Med. 2008;23(12):2000–9.

McDonald EA, Gartland D, Small R, Brown SJ. Dyspareunia and childbirth: a prospective cohort study. BJOG. 2015;122(5):672–9. doi:10.1111/1471-0528.13263. Epub 2015 Jan 21.

Murphy R. Lichen sclerosus. Dermatol Clin. 2010;28(4):707–15. doi:10.1016/j.det.2010.07.006. Review.

NAMS. Management of symptomatic vulvovaginal atrophy: 2013 position statement of The North American Menopause Society. Menopause. 2013;20(9):888–902.

Parish SJ, Nappi RE, Krychman ML, et al. Impact of vulvovaginal health on post-menopausal women: a review of surveys on symptoms of vulvovaginal atrophy. Int J Womens Health. 2013;5:437–47.

Paterson L, Davis SN, Khalife S, Amsel R, Binik YM. Persistent genital pain and pelvic pain after childbirth. J Sex Med. 2009;6:215–21.

Powell J, Wojnarowska F. Childhood vulvar lichen sclerosus. The course after puberty. J Reprod Med. 2002;47:706.

Reed BD, Crawford S, Couper M, Cave C, Haefner HK. Pain at the vulvar vestibule: a web-based survey. J Low Genit Tract Dis. 2004;8:48–57.

Reed BD, Haefner HK, Harlow SD, Gorenflo DW, Sen A. Reliability and validity of self-reported symptoms for predicting vulvodynia. Obstet Gynecol. 2006;108:906–13.

Reed BD, Harlow SD, Sen A, et al. Prevalence and demographic characteristics of vulvodynia in a population-based sample. Am J Obstet Gynecol. 2012a;206:170.e1–9.

Reed BD, Harlow SD, Sen A, Edwards R, et al. Relationship between vulvodynia and chronic comorbid pain conditions. Obstet Gynecol. 2012b;120:145–51.

Reed BD, Legocki LJ, Plegue MA, Sen A, Haefner HK, Harlow SD. Factors associated with vulvodynia incidence. Obstet Gynecol. 2014;123:225–31.

Salonia A, Clementi MC, Graziottin A, Nappi RE, Castiglione F, Ferrari M, Capitanio U, Damiano R, Montorsi F. Secondary provoked vestibulodynia in sexually-active women with recurrent uncomplicated urinary tract infections. J Sex Med. 2013;10(9):2265–73.

Schneidewind-Skibbe A, Hayes RD, Koochaki PE, Meyer J, Dennerstein L. The frequency of sexual intercourse reported by women: a review of community-based studies and factors limiting their conclusions. J Sex Med. 2008;5(2):301–35.

Smith SD, Fischer G. Childhood onset of vulvar lichen sclerosus does not resolve at puberty: a prospective case series. Pediatr Dermatol. 2009;26:725.

Spinosa JP, de Bisschop E, Laurencon J, Kuhn G, Dubuisson JB, Riederer BM. Sacral staged reflexes to localize the pudendal compression: an anatomical validation of the concept. Rev Med Suisse. 2006;2:2416–8, 2420–1.

Thomas TG. Practical treatise on the diseases of women. Philadelphia: Henry C. Lea; 1874.

Williams A, Herron-Marx S, Knibb R. The prevalence of enduring postnatal perineal morbidity and its relationship to type of birth and birth risk factors. J Clin Nurs. 2007;16:549–61.

World Health Organization. Eliminating female genital mutilation: an inter-agency statement. Geneva: WHO, OHCHR, UNAIDS, UNDP, UNECA, UNESCO, UNFPA, UNHCR, UNICEF, UNIFEM, WHO; 2008.

Xie Y, Shi L, Xiong X, Wu E, Veasley C, Dade C. Economic burden and quality of life of vulvodynia in the United States. Curr Med Res Opin. 2012;28:601–8.

The Pathophysiology of Vulvar Pain 3

Vulvar pain affects an area of the body that is hidden by taboo and fraught with misinformation. It is an area rich of secret and seducing pleasures but also a source of potential excruciating and invalidating pain (Graziottin and Gambini 2015). The vulvar organ, its erotic meaning, and the many symptoms that may affect it have been too long neglected by the medical establishment. Discussing vulvar symptoms may be perceived as very challenging both for patients and healthcare providers, as they seem to be "too intimate to be spoken of."

Patients may present with a variety of vulvar symptoms (pain, burning, itching, irritation, dryness, soreness) and patterns of symptoms (continuous or intermittent, localized, or generalized). Different comorbidities, pelvic and systemic, may further complicate the clinical scenario when women finally dare to ask for help (Graziottin and Murina 2011).

3.1 The Vulva: Anatomical and Physiological Considerations

The vulva refers to the female external genitalia comprising *the mons pubis*, *clitoris*, *labia majora*, *labia minora*, and *perineum* (Fig. 3.1). They are supported by superficial and deep muscles of the perineum and their fasciae (Yavagal et al. 2011).

The cutaneous epithelium covering the *mons pubis* and labia majora is derived from the embryonic ectoderm. It exhibits a keratinized, stratified, squamous structure with sweat gland, sebaceous glands, and hair follicles.

The *labia minora* are two small cutaneous folds 3–4 cm long, situated between the labia majora and extended from the clitoris anteriorly to the fourchette posteriorly (Putz and Pabst 2008). Anteriorly each labium is divided into two portions: the upper division passes above the glans of the *clitoris* to fuse with the opposite part and form the *preputium clitoridis*; the lower division passes under the *clitoris* forming the *frenulum* of the *clitoris* with its contralateral part. The *labia minora* are rich in sebaceous glands, connective tissue, and vascular erectile tissue with a considerable

A. Graziottin, F. Murina, *Vulvar Pain*, DOI 10.1007/978-3-319-42677-8_3

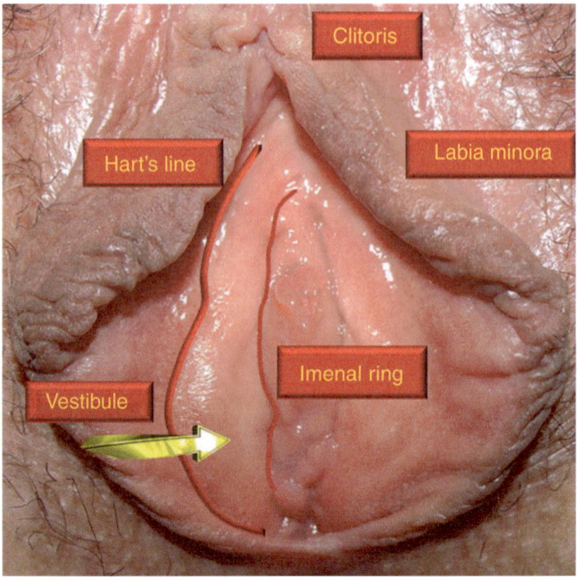

Fig. 3.1 The vulva: anatomical aspect

number of sensory nerve endings and receptors (Netter 2010). They are covered with keratinized skin that contains sebaceous glands but lacks sweat glands or hair follicles. The *epidermis* is thinner than on the *labia majora*, and the degree of keratinization diminishes gradually. From the inner third of the *labia minora* toward the vestibule, the epithelium is nonkeratinized, endodermal-originated mucosal tissue.

The *vestibule* of the vagina extends from the *glans clitoridis* to the posterior fourchette between the *labia minora*, up to their internal border. It contains the vaginal orifice, external urethral meatus, vestibular bulbs, and the openings of the greater vestibular glands (also known as Bartholin's glands). The vaginal orifice is below the opening of the urethra, and it is characterized by the presence of the hymen (a circumferential hairless skin with variable shape) (Standring 2008). The urethral orifice (lower third of the urethra) is surrounded by the erectile tissue of the clitoral bulbs, partly considered the equivalent of the male urethral corpus spongiosum (O'Connel and DeLancey 2005). It has both a sexual and protective function. It gets very congested during physiologic sexual arousal, contributing to genital congestion and the formation of the so-called orgasmic platform (Masters et al. 1986). Meanwhile, it constitutes a kind of physiologic airbag, protecting the urethra from the "mechanical" trauma of repeated sexual thrusting at intercourse. When women suffer from vaginal dryness and/or inadequate genital arousal due to different etiologies, including low desire, poor foreplay and/or vestibular pain with dyspareunia, and/or hyperactive pelvic floor mechanically narrowing the vaginal entrance, the lack of this protective cuff increases the urethral and bladder vulnerability to the "mechanical" trauma of the intercourse, contributing to recurrent cystitis (r-UTIs). Sixty percent of r-UTIs are complained of 24–72 h after the intercourse and are referred to as "postcoital cystitis," a powerful contributor of chronic bladder pain syndrome (Graziottin et al. 2014b). The vestibular bulbs (recently renamed as "bulbs of the clitoris" (O'Connel and DeLancey 2005) are two erectile organs situated laterally to the vaginal orifice directly beneath the skin of the *labia minora* and joined together (*pars intermedia*) and extended to the base of the glans. They are in contact with the greater vestibular glands posteriorly and covered by the bulbocavernosus muscles superficially. The greater vestibular glans (Bartholin's) are two small glands situated one on either side of the vaginal orifice and through a 2 cm long duct opened between the hymen, and the *labia minora* (Standring 2008) extends anteroposterior from the frenulum of the clitoris to the fourchette and laterally to the labium minus on each side. The vestibule is covered by endodermal-originated mucosa. Its border is referred to as the Hart line, which is the junction between the keratinized and nonkeratinized *labia majora*. Numerous mucous glands, called the minor vestibular glands, open in the vestibule. It exhibits a high concentration of sensory free ends with a dense and shallow ramification.

The *clitoris* is an erectile structure, homologue to the male penis, formed by two *corpora cavernosa* and the glans, covered by the prepuce. Only a fifth (or less) is visible (glans), while the rest is hidden under the skin (O'Connel et al. 1998, 2008; O'Connel and DeLancey 2005). The corpora cavernosa are made of cavernous erectile tissue and diverge and follow the pubic rami on each side, forming the crura. It represents the hidden part of the clitoris which is covered by the ischiocavernosus muscle: it may reach 7 or more cm in length. The glans of the clitoris is the free extreme of it. It's 4–7 mm long and covers the distal part of the corpora cavernosa from which it is not dependent (Williams and Bannister 2008). It represents the most innervated part of the clitoris, full of free nerve endings, Krause-finger corpuscles, and corpuscles of Pacini and Meissner (Yang et al. 2006). The clitoris is connected to the mons pubis and pubic symphysis by the suspensory ligament which influences the clitoridis stability during sexual intercourse. The urethra lies surrounded by this complex with the body directly anterior to it, flanked superficially by the bulbs and deeply by the crura. In anatomy texts the bulbs are referred to as the bulbs of the vestibule and appear as if they form an erectile structure of the *labia minora* (Standring 2008; Netter 2010). However, according to most recent studies, the bulbs relate most closely to the clitoris and urethra so that they would be renamed the bulbs of the clitoris (O'Connel and DeLancey 2005). O'Connell refers to the "clitoral complex," composed of the distal vagina, urethra, and clitoris, as "the" location of female sexual activity (O'Connell et al. 2008). Recently, the term clitoral-urethral-vaginal complex (CUV) (Jannini and d'Amati 2006) has been proposed, to include the specialized area called the "G-spot," encompassing the anterior vaginal wall and the embedded structures. The vagina is related anteriorly to the base of urinary bladder and urethra, so strictly that some anatomists recently wrote that "the urethra is embedded in the vaginal wall" (O'Connel and DeLancey 2005). This very close relationship contributes to the high comorbidity between the bladder, vaginal, and sexual symptoms.

The vestibule *and the* vulva *"receive" secretions from the vagina*. Their health is modulated (also) by the vaginal microbiota, i.e., the microorganisms living in a specific organ or tissue. Lactobacilli are the microorganism typical of the fertile age.

Lactobacilli, Gram-positive bacilli, the so-called Doderlein's bacilli, represent the most prevalent microorganisms (up to 90 %) in the normal vaginal ecosystem, and they present two mechanisms to interfere with pathogens: (1) adherence to the mucus, forming a barrier which prevents colonization by pathogens; (2) production of antimicrobial compounds such as lactic acid, hydrogen peroxide, and bacteriocin-like substances (Boris and Barbés 2000). The vaginal acid system is facilitated by Lactobacilli, that metabolizes glycogen into lactic acid lowering vaginal pH to a normal value of 4.2. In physiologic conditions, lactobacilli include 90 % of the vaginal ecosystem during the fertile age, the remaining 10 % being composed by different commensal germs. The ecosystem is important for limiting the growth of pathogenic bacteria (Stumpf et al. 2013). The concept of "pathogenic biofilms" (Graziottin and Zanello 2015) is currently referring to structured germ communities living inside a self-produced polysaccharidic network adhering to the vaginal mucosa and/or to inert medical devices. They can contribute to recurrent vaginitis and cystitis with their associated sexual comorbidities, such as introital dyspareunia and postcoital cystitis.

3.2 The Pelvic Floor Muscles

"There is no considerable muscle in the body whose form and function are more difficult to understand than those of the levator ani, and about which such nebulous impressions prevail" (Dickinson 1889). Despite a century of medical progress since Dickinson offered this observation, the details of levator ani muscle anatomy remain poorly understood (Lawson 1974; Bustami 1988–1989; Kearney et al. 2004).

The pelvic floor consists of different muscles' layers: the pelvic diaphragm, the urogenital diaphragm, the superficial trigonal muscles and the lateral muscles (Standring 2008). The pelvic floor is important for the support of the pelvic organs, to assist fecal and urinary continence and to improve pelvic-spinal stability; furthermore, it plays a key role for sexual pleasure. The pelvic diaphragm is formed by the levator ani and the coccygeus muscles (Kearney et al. 2004).

The coccygeus muscle forms a triangular structure attached to the spine of the ischium and to the lateral surface of the coccyx and S5. This muscle does not contribute to active movement of the pelvic floor; in fact the effective contractile support structure is represented by the levator ani muscle. The components of the levator ani muscle are the puborectal, iliococcygeal, and pubovisceral (pubococcygeus) muscles, further subdivided into pubovaginal, puboperineal, and puboanal. This terminology was accepted in 1998 by the Federative Committee on Anatomical Terminology (International Anatomical Nomenclature Committee 1983).

The iliococcygeus originates from the tendinous arch of levator ani and forms a diaphragm between the anus and the coccyx. The puborectalis originates from the pubic bone forming a ring around the rectum. The pubococcygeus with its three branches originates from the pubic bone and insert into the perineal body, the vaginal wall, and into the tissue between the internal and external anal sphincter. In the axial plane, the puborectal muscle can be seen lateral to the pubovisceral muscle and decussating dorsal to the rectum. The course of the puboperineal muscle near the perineal body is visualized in the axial plane. The coronal view is perpendicular to the fiber direction of the puborectal and pubovisceral muscles and shows them as "clusters" of muscle on either side of the vagina. The sagittal plane consistently demonstrates the puborectal muscle passing dorsal to the rectum to form a sling that can consistently be seen as a "bump." This plane is also parallel to the pubovisceral muscle fiber direction and shows the puboperineal muscle (Margulies et al. 2006).

The urogenital diaphragm consists of the deep transverse perineal muscle with the superior and inferior fascia. The perineal membrane is composed of two regions, one dorsal and one ventral. The dorsal portion consists of bilateral transverse fibrous sheets that attach the lateral wall of the vagina and perineal body to the ischiopubic ramus. This portion is devoid of striated muscle. The ventral portion is part of a solid 3-dimensional tissue mass in which several structures are embedded. It is intimately associated with the compressor urethrae and the urethrovaginal sphincter muscle of the distal urethra, with the urethra and its surrounding connective tissue. In this region the perineal membrane is continuous with the insertion of the arcus tendineus fascia pelvis. The levator ani muscles are connected with the cranial surface of the perineal membrane. The vestibular bulb and clitoral crus are fused with the membrane's caudal surface (Stein and DeLancey 2008). The superficial trigonal muscle is composed of the bulbocavernosus, ischiocavernosus, and the superficial transverse perineal muscles in the anterior triangle and the anal sphincter in the posterior triangle. The superficial transverse perineal originates from the ischial tuberosity and insert on the perineal body (Stein and DeLancey 2008). The ischiocavernosus muscle extends from the ischial tuberosity to the clitoral *crura* inserting on to the body of the *clitoris* (this muscle compresses the *crura* of the *clitoris* and retard the return of blood through the veins contributing to maintain the erection). The bulbocavernosus muscle occupies each lateral side of vagina between the perineal body and the *clitoris* body (it diminishes the orifice of the vagina and with its anterior fibers contributes to the erection of the clitoris) (Standring 2008). Female longitudinal anal muscles or conjoint longitudinal coats (CLCs) are attached to the subcutaneous tissue along the vaginal vestibule on the anterior side of the external anal sphincter. Lateral to the CLCs, the external anal sphincter also extends anteriorly toward the vaginal side walls. The anterior part of the CLCs originates from the perimysium of the levator ani muscle. In terms of topographical anatomy, the female anterior CLCs are likely to correspond to the lateral extension of the perineal body (a bulky subcutaneous smooth muscle mass present in adult women), supporting the vaginal vestibule by transmission of force from the levator ani (Kinugasa et al. 2013).

The lateral walls of the pelvis are composed of the piriformis and obturator internus (muscles of the lower limb). The *perineum* is a diamond-shaped area limited by the pubic symphysis, ischiopubic rami, sacrotuberous ligaments, and the coccyx. A line that passes through the two ischial tuberosities divides the perineum into two triangles: the anterior urogenital and the posterior anal.

3.3 The Connective System

In addition to muscles, the pelvic organs are supported by connective tissue organized in different layers of fasciae and ligaments. Magnetic resonance studies offer new insights to the traditional anatomic readings (Tunn et al. 2001, 2003).

The endopelvic fascia covers the pelvic organs and connects them to the lateral pelvic wall. It's made up of a combination of elastin, collagen, mucopolysaccharides, and adipose and neurovascular tissue. The fascia covering the levator ani muscle continues with the endopelvic fascia above, perineal fascia below, and obturator fascia laterally (Yavagal et al. 2011). The levator ani muscles and their superior and inferior fascia combined together form the so-called pelvic diaphragm (Ashton-Miller and DeLancey 2007).

The broad ligaments connect the uterus to the lateral pelvic walls on both side, and on its upper end it encases the fallopian tubes, round ligaments, utero-ovarian ligaments, and the ovaries (Standring 2008).

The round ligaments extend from the lateral side of the uterine body and passing through the inguinal canal insert into the labia majora (Standring 2008).

The uterosacral ligaments support the cervix and the upper part of the vagina by their attachment to the sacrum, having also an important role of contention function in sexual intercourse.

The cardinal ligaments, or Mackenrodt's ligaments, extend from the cervix to the posterolateral pelvic wall (Ramanah et al. 2012).

The fascia of the obturator internus covers the pelvic surface of the muscle; it arches beneath the obturator vessels and nerve, completing the obturator canal, and at the front of the pelvis is attached to the back of the superior ramus of the pubis. Below it's attached to the falciform process of the sacrotuberous ligament and to the pubic arch. Thickening in the obturator fascia is called the arcus tendinous fascia pelvis, extended from the pubis anteriorly to the ischial spine (Ziouziou et al. 2013). Alcock's canal syndrome or pudendal nerve entrapment (Labat et al. 2008) is a condition caused by the compression of the pudendal nerve in the canal, resulting in a neuralgia in the area of distribution of the pudendal nerve (vulva, vagina, clitoris) (Oelhafen et al. 2013).

3.4 The Vascular System

The arterial supply of the vulva is derived from the external and internal pudendal arteries. The internal pudendal artery is a branch of the anterior division of the internal iliac artery, and the veins drain into the internal iliac vein (Netter 2010). The inferior rectal artery supplies the anal canal; the perineal artery supplies the superficial perineal muscles; and the posterior labial branch gives artery to the bulbs of the vestibule and dorsal and deep arteries of the clitoris. The superficial and deep external pudendal arteries are branches of the femoral artery, and they supply the *labia majora* with branches of the pudendal artery (Beech and Adams 2009). The internal pudendal arteries are the key resistance vessels controlling the peripheral circulatory component of sexual responses in both male and females. Structurally, the pudendal artery has a smaller lumen diameter and wall thickness and much lower wall-to-lumen ratio compared to that of the male. The lumen of this artery also tapers as it travels distally and becomes the clitoral artery. Based on its smaller wall thickness, as expected, the female pudendal artery does not contract to the same magnitudes attained by the male pudendal. However, the sensitivity to adrenergic-mediated contraction is not different between male and women (Hannan et al. 2012).

Many of the differences between the male and female pudendal arteries can be explained by the hemodynamic demands of their genital organs. The volume of blood and inflow pressures required to fill the penis are much greater than the demands of the female genitalia, when sexual purposes are considered. Furthermore, various clinical studies have confirmed the difference in the volume of blood as well as the pressures achieved by the genital organs during orgasm in both sexes. In fact, the volume of blood required to fill the clitoral tissue during a sexual response is one tenth than that required to fill the penis (10 ml vs 100 ml) (Maravilla and Yang 2008). Furthermore, the intracavernosal pressure within the penis reaches suprasystolic values during orgasm/ejaculation, whereas the vaginal, clitoral, and labial pressures only increase approximately 30–40 mm/Hg at peak sexual response (Kandeel et al. 2001; Sommer et al. 2001). Thus, the male pudendal artery needs to be able to withstand greater inflow of blood at higher pressures, and these requirements are reflected in the increased wall-to-lumen ratio of the pudendal artery. The pudendal artery in the female rat is very similar anatomically to that of women. In women, the origin of the internal pudendal artery is also located on the internal iliac artery but appears to arise much further down after the obturator, vesicular, and inferior gluteal branches (Beech and Adams 2009). In both species, the internal pudendal artery gives off branches supplying the *labia* and distal vaginal wall and terminates as the common clitoral artery with branches forming the clitoral cavernous and dorsal clitoral arteries (Fătu et al. 2006; O'Connel and DeLancey 2005). There is also evidence in both men and women of accessory pudendal arteries which arise off the inferior vesical, obturator, and external pudendal arteries and supply the genital tissues.

The internal pudendal artery has markedly heightened susceptibility to vascular damage compared to other vessels in the body. Evidence suggests that the female may also be susceptible to vascular pathologies contributing to sexual dysfunction. Indeed, vaginal/clitoral engorgement is a central nervous system-driven event leading to increases in blood flow to the genital organs: an event that precedes arousal (Traish et al. 2010). This increased blood flow to the vagina, *clitoris*, and *labia* is responsible for the vasocongestion, engorgement, and lubrication in the sexual arousal response.

3.5 The Innervation of Genitals and Pelvic Floor System

The pudendal nerve arises from the sacral plexus; it is formed by the second, third, and fourth sacral nerve roots. It passes between the piriformis and coccygeus muscles and leaves the pelvis through the lower part of the greater sciatic foramen. It then crosses the spine of the ischium being situated between the sacrospinous and the sacrotuberous ligament (Robert et al. 1998) and reenters the pelvis through the lesser sciatic foramen. It goes along the lateral wall of the ischiorectal fossa with the internal pudendal vessels (the pudendal artery lies on its medial side), contained in a duplication of the obturator fascia called Alcock's canal (Schraffordt et al. 2004) and divides at the level of the perineum in three terminal branches: the dorsal nerve of the clitoris, the perineal nerve, and the inferior rectal nerve, providing the sensory branches to the skin of the perineal area, labia majora, and clitoris (Tagliafico et al. 2014; Mahakkanukrauh et al. 2005). It also innervates the external anal sphincter (inferior rectal nerve) and deep muscles of the urogenital triangle (perineal nerve). The perineal nerve is situated below the internal pudendal artery and divides into a posterior labial branch and a muscular branch. The dorsal nerve of the clitoris is the deepest division of the pudendal nerve. Considering the relatively small size of the clitoris, even inclusive of the crura and bulbs, in comparison to the penis, the size of the dorsal nerve of the clitoris is proportional to its extraordinary sensory capacity, albeit it is small in absolute terms. The dorsal nerve supplies the clitoris. The pudendal nerve is the most important human nerve in terms of pleasure perception. At the same time, it is also critical in sexual pain disorders, namely, introital dyspareunia and vaginismus.

The lumbar plexus is formed by the loops of communication between the anterior division of the first three and the greater part of the fourth lumbar nerves; it is situated in the posterior part of the psoas major, in front of the transverse processes of the lumbar vertebrae. It divides into many branches, giving origin to the ileoinguinal nerve and genitofemoral nerve which are important for pelvic innervation. The ileoinguinal nerve arises from the first lumbar nerve giving branches to the obliquus internus muscle and to the skin covering the mons pubis and labia majora. The genitofemoral nerve arises from the first and second lumbar nerves, and it divides into the external spermatic nerve (it accompanies the round ligament of the uterus and it gets lost upon it) and into the lumboinguinal nerve (it supplies the skin of the anterior surface of the upper part of the thigh) (Standring 2008).

Women use the term pain to include *a variety of unpleasant symptoms* including burning, soreness, and throbbing, and some women insist that they do not have pain but describe the sensation with one of these words, which can be misleading for clinicians. It is not surprising that the etiology of the pain can be difficult to pinpoint.

Vulvar pain has *several common etiologies*, but a very common cause of chronic vulvar symptoms is *vulvodynia*. Most often, the discomfort of vulvodynia is characterized as perceptions of burning, rawness, or irritation, and dyspareunia is nearly always present as well.

The International Society for the Study of Vulvovaginal Disease (ISSVD), the International Society for the Study of Women's Sexual Health (ISSWSH), and the International Pelvic Pain Society (IPPS) recently defined *a revision* of persistent vulvar pain (Bornstein et al. 2016) (Table 3.1).

Table 3.1 2015 consensus terminology and classification of persistent vulvar pain

Vulvar pain caused by a specific disorder
Infectious (e.g., herpes)
Dermatoses (e.g., lichen sclerosus and lichen planus)
Neoplastic (e.g., Paget disease, squamous cell carcinoma)
Neurologic (e.g., post-herpetic neuralgia, nerve compression or injury)
Trauma (e.g., female genital cutting, obstetrical)
Iatrogenic (e.g., post-operative, chemotherapy, radiation)
Hormonal deficiencies (e.g., genitourinary syndrome of menopause)
Vulvodynia
Vulvar pain of at least 3 months duration, without clear identifiable cause, which may have potential associated factors
Descriptors:
Localized (e.g., vestibulodynia: about 80 %; clitorodynia)
Generalized

Modified from Bornstein et al. (2016)

Two main elements characterize this new classification:

- The *division to sections*, with the first being: "Vulvar pain caused by a specific disorder." This section contains vulvar pain conditions for which a cause has been clearly identified.
- The 2003 definition of *vulvodynia* ("Chronic vulvar discomfort, mainly described as burning, occurring in the absence of visible relevant findings") has been changed in 2015 to: "Vulvar pain of at least 3 months duration, without clear identifiable cause, which may have potential associated factors" (Table 3.2).

Vulvodynia is not a specific entity but a multifactorial condition, and we believe that associated factors are themselves *pathophysiological components of the disease*, with a different relevance in each individual.

3.6 The Vulvar Pain Transmission into the Central Nervous System

Recent evidence from human studies has significantly expanded the understanding of pain perception and has demonstrated that *a complex series of spinal, midbrain, and cortical structures are involved in pain perception.*

Pain transmission from the periphery to the higher brain centers via the spinal cord is not a simple, passive process involving exclusive pathways (Fig. 3.2). The relationship between a stimulus causing pain and the way it is perceived by an individual is dramatically affected by circuitry within the spinal cord and the brain. The sensation of pain is modulated as it is transmitted upward from the periphery to the cortex. It is modulated at a segmental level and by descending control from higher centers, with the main neurotransmitters involved being serotonin, norepinephrine (noradrenaline), and the endogenous opioids.

Table 3.2 Potential factors associated with vulvodynia

Neurologic central mechanisms: spine and brain
Inflammation
Neural proliferation
Musculoskeletal pattern (e.g., pelvic muscle overactivity, myofascial, biomechanical)
Genetic predisposition
Hormonal factors
Psychosocial factors (e.g., mood, interpersonal, coping, role, sexual function)

Modified from Bornstein et al. (2016)

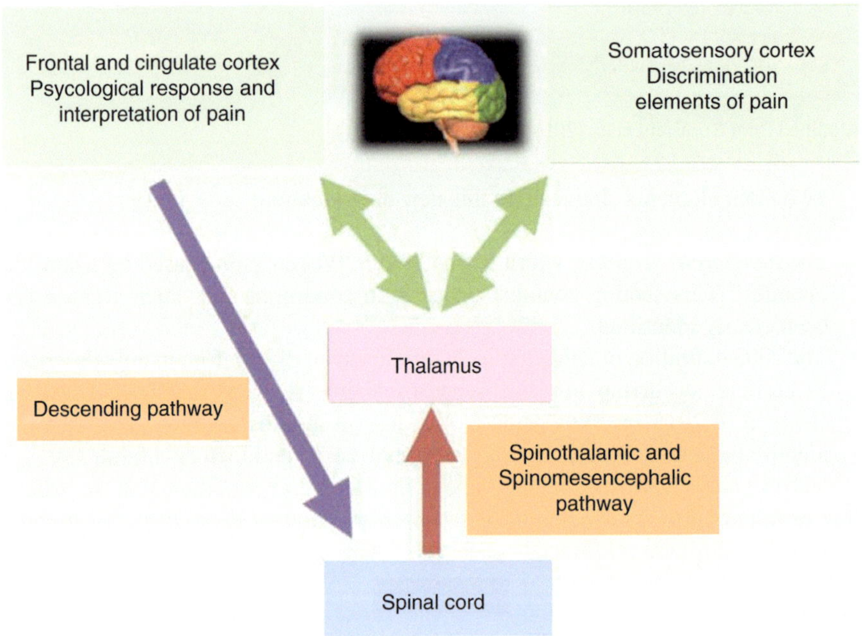

Fig. 3.2 Schematic representation of pain pathways (Graziottin and Murina 2011)

3.6.1 Peripheral Nociceptors

They are simple bare-ending nerve fibers that are widespread in the superficial layers of the skin. Nociceptors are classified as Aδ, which are small diameter, lightly myelinated, and C-fibers, which are not myelinated. Neurons originating at the nociceptors pass into the peripheral nerves and enter the spinal cord at the dermatomal level ascribed by their insertion. Innervation to the vulva is via the pudendal nerve which originates from the S2–4 nerve roots and the ilioinguinal and genitofemoral nerves, arising from L1–2. The latter two nerves are predominantly sensory, but the pudendal nerve contains motor, sensory, and sympathetic fibers which supply the complex autonomic reflexes of the pelvic organs. The vagina itself is relatively insensitive to pain, while the vulva and particularly the vulvar vestibule have a high level of free nerve endings (Schober et al. 2015).

3.6.2 Spinal Cord

Following spinal cord integration of afferent inputs, there are neurons (second-order neurons) that transmit the information to the higher centers via ascending pathways. The classical ascending pathway ascribed to pain is the spinothalamic one; other pathways relevant in pain modulation include the spinomesencephalic, spinoreticular, and dorsal column pathways.

3.6.3 Cerebral Cortex

Functional imaging studies over the last decade have revealed several neuroanatomical pain-related structures, including primary and secondary somatosensory cortices, insula, prefrontal cortex and parietal association cortices, thalamus, and brain stem nuclei, thus corroborating this multidimensional concept of pain. Consequently, these brain areas are often referred as the "neuronal matrix of pain." This pain neuromatrix is often divided into a lateral (primary and secondary sensory cortex and posterior insula) and a medial (anterior gyrus cinguli, prefrontal cortex, anterior insula). The lateral system appears to encode the sensory discriminative component and, the medial system, the affective and motivational dimensions.

3.6.4 Descending Pathways

Some of the spinothalamic fibers project to the periaqueductal gray (PAG) and hypothalamus and then to the dorsal horn of the spinal cord. The PAG is an area of the brain that is rich in opioid receptors and is thus involved in the endogenous opioid system. The descending pathways are, therefore, inhibitory at the dorsal horn, reducing ascending nociceptive inputs.

3.7 Pain Pathophysiology

Pain can be categorized as nociceptive, inflammatory, and pathological/neuropathic.

Nociceptive pain is produced by repetitive, prolonged, and/or excessive stimulation of pain receptors that results in receptor or nerve damage. It could originate from nociceptors located in the skin, musculoskeletal tissue, external or internal organs, or anatomical structures. Stabbing and burning characterize vulvar pain. Nociceptive pain reflects our capacity to detect the presence of potentially damaging stimuli; it is an essential early warning mechanism (Haanpää et al. 2011). It quickly indicates damaging factor(s) the body should withdraw from and/or avoid, while the resulting inflammatory process is finalized to repair and heal-

This sensation is mediated in the periphery by high threshold primary sensory neurons, the nociceptors, which transmit information via nociceptive pathways in the spinal cord to the brain. Following peripheral tissue injury or inflammation, reversible adaptive changes in the sensory nervous system lead to the generation of pain hypersensitivity, a protective mechanism that ensures proper healing of damaged tissue. The noxious stimulus is transmitted by nociceptors to the dorsal root ganglion of the spinal cord. Thinly myelinated A-δ nociceptors transmit immediate sharp pain, whereas unmyelinated C-fibers transmit delayed and longer-lasting pain.

By contrast, chronic pain, which is persistently inflammatory until it becomes neuropathic, is the results of aberrant functioning of peripheral or central nervous systems that have been pathologically modified (Watson and Sandroni 2016).

Inflammatory pain also has an adaptive function to protect healing tissues. Tissue damage triggers reversible changes of hypersensitivity in the sensory system, which last as long as inflammation persists. The mast cell is the director of the inflammatory orchestra, the leading protagonist of the tissue response to high variety of damaging factors (Fig. 3.3). Mast cells, degranulated mast cells, and mast cells close to pain fibers are significantly increased in the vestibular tissue (Bohm-Starke et al. 1999; Bornstein et al. 2004; Graziottin 2009; Graziottin et al. 2013, 2014a; Graziottin and Gambini 2016).

Inflammatory pain:

- Is *physiologic* when:
  - It is "*resolving*," i.e., *finalized* to restore the normal cytoarchitecture and functions:
    - Of tissues undergoing cyclical functional changes, such as the ovary at ovulation, the endometrium at menstruation, and the whole uterus during and after delivery
    - Of damaged tissues, because of traumas and chemical, physical, infective, and autoimmunitary lesions
  - It is of *limited duration*, adequate to restore normality ("restitutio ad integrum," according to ancient physicians)
  - It is of *intensity adequate and proportionate to restore normality*
- Is *pathologic* when:
  - It is *not finalized, i.e., non-resolving*, with progressive loss of the tissue's cytoarchitecture and function: endometriosis is a typical example.
  - It tends to become *chronic*.
  - *The intensity becomes disproportionate* in comparison to the triggering factors of inflammation (please see Chap. 6 for further details).

Acute vulvar pain of whatever cause is typically first nociceptive and rapidly turns into inflammatory. When the peripheral vestibular/genital tissue's *inflammation*

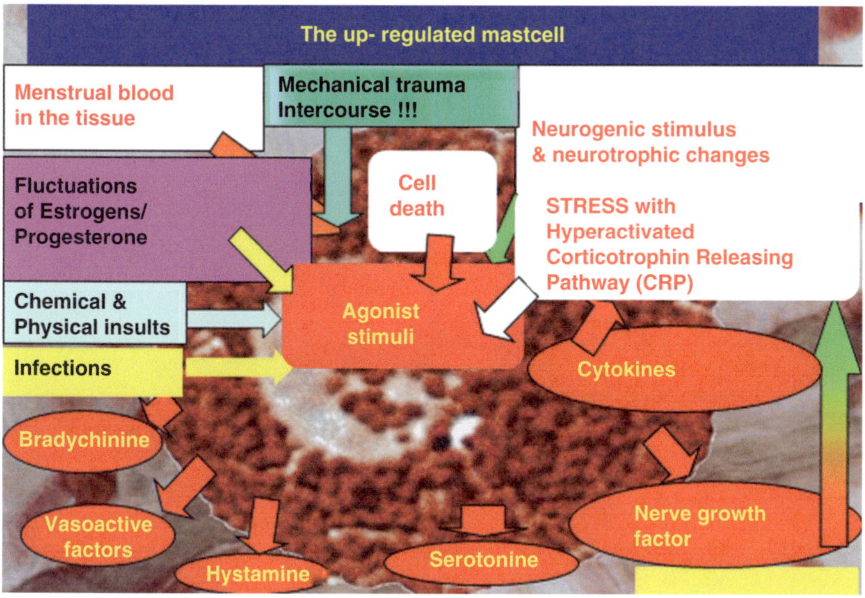

Fig. 3.3 The upregulated mast cell. Agonist factors that induce the mast cell to degranulate, i.e., to activate the inflammatory response, include infections, chemical and physical insults, fluctuations of estrogens and progesterone (typical of the menstrual period), the vestibular trauma induced by intercourse (a specific precipitating and perpetuating cause of vestibular trauma), inflammation and shift to pathologic/neuropathic pain, cell death, typical of vulvar traumatic lesion, spontaneous or iatrogenic, neurogenic stimuli induced by neuroinflammation, and chronic stress, via the hyperactivation of the corticotrophin releasing pathway. The content of the vesicle strategically and timely released in the tissue include, among others, bradykinin, vasoactive factors, histamine, serotonin, nerve growth factor (NGF), cytokines, tryptase, heparanase (Graziottin 2015)

persists, a progressive cytokines' flooding of the central nervous system takes play. Cytokines, interleukin 1 beta, tumor necrosis factor alpha, and other inflammatory molecules cross the brain barrier, hyperactive the glial cells, and particularly the microglia.

The *microglia's* role shifts progressively from neuroplastic to neurotoxic, with *neuroinflammatio*n leading to *sickness behavior*, with changes in mood, energy, sleep patterns, cognition, and memory. Sickness behavior is initially protective, aimed at sparing energy to optimize the healing process. When the *inflammatory pain becomes chronic*, *sickness behavior* becomes *maladaptive* with more persistent behavioral changes (Xanthos et al. 2011; Graziottin et al. 2013, 2014a).

Critical changes consequent to central *neuroinflammation* include:

- Neurogenic neuroinflammation (within the brain)
- Neurogenic peripheral inflammation
- Central sensitization

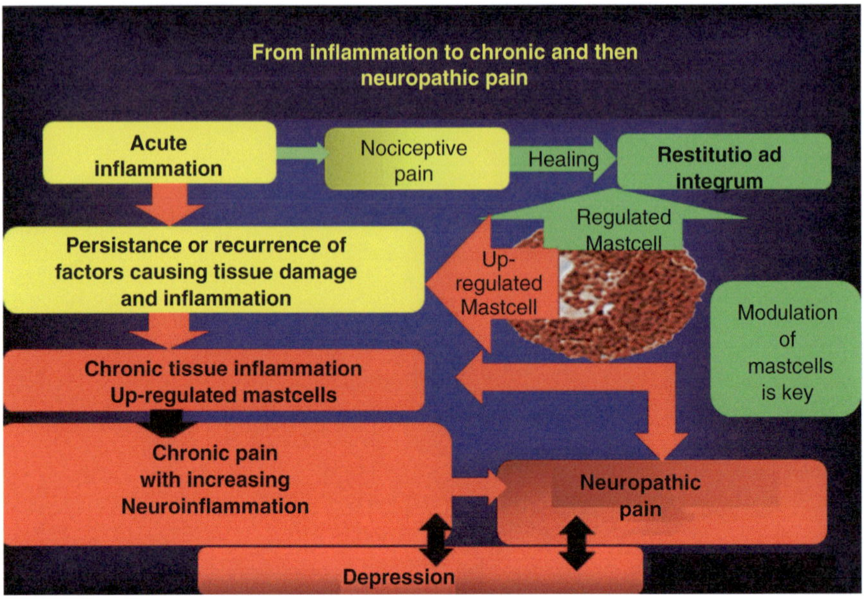

Fig. 3.4 The figure summarizes the leading characteristics and cascade of events starting with acute vulvar inflammation. The physiologic inflammation leads to the healing process. The pathological inflammation, with upregulated mat cells, leads to the worsening of vestibular/vulvar pain, with shift to other sensations and perceptions. Persistent inflammation contributes to neuroinflammation and neuropathic pain, when pain becomes a real disease per se. Hyperalgesia and allodynia are part of the pathologic, neuropathic pain process (Graziottin 2010)

- Depression (the behavioral and perceptive correlate of neuroinflammation) (Graziottin et al. 2013, 2014a; Graziottin and Gambini 2015, 2016) (Fig. 3.4)

All these changes cause a progressive shift of pain from acute nociceptive and inflammatory, to chronic inflammatory, to pathological/neuropathic (Graziottin et al. 2013, 2014a; Walker et al. 2013). Figure 3.4 summarizes the key concepts on the relationship between mast cell-mediated inflammation, mood disorders, and vulvar pain.

Pathological pain is caused by structural damage to the nervous system (*neuropathic pain*) or abnormal function of the nervous system (*dysfunctional pain*). When pain continues after noxious stimuli or inflammation in the peripheral tissue resolves, it is maladaptive and therefore pathological. In pathological pain, the nervous system itself is injured by *persistent neuroinflammation*. Changes in its sensitivity can become persistent: pain can occur spontaneously, its threshold may fall dramatically such that innocuous stimuli produce pain, and the duration and amplitude of its response to noxious stimuli are amplified. Because these neural changes in susceptible individuals can be irreversible, neuropathic pain, once established, should be regarded as an *autonomous disease state of the nervous system* in its own right (Treede et al. 2008).

The Neuropathic Pain Special Interest Group of the International Association for the Study of Pain (NeuPSIG) revised the definition of neuropathic pain in 2009 (Cruccu et al. 2010).

It is now defined as "pain arising as direct consequence of a lesion or disease affecting the somatosensory system." This implies that neuropathic pain can arise from a lesion affecting either the peripheral or the central nervous system. The new definition proposed by NeuPSIG replaces "dysfunction" with "disease" to distinguish neuropathic pain from pain such as that caused by neuroplastic changes in response to strong nociceptive stimulation.

Neuropathic pain can include peripheral and central nervous system components.

3.7.1 Peripheral Nervous System

Noxious insults trigger inflammatory mediators, neurotransmitters, and growth factor activity, which can result in nociceptor sensitization or ectopic excitability of afferent neurons. This results in innocuous stimuli at the site of inflammation, such as light touch, warm or cool temperatures, being perceived as painful (*allodynia*), and stimuli that usually are felt as uncomfortable or slightly painful, such as a pinprick, becoming extremely painful (*hyperalgesia*).

Peripheral sensitization characteristically occurs after peripheral inflammation and comprises a reduction in threshold and an increase in the excitability of the peripheral terminals of nociceptors in response to sensitizing inflammatory mediators.

Inflammation has been suggested to be pivotal to the development of peripheral sensitization. *Nerve grow factor* (NGF) appears to be a key molecule in the orchestration of peripheral inflammation. NGF is released from many cells after tissue injury and has several pro-inflammatory roles. Indeed, NGF has significant action on the expression of other inflammatory mediators (interleukin-1ß, tumor necrosis factor, etc.), and it is also capable of direct and indirect sensitization of nociceptors. Inflammation-driven release of cytokines from immune cells provokes hyperalgesia through stimulation and production of other pro-inflammatory agents (Schaible 2015).

Peripheral *mast cell activation* is generally considered *pro-inflammatory* and *pro-nociceptive*. These peripheral cell types are located in the dermis, adjacent to blood vessels, nerve endings, and glandular ducts, and have a cytoplasm filled with spherical granules. Mast cell granules contain many factors implicated in *neurogenic inflammation*, such as NGF, tumor necrosis factor (TNF), proteases, and cytokines (Fig. 3.3).

Physical, chemical, and mechanical stimuli activate local mast cells, causing degranulation and secretion of mediators that have been found to sensitize and induce the proliferation of C-afferent nerve fibers. *These nerve fibers release inflammatory mediators, including NGF*, which increase the proliferation and degranulation of mast cells, causing hyperesthesia, and enhance the inflammatory response. Mast cells show particular complexity in relation to the inflammatory response, and their density in inflamed tissue changes over time. In tissue where there is an acute inflammatory response, the concentration of mast cells is high. As the inflammation becomes more chronic, the number of mast cells decreases and there is a parallel increase in neuronal proliferation. At this stage of the inflammatory process, neuropathic symptoms became prominent, but mast cell reactivation can occur at any time, with an exacerbation of symptoms or an acceleration of *neurogenic inflammatory processes* (Xanthos et al. 2011).

3.7.2 Central Nervous System Components

The dorsal horn is now known to play a key role in the modulation of pain and the development of chronic pain states. Pain is perceived only if this electrical activity reaches the brain, and, hence, any modulation or alteration within the dorsal horn can have profound effects on pain sensation.

Laminas IV and V of the dorsal horn contain a peculiar type of neuron called wide dynamic range (WDR). Repetitive stimulation by C-fibers causes some WDR cells in the dorsal horn to augment their response. Thus, for a given input stimulus, the output is enhanced; this process is referred to as "windup." Windup is a part of a process termed "central sensitization."

Cortical functioning has localizing, emotional, and memory components. Descending modulatory control is bidirectional in nature. These descending control systems link the brain cortex to the dorsal horn, acting either directly on primary afferents or indirectly via inhibitory and excitatory interneurons. *Central sensitization involves changes from neuroplastic to neurotoxic in the microglia activity,* within the spinal cord and the brain in response to damage to the peripheral somatosensory nervous system. Neuroimaging demonstrates increased sensitivity and activity of neurons in the thalamus and somatosensory cortex in response to chronic pain (Baron et al. 2013) (Box 3.1).

Box 3.1 Pain Glossary and Anatomofunctional Correlates

- *Allodynia*: pain due to a stimulus that does not normally provoke pain, such as touch or light pressure. In the vestibular mucosa, it is the functional/perceptive result of a dislocation of pain fibers from the deep layers of submucosal tissue, passing across the basal membrane through micro-tunnels excavated by heparanase and tryptase enzymes produced by the mast cells, to a progressive superficialization among the mucosal cells. This location's change of pain fibers induces the brain to read as "burning pain" a tactile stimulus (Fig. 3.5).
- *Hyperalgesia*: increased pain response from a stimulus that normally provokes pain. It is due to the proliferation of peripheral pain nerve fibers induced by the NGF and other neurotrophins.

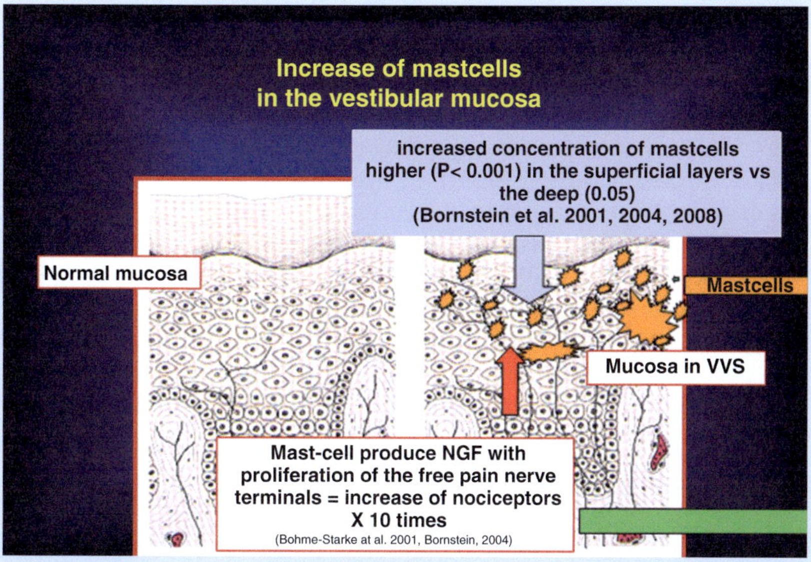

Fig. 3.5 Increase of mast cells in the inflamed and "burning" vestibular mucosa. On the right part of the drawing, the number of mast cells and activated mast cells is significantly increased in the superficial layers of the inflamed vestibular mucosa in comparison to controls: this justifies the name "vulvar vestibulitis," in the acute inflammatory phase of the pain process. With persistent, chronic inflammation, the mast cell production of NGF induces the proliferation of pain nerve fibers. Their number is significantly increased leading to hyperalgesia. Inflammation progressively shifts from physiologic to pathologic. Pain fibers cross the basal membrane along the microtunnels excavated by heparanase and tryptase enzymes produced by the mast cells. Pain fibers superficialize and this gives the brain a wrong signal as if the pain fiber were stimulated deep in the tissue: this is the anatomofunctional correlate explaining the perceptive shift from a tactile stimulus (such as a gentle touch) into a burning feeling (a pain signal), a shift called "allodynia" (Graziottin and Vincenti 2004)

- *Peripheral sensitization*: increased responsiveness and reduced threshold of nociceptive neurons in the periphery to the stimulation of their receptive fields.
- *Central sensitization*: increased responsiveness of nociceptive neurons in the central nervous system to their normal or subthreshold afferent input (in simple words, it causes a reduced pain threshold within the brain). Central sensitization is the result of a progressive, maladaptive, non-resolving, and neuroinflammation.
- *Neuroplasticity*: adaptive, when positive, or maladaptive changes ("neurotoxicity") in the nervous system.

Modified from Baron et al. (2013)

3.8 Factors Associated with Vulvodynia or Pathophysiological Components of the Disease

3.8.1 Vestibular Neuroproliferation

In 1997, Westrom first reported a nerve fiber proliferation in the vestibular mucosa in women with vestibulodynia. Since then, many studies have reported similar findings. Currently, the nerve hyperplasia is the main marker of vestibulodynia.

Immunohistochemistry has shown altered density of nerve endings such as the vanilloid receptor VR1 (TRPV1), which is expressed by nociceptors, and is triggered by capsaicin, noxious heat, and chemicals produced during inflammation, as well as increased number of intraepithelial free nerve endings, calcitonin-related gene peptide (peptide found in nerve fibers), lowered tactile and pain thresholds, nociceptor sensitization, and overall peripheral nerve hyperplasia (Reed et al. 2014).

3.8.2 Inflammation

Pro-inflammatory cell migration and activation to the vulvar vestibule and local production, and release of pro-inflammatory pain-inducing substances, are pivotal elements in vestibulodynia patients.

Studying vulvodynia immune-histology, several groups report *mast cell predominant inflammation*. Their activation is associated with the discharge of various mediators from the granules, such as NGF, tryptase, and bradykinin. Vestibular changes in the biochemical milieu could alter ion channel activity of the peripheral preterminal axon. This could lead to a lowering of mechanical, thermal, or chemical threshold in the primary nociceptors (Regauer et al. 2015).

Elevated concentrations of IL-1 beta and TNF-alpha have been found in women with vestibulodynia relative to asymptomatic controls and changes in IL-1 beta-receptors have also been demonstrated (Foster et al. 2007).

Local organized vestibule-associated lymphoid tissue (VALT), analogous to mucosa-associated lymphoid tissue, was found in vestibulodynia. While protecting against local infection, an *activated VALT* could cause an exaggerated inflammatory reaction and contribute to the sensitized pain perception in the vestibular mucosa. This suggests a link between the *mast cell activation and vascular hyperemic response* and possibly the interplay with neurons as well (Tommola et al. 2015).

Bohm-Starke et al. (2001) provided data indicating that vestibular pain is not mediated by classic inflammatory mechanisms, explaining why treatments that target the cyclooxygenase or nitric oxide systems are not effective. Neurogenic inflammation is the most appropriate definition of this series of events.

3.8.3 Neurologic Central Mechanisms

Several lines of investigation support the elements of central sensitization in vulvodynia patients. Structural and functional magnetic resonance imaging (fMRI) studies have revealed that using pressure (perceived as painful in patients but not in controls) to the posterior portion of the vulvar vestibule as a stimulus in women with vestibulodynia and healthy controls, women with vestibulodynia showed significantly higher activation levels in the insular and frontal cortical regions than did controls, mirroring activation patterns observed in other chronic pain conditions.

In addition, it has been shown that vestibulodynia is associated with increased gray matter density in pain modulatory and stress-related brain regions. It has been speculated that increased gray matter density could be caused by microglial proliferation maybe due to excess excitatory neural activity (Hampson et al. 2013) (Box 3.2).

Box 3.2 Central Sensitization and Vulvodynia

- Increased pressure sensitivity in both the vulva and peripheral body regions
- Increased pain intensity and unpleasantness in response to tender-point examination in nongenital sites
- Higher levels of brain activity in primary and secondary somatosensory cortices during application of pressure to the posterior vestibule
- Lower pain pressure thresholds to noxious cold stimulation, suggesting a systemic hypersensitivity
- Higher gray matter density in pain modulatory and stress-related areas

Modified from Vulvodynia: National Vulvodynia Association, Integrating Current Knowledge into Clinical Practice

3.8.4 Musculoskeletal Pattern

It has long been recognized that many vulvar pain conditions are often associated with some degree of pelvic floor muscle (PFM) dysfunction, and hypertonic dysfunction is found in 80–90 % of patients with vulvodynia (Graziottin and Murina 2011; Graziottin and Gambini 2016).

High-resting tension, muscle irritability, tenderness to palpation, and overall weakness are the hallmark of pelvic floor muscle dysfunction in vestibulodynia patients.

Study on hypertonicity of pelvic floor muscle dysfunction in women with vestibulodynia demonstrated that these women exhibited significantly more hypertonicity in the superficial PFM layer, less PFM strength, less ability to relax the PFM, and a smaller degree of vaginal opening than non-affected women (Gentilcore-Saulnier et al. 2010).

Women with vestibulodynia display differences in transperineal 4D ultrasound PFM morphometry at rest and during maximal contraction, suggesting higher tone, lower strength, and poor control (Morin et al. 2014).

A relevant topic to be investigated is whether vulvodynia reflects pelvic floor dysfunction with trigger points of pain, or whether it is a form of referred pain, or a result of dysfunctional nerve fibers in the pelvis.

It is hypothesized that vestibular pain and inflammation trigger a protective defense mechanism of the pelvic floor muscles in addition to poor muscle control and hypertonicity pelvic floor muscles; hypertonicity may also act as an initiator of vestibular sensory changes and inflammation.

The leading opinion indicates that vulvar pain can produce spasm of the levator ani muscle, and pelvic floor hypertonicity contributes to self-maintenance of pain.

In summary, the levator ani muscles are innervated by the levator ani nerve, while no evidence of innervation by the pudendal nerve can be found. The levator ani motor neurons are diffusely distributed in the sacral ventral horn, while the pudendal motor neurons are concentrated in Onuf's nucleus (a group of neurons located in the ventral part of laminae IX of the anterior horn). However, there is a deal of overlap between the dendrites of levator ani motor neurons and pudendal motor neurons, and both nerves contain primary afferent fibers that project into the sacral spinal cord. Thus, there is great potential for interaction between the sensory and motor nerve fibers that controlled the levator ani muscle, the vulva, and the vestibule.

Key Points

- It is not important what starts the process (muscle or nerve), but it is important how alteration of the pelvic muscles is responsible for the severity of symptoms.
- Indeed, "the weight of the muscle" may be different between patients with vulvodynia, and this is the only important target of the treatment program.

3.8.5 Genetic Predisposition

A genetic predisposition to pain sensitivity may be a causative/contributing factor in vulvodynia. Recent lines of evidence highlight a potential genetic predisposition to chronic inflammation among vestibulodynia-afflicted women. These genetic polymorphisms lead to a reduced capacity to terminate ("resolving inflammation") and to an exaggerated inflammatory response ("non-resolving, chronic inflammation" with inflammatory pain progressively shifting to pathological/neuropathic pain).

There is great frequency of polymorphisms in genes for interleukin (IL)-1 beta and IL-1 receptor antagonist, factors associated with an increased and prolonged inflammatory response (Gerber et al. 2003).

Variant alleles encoding molecules involved in immune responses to *Candida* infection such as mannose-binding lectin and NALP3 inflammasome are more frequent in vulvodynia patients. This suggests that defective clearance of the organism or altered inflammatory patterns contribute to the development of vulvodynia.

A study based upon the Utah Population Database shows a genetic predisposition to the disease in families of patients who underwent vestibulectomy due to chronic vulvar pain. These findings, as well as a strong family history of symptoms of vulvodynia among those patients, suggest a possible genetic origin for vulvodynia (Reed et al. 2012).

Key Points
A genetic predisposition to the development of vestibulodynia is potentially based on three mechanisms:

- Influence on the risks of recurrent vulvovaginal candidiasis
- Altered inflammatory response
- Increased sensitivity to pain

3.8.6 Hormonal Factors

Some studies have concentrated on the effects of estrogens and progesterone on peripheral nervous system pathways, emphasizing those that pertain to vulvar pain. A review of the literature reveals a somewhat common idea that there is a relationship between estrogen and sensation and that a decrease in threshold occurs with increased estrogen levels, such as during the menstrual cycle (Graziottin 2015), during pregnancy, and estrogen replacement. This may explain a change in symptoms during the menstrual cycle; in fact many vulvodynia patients can have an exacerbation of symptoms during the premenstrual period. Furthermore some vestibulodynia patients presented with dyspareunia and signs of vestibular atrophy including a thinned, dry, fragile or pale mucosa, quite similar to menopausal women (Fig. 3.6).

Autonomic and sensory neurons express estrogen receptors and are responsive to estradiol in culture, supporting the idea that estrogens can act directly on neurons. Estrogen is known to affect inflammatory neuropeptides involved in chronic pain, in which the lack of estrogen is associated with an increased density of sympathetic, parasympathetic, and sensory nerve fibers in the vulva (Ting et al. 2004).

We can conclude that between the level of estrogen and vaginal innervation, there is an inverse proportionality relationship.

It was demonstrated that progesterone increases neurite outgrowth by small unmyelinated sensory neurons, and pre-treatment of ganglion with progesterone also increased neurite outgrowth in response to vaginal target explants (Liao and Smith 2014).

Results from studies investigating the expression of the estrogen receptor alpha (ERα) in women with vestibulodynia are contradictory. Initially, decreased expression of ERα in the vestibular mucosa was reported. In a more recent study, biopsies were taken in the same phase of the menstrual cycle, and a significant increase in ERα was found in patients compared to controls. Furthermore, the vulvar vestibule is embryologically analogous to the urogenital gland in males. These glands have

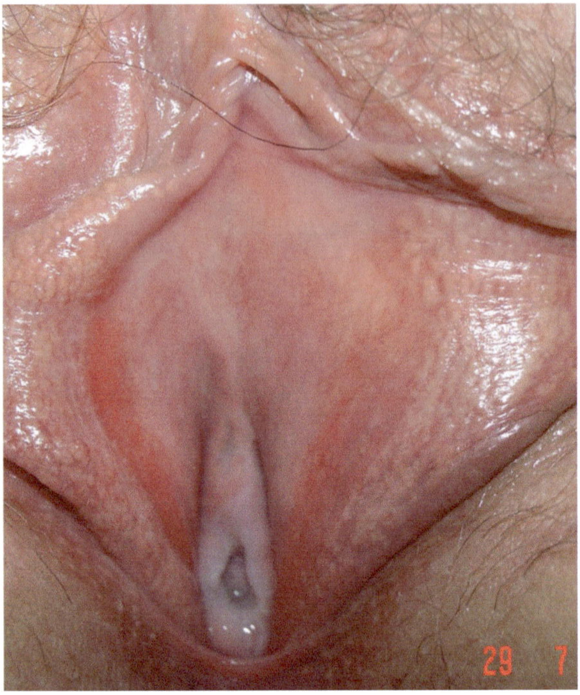

Fig. 3.6 Trophic changes in vestibulodynia patient

a high density of androgen receptors, which implies that adequate testosterone levels are essential for the maintenance of healthy vestibular tissue (Goldstein et al. 2009).

One potential claimed cause of vestibulodynia is use of combined hormonal contraceptives (CHCs) (Reed et al. 2013). Some studies suggest increased risk for vulvodynia among users of oral contraceptives that may be related to age of first use, duration of use, or strength of hormonal composition. CHCs use has been associated with a sevenfold increase in the risk of developing vestibulodynia. The risk is higher with current, long term or early use, and with use of CHCs of high progestogenic potency and low estrogenic and androgenic potency (Bouchard et al. 2002).

It should be noted that the bias of some studies is the lack of a clear evaluation of patients pre-existing conditions. The vestibular mucosa of women with CHCs displays an altered morphological pattern with shallow and sparse dermal papillae compared with the follicular phase. Similar findings are seen in women without CHCs during the luteal phase which indicate a gestagenic effect on the mucosa. These findings are thought to be reflective of a gestagenic effect, and they support the data pointing to an increased risk of developing vestibular pain from using pills with high gestagenic potency. It has also been reported that women without dyspareunia who use CHCs have lower vestibular pain thresholds to mechanical stimuli (Johannesson et al. 2007).

Key Points

- Progesterone exposure may contribute to vestibulodynia by eliciting persistent genital hyperinnervation via a direct effect on unmyelinated sensory nociceptor neurons, and estradiol may alleviate symptoms in part by reducing progesterone-induced sensory hyperinnervation
- It is unclear whether CHCs play a role in the development of vulvodynia. The current recommendation is to continue to prescribe the pill when needed, but prescribers should be aware of side-effects, and the selection of the most appropriate formulation is needed

3.8.7 Psychosocial Factors

Psychological morbidity is significantly higher in women with vulvodynia compared with asymptomatic women. Many studies demonstrate high degrees of anxiety, depressive symptoms, somatization disorders, and hypochondriacal symptoms in vulvodynia patients (Bergeron et al. 2014).

While someone proposes that the syndrome has a purely psychogenic origin, the leading opinion suggests that sexual dysfunction and psychological distress are the consequence rather than the cause of vulvodynia. However, this concept is still under debate.

The anterior cingulate brain cortex (ACC) contributes to the control of the state of conscious arousal and attention based on prefrontal cortical innervations. Anxiety-dependent pain exacerbation is also mediated by other limbic structures, such as the hippocampus. A history of abuse or trauma is common in chronic pelvic pain patients, and this is also mediated by limbic dysfunction, particularly of the ACC, hippocampus, and amygdala.

It has been observed that vulvodynia patients have higher rates of sexual abuse, including threatened sex, forced intercourse, lifetime sexual victimization, and severe child sexual abuse, an association that appears to hold true for other vulvodynia comorbidities such as irritable bowel syndrome and interstitial cystitis (Khandker et al. 2014).

Although there is a degree of association, several studies have refuted the notion that prior sexual and/or physical abuse is a predisposing factor for vulvodynia. Regardless of the sequence of events, physical and psychological factors produce a continuum with multiple dimensions of pain. Studies show lower frequency of intercourse, decrease in desire, and increased difficulty achieving orgasm, and many patients with vulvodynia who do have intercourse do so out of a sense of obligation rather than desire.

In conclusion, it is still impossible to say whether psychosexual factors are involved in the development or maintenance of vestibulodynia or whether they are the consequence of an undiagnosed, persistent, and debilitating pain. Pain modulation by psychological factors is one of the most complex problems: in vulvodynia patients, psycho-neurobiological vulnerability plays a relevant role, and the experience of pain varies depending on the patient's psychological state.

3.9 Triggers

In addition to the possible underlying causes or potential factors associated with vulvodynia, various triggers causing vestibular inflammation and vestibular pain have been identified. They progressively shift acute vulvar pain to chronic and neuropathic, with hyperalgesia and allodynia in the vestibule and vulva.

These associations include *infections* such as sexual factors (Box 3.3 and 3.4), recurrent vulvovaginal candidiasis (please see Chap. 6), urinary tract infection, bacterial vaginosis, and allergic reactions or atopy; neurological and neoplastic etiology need to be adequately considered as well, when a careful clinical history and competent clinical examination is suggestive of these specific, more complex etiologies.

Box 3.3. Sexual Factors and Vestibular Pain

Sexual factors may act as:

- *Predisposing to vestibular trauma*: vaginismus, with the associated hyperactived, defensively contracted pelvic floor, predisposes to introital microtraumas at every intercourse attempt
- *Precipitating vestibular trauma, pain, and inflammation when intercourse causes introital damage*, in case of fear of intercourse, poor sexual arousal, defensive pelvic floor contraction, hyperactive pelvic floor, larger than average penis dimension, and recurrent *Candida* vaginitis
- *Perpetuating vestibular trauma, when intercourse is repeatedly accepted in spite of worsening introital pain (introital dyspareunia)* with progressive shift of inflammation from physiologic, resolving, of limited duration and appropriate intensity, to pathologic, non-resolving, of prolonged duration, i.e., chronic, and inappropriate intensity until pathological neuropathic pain is in play

Box 3.4. Vaginismus and Dyspareunia: How Can They Contribute to Vulvar Pain?

Although there is a long-standing tradition of distinguishing female sexual pain disorders into vaginismus and (superficial) dyspareunia, recent research has demonstrated persistent problems with the sensitivity and specificity of the differential diagnosis of these two phenomena (Graziottin 2006).

Both complaints may comprise, to a smaller or larger extent (Fig. 3.7):

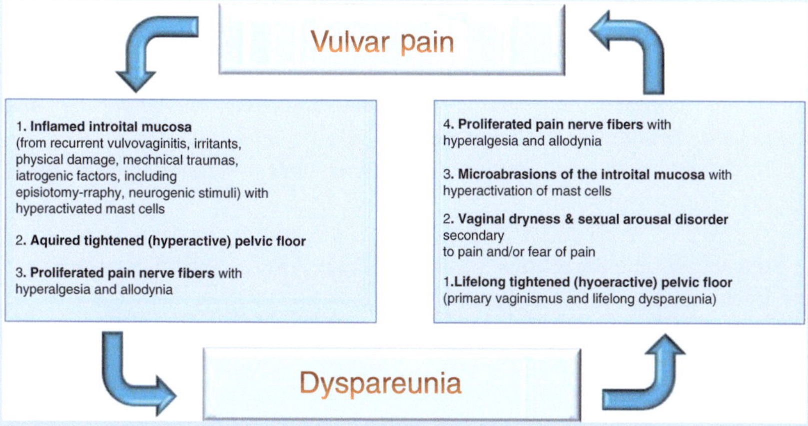

Fig. 3.7 Coital pain is associated with an inflamed introital mucosa, for different reasons. HCPs can observe a defensive hyperactive pelvic floor (myogenic hyperactivity) followed by hyperalgesia and allodynia due to the proliferation of pain nerve fibers. In a woman with a normal vestibular mucosa, if the initial symptom is coital pain, the first consequence will be the defensive contraction of the levator ani (like in primary vaginismus and lifelong dyspareunia). This predisposes the introital vestibular mucosa to microabrasions resulting from the mechanical damage that can occur at attempts of sexual intercourse. Microtraumas of the introital mucosa with hyperactivation of mast cells and proliferation of nerve fibers lead to pathological vulvar pain, while neuroinflammation becomes prominent (Graziottin and Murina 2011)

(a) Problems with muscle tension: voluntary, involuntary, limited to vaginal sphincter, the bulbocavernous muscle, or extending to the pelvic floor, adductor muscles, back, jaws, or entire body.
(b) Pain upon genital touching: superficially located at the vaginal entry, the vulvar vestibulum and/or the perineum; either event-related (to the duration of genital touching/pressure), or more chronic (lasting for minutes/hours/days after termination of touching); ranging from unique association with genital touching during sexual activity to more general association with all types of vulvar/vaginal/pelvic pressure (e.g., sitting, riding a horse or bicycle, wearing tight trousers).
(c) Fear of sexual pain: either specifically associated with genital touching/intercourse or more generalized fear of pain or fear of sex.
(d) Propensity for behavioral approach or avoidance: despite painful experiences with genital touching/intercourse, a subgroup of women continues to be receptive to sexual interaction initiated by a partner or by themselves. This continuation of sexual interaction may have very different psychodynamic meanings. Whether a conscious or unconscious choice, it may help to maintain closer bonding, but at the price of worsening mucosal inflammation. On the other hand, it may be perceived as frank abuse if it is imposed by the partner. The majority of patients affected by dyspareunia and/or vulvodynia tend, however, to progressively avoid intercourse.

Key Points

Vaginismus, which may contribute to lifelong dyspareunia, when mild/moderate, and may prevent intercourse, when severe, needs to be better understood in its complex neurobiologic, muscular, and psychosexual etiology and addressed via a multimodal approach.

In patients with vaginismus, the diagnosis and prognosis may be made based on three variables:

- Intensity of phobic attitude (mild, moderate, severe) toward penetration
- Intensity of pelvic floor hypertonicity
- Coexisting personal and/or relational psychosexual problems

Relationship issues should be diagnosed and appropriate referral considered when the male partner presents with a concomitant male sexual disorder.

Vestibular traumas include *precipitating factors* such as:

- *Intercourse*, when *vaginismus, poor genital arousal, vaginal dryness, and/or hyperactive pelvic floor* predispose the vestibular mucosa to microtraumas leading to vestibular nociceptive and inflammatory pain ("introital dyspareunia" or "painful intercourse") in the short term. Intercourse may cause pathological/neuropathic pain when the vestibular trauma is persistently repeated for more than three to six months (please see Chap. 6 for details).
- *Vaginal birth, instrumental delivery including episiotomy*. The role of these preceding events in the pathogenesis of vulvodynia is complex, but each may trigger vestibular and vulvar traumas and microtraumas with vulvar and genital inflammation. When chronic and non-resolving, this may cause sensitization of the nervous system either directly through nerve damage or indirectly through neurogenic inflammation (please see Chap. 7).

Attempting to identify a single causative factor for an individual patient's vulvodynia is unhelpful. Instead, a multifactorial and multidisciplinary approach is preferred, including addressing contributory elements and counseling the patient about the multifactorial etiology of the condition.

3.9.1 The Role of Recurrent Vulvovaginal Candidiasis

Women with vestibulodynia are more likely to report a history of vulvovaginal candidiasis (VVC), recurrent VVC, and an association between *Candida* infection and pain symptom initiation.

Mimicking repeated vaginal candidiasis that some women report experiencing vestibulodynia, a rodent model of long-lasting mechanical allodynia, after repeated exposure of the vulva to *Candida albicans*, has been developed in mice. Allodynia persists for at least 3 weeks after resolution of infection in a subset of female mice in this model and produces hyperinnervation (Farmer et al. 2011).

It has also been demonstrated that women with vulvodynia more frequently react to patch tests for *Candida albicans*, and it was postulated that exposure to *Candida albicans* at low concentrations may involve neurotransmitters that have been shown to influence contact hypersensitivity (Ramirez De Knott et al. 2005).

Selective sampling of fibroblasts from painful and adjacent nonpainful sites demonstrates enhanced pro-inflammatory cytokine production after yeast extract stimulation (Foster et al. 2015).

As mentioned above, a polymorphism in the gene coding for mannose-binding lectin, an innate immune antimicrobial protein that inhibits *Candida* proliferation, and polymorphisms in the genes coding for inflammasomes (macromolecules that regulate the release of interleukin IL-1ß) reduce the production of active IL-1ß, necessary for recruitment of immune cells that inactivate yeast, are more common in vestibulodynia patients with recurrent VVC (Babula et al. 2008).

Key Points

A genetic susceptibility to *Candida* infection, coupled with reduced capacity to terminate the resulting inflammation, could initiate an inflammatory cascade that triggers neurogenic changes in the vestibule leading to a persistently altered pain response.

3.9.2 What Is the Relationship Between Vestibulodynia and Generalized Vulvodynia?

Some clinicians think that vestibulodynia (about 80 % of vulvodynia patients) and generalized vulvodynia may be variations in severity of the same disorder. The etiopathological process has been suggested to first result in the localized pain of vestibulodynia then progress to the chronic, generalized vulvar pain; *instead, our experience suggests that the two conditions may be two distinct disorders*.

The two subtypes of vulvodynia can be clearly distinguished by some characteristics such as age, symptoms, and triggering inflammatory factors. Nevertheless, individuals may have aspects of both vestibulodynia and generalized vulvodynia, with overlapping symptoms. The morphological findings of vestibular nerve-ending proliferation have not been demonstrated for generalized vulvodynia, but new elements have been identified in this subtype of disease where there is a scarcity of research on the pathophysiology. As with patients with neuropathic pain, women with generalized vulvodynia exhibit hyperalgesia and/or allodynia, which can be considered a functional effect corresponding to neural hyperplasia.

Our study indicates that the current perception threshold (CPT) values were lower in women affected by vulvodynia than those in controls, suggesting a hypersensitivity (Murina et al. 2010).

The CPT measures provide objective and quantitative determinations of the sensory nerve conduction and nerve functional integrity, and it uses an electrical stimulus selective for the large and small myelinated and unmyelinated fibers that are involved in the transmission of painless and painful sensation.

Each of the three major sensory fiber types has a characteristic neurophysiological profile, sensory function, sensation evoked by electrical stimulation, and conduction block susceptibility.

Because findings of enhanced pain perception are typical of neuropathic pain syndromes, our results add strength to a neuropathic hypothesis for pain also in generalized vulvodynia.

In our opinion a different subtype of vestibulodynia exists that is distinguishable by certain characteristics such as trigger factors, age, pelvic floor dysfunction, and comorbidities, rather than two diseases classified upon the vulvar symptoms localization and characteristics of pain (provoked or unprovoked).

Conclusions

Acute vulvar pain is the subjective experience of a vulvar damage/insult/trauma of different etiology. Nociceptive pain is its first correlate, rapidly shifting into inflammatory pain, physiologic in the first part of the process, when it is resolving (i.e., finalized to heal the tissue), of limited duration and appropriate intensity.

Inflammatory pain becomes chronic and progressively pathologic when it is non-resolving, of persistent duration and of disproportionate intensity in comparison to the initial trauma. Inflammation progressively involves the neighboring organs ("pelvic comorbidity"), gradually become systemic and involves the brain ("neuroinflammation") leading to the typical features of pathological/neuropathic pain.

We believe that vestibulodynia results from many predisposing, precipitating, and perpetuating factors that ultimately promote and maintain neurogenic neuroinflammation and neurogenic peripheral inflammation, with a persistent pain response. An immune cell-mediated inflammatory cascade may be a common pathway through which neurogenic vestibular pain becomes established (Fig. 3.8).

Neuropathic pain is an indicator of disorganized sensory motor and reference frames that an evolved adaptive system in the peripheral and central nervous system responds to as an indication of multiple trigger factors.

IASP has recently published a new definition of neuropathic pain according to which the condition is defined as "pain caused by a lesion or disease of the somatosensory system."

In vulvodynia we can find allodynia and hyperalgesia, neurogenic inflammation, and peripheral ad central sensitization, all typical items of neuropathic pain syndrome.

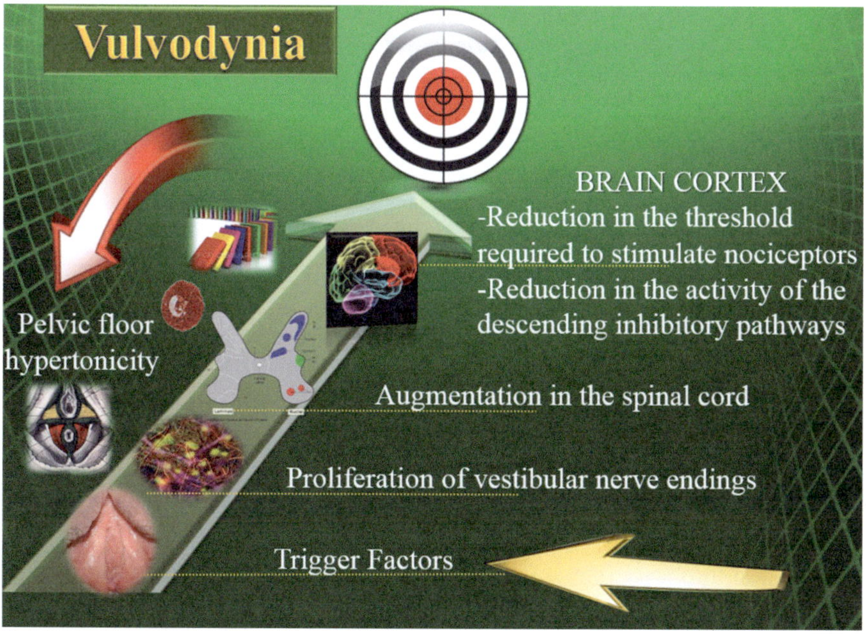

Fig. 3.8 The pathophysiology of vulvodynia

Is it right to define vulvodynia a dysfunctional pain syndrome with an unclear etiology only because a clear lesion or disease of the somatosensory system has not been demonstrated (yet)? A more pathophysiologically oriented reading may clarify its many biological peripheral and central component, anatomic/morphologic and not only "dysfunctional."

References

Ashton-Miller JA, De Lancey JO. Functional anatomy of the female pelvic floor. Ann N Y Acad Sci. 2007;1101:266–96. Epub 2007 Apr 7. Review.

Babula O, Linhares IM, Bongiovanni AM, Ledger WJ, Witkin SS. Association between primary vulvar vestibulitis syndrome, defective induction of tumor necrosis factor-alpha, and carriage of the mannose-binding lectin codon 54 gene polymorphism. Am J Obstet Gynecol. 2008;198:101.e1–4.

Baron R, Hans G, Dickenson AH. Peripheral input and its importance for central sensitization. Ann Neurol. 2013;74(5):630–6.

Beech SLI, Adams MA. Comparative anatomic investigation of the vasculature architecture of the internal pudendal artery in men and women. J Sex Med. 2009;6:105.

Bergeron S, Likes WM, Steben M. Psychosexual aspects of vulvovaginal pain. Best Pract Res Clin Obstet Gynaecol. 2014;28:991–9.

Bohm-Starke N, Hilliges M, Falconer C, et al. Neurochemical characterization of the vestibular nerves in women with vulvar vestibulitis syndrome. Gynecol Obstet Invest. 1999;48(4):270–5.

Bohm-Starke N, Falconer C, Rylander E, et al. The expression of cyclooxygenase 2 and inducible nitric oxide synthase indicates no active inflammation in vulvar vestibulitis. Acta Obstet Gynecol Scand. 2001;80:638–44.

Boris S, Barbés C. Role played by lactobacilli in controlling the population of vaginal pathogens. Microbes Infect. 2000;2(5):543–6.

Bornstein J, Maman M, Abramovici H. "Primary" versus "secondary" vulvar vestibulitis: One disease, two variants. Am J Obstet Gynecol. 2001;184:28–31.

Bornstein J, Goldschmid N, Sabo E. Hyperinnervation and mast cell activation may be used ashistopathologic diagnostic criteria for vulvar vestibulitis. Gynecol Obstet Invest. 2004;58(3):171–8. Epub 2004 Jul 9.

Bornstein J, Cohen Y, Zarfati D, Sela S, Ophir E. Involvement of heparanase in the pathogenesis of localized vulvodynia. Int J Gynecol Pathol. 2008;27:136–41.

Bornstein J, Goldstein AT, Stockdale CK, Bergeron S, Pukall C, Zolnoun D, Coady D. 2015 ISSVD, ISSWSH, and IPPS consensus terminology and classification of persistent vulvar pain and vulvodynia. J Sex Med. 2016;13:607–12.

Bouchard C, Brisson J, Fortier M, Morin C, Blanchette C. Use of oral contraceptive pills and vulvar vestibulitis: a case control study. Am J Epidemiol. 2002;156:254–61.

Bustami FM. A reappraisal of the anatomy of the levator ani muscle in man. Acta Morphol Neerl Scand. 1988–1989;26(4):255–68.

Cruccu G, Sommer C, Anand P, Attal N, Baron R, Garcia-Larrea L, Haanpaa M, Jensen TS, Serra J, Treede RD. EFNS guidelines on neuropathic pain assessment: revised 2009. Eur J Neurol. 2010;17(8):1010–8. doi:10.1111/j.1468-1331.2010.02969.x. Epub 2010 Mar 8.

Dickinson WH. The past and future of pathology. Br Med J. 1889;1(1466):238–40.

Farmer MA, Taylor AM, Bailey AL, Tuttle AH, MacIntyre LC, Milagrosa ZE, et al. Repeated vulvovaginal fungal infections cause persistent pain in a mouse model of vulvodynia. Sci Transl Med. 2011;3:101ra91.

Fătu C, Puişoru M, Fătu IC. Morphometry of the internal iliac artery in different ethnic groups. Ann Anat. 2006;188(6):541–6.

Foster DC, Piekarz KH, Murant TI, LaPoint R, Haidaris CG, Phipps RP. Enhanced synthesis of proinflammatory cytokines by vulvar vestibular fibroblasts: implications for vulvar vestibulitis. Am J Obstet Gynecol. 2007;196:346.e1–8.

Foster D, Falsetta M, Woeller C, Pollock S, Song K, Bonham A, et al. Site-specific mesenchymal control of inflammatory pain to yeast challenge in vulvodynia afflicted and pain-free women. Pain. 2015;156:386–96.

Gentilcore-Saulnier E, McLean L, Goldfinger C, et al. Pelvic floor muscle assessment outcomes in women with and without provoked vestibulodynia and the impact of a physical therapy program. J Sex Med. 2010;7:1003–22.

Gerber S, Bongiovanni AM, Ledger WJ, et al. Interleukin-1beta gene polymorphism in women with vulvar vestibulitis syndrome. Eur J Obstet Gynecol Reprod Biol. 2003;107:74–7.

Goldstein AT, Pukall CF, Goldstein I, editors. Female sexual pain disorders: evaluation and management. Oxford, UK: Wiley- Blackwell; 2009.

Graziottin A. Sexual pain disorders: dyspareunia and vaginismus. In: Porst H, Buvat J, editors. ISSM (International Society of Sexual Medicine) standard committee book, standard practice in sexual medicine. Oxford, UK: Blackwell; 2006. p. 342–50.

Graziottin A. Mast cells and their role in sexual pain disorders. In: Goldstein A, Pukall C, Goldstein I, editors. Female sexual pain disorders: evaluation and management. Chichester: Blackwell Publishing; 2009. p. 176–9.

Graziottin A. "The shorter, the better": a review of the evidence for a shorter contraception hormone-free interval. Eur J Contracept Reprod Health Care. 2015;20:1–13 [Epub ahead of print].

Graziottin A, Gambini D. Evaluation of genito-pelvic pain penetration disorder. In: Waguih WI, editor. The textbook of sexual medicine. Philadelphia: Springer Verlag; 2016.

Graziottin A, Murina F. Vulvodynia – tips and tricks. Milan: Springer; 2011.

Graziottin A, Zanello PP. Pathogenic biofilms: their role in recurrent cystitis and vaginitis (with focus on D-mannose as a new prophylactic strategy). In: Studd J, Seang LT, Chervenak FA,

editors. Current progress in obstetrics and gynaecology, vol. 3. 2nd ed. Mumbai: Kothari Medical; 2015. p. 218–38.
Graziottin A, Skaper S, Fusco M. Inflammation and chronic pelvic pain: a biological trigger for depression in women? J Depress Anxiety. 2013;3:142–50.
Graziottin A, Skaper S, Fusco M. Mast cells in chronic inflammation, pelvic pain and depression in women. Gynecol Endocrinol. 2014a;30(7):472–7.
Graziottin A, Zanello PP, D'Errico G. Recurrent cystitis and vaginitis: role of biofilms and persister cells. From pathophysiology to new therapeutic strategies. Minerva Ginecol. 2014b;66(5):497–512.
Graziottin A, Gambini D. Anatomy and physiology of genital organs - Women. In: Vodusek D, Boller F, editors. Neurology of sexual and bladder disorders, Handbook of clinical neurology, vol. 130, 3rd series. Edinburgh: Elsevier; 2015. p. 39–60.
Haanpää M, Attal N, Backonja M, Baron R, Bennett M, Bouhassira D, Cruccu G, Hansson P, Haythornthwaite JA, Iannetti GD, Jensen TS, Kauppila T, Nurmikko TJ, Rice AS, Rowbotham M, Serra J, Sommer C, Smith BH, Treede RD. NeuPSIG guidelines on neuropathic pain assessment. Pain. 2011;152(1):14–27. doi:10.1016/j.pain.2010.07.031. Epub 2010 Sep 19.
Hampson JP, Reed BD, Clauw DJ, et al. Augmented central pain processing in vulvodynia. J Pain. 2013;14:579–89.
Hannan JL, Cheung GL, Blaser MC, Pang JJ, Pang SC, Webb RC, Adams MA. Characterization of the vasculature supplying the genital tissues in female rats. J Sex Med. 2012;9(1):136–47. doi:10.1111/j.1743-6109.2011.02508.x. Epub 2011 Oct 24.
International Anatomical Nomenclature Committee. Nomina anatomica. 5th ed. Baltimore: Williams & Wilkins; 1983.
Jannini EA, d'Amati G. Histology and immunohistochemical studies of female genital tissue. In: Goldstein I, Meston C, editors. Women's sexual function and dysfunction: study, diagnosis and treatment. London: Taylor and Francis; 2006. p. 125–33.
Johannesson U, Blomgren B, Hilliges M, Rylander E, Bohm-Starke N. The vulval vestibular mucosa-morphological effects of oral contraceptives and menstrual cycle. Br J Dermatol. 2007;157:487–93.
Kandeel FR, Koussa VK, Swerdloff RS. Male sexual function and its disorders: physiology, pathophysiology, clinical investigation, and treatment. Endocr Rev. 2001;22(3):342–88.
Kearney R, Sawhney R, DeLancey JO. Levator ani muscle anatomy evaluated by origin-insertion pairs. Obstet Gynecol. 2004;104(1):168–73. Review.
Khandker M, Brady SS, Stewart EG, Harlow BL. Is chronic stress during childhood associated with adult-onset vulvodynia? J Womens Health. 2014;23:649–56.
Kinugasa Y, Arakawa T, Abe H, Rodríguez-Vázquez JF, Murakami G, Sugihara K. Female longitudinal anal muscles or conjoint longitudinal coats extend into the subcutaneous tissue along the vaginal vestibule: a histological study using human fetuses. Yonsei Med J. 2013;54(3):778–84. doi:10.3349/ymj.2013.54.3.778.
Labat JJ, Riant T, Robert R, Amarenco G, Lefaucheur JP, Rigaud J. Diagnostic criteria for pudendal neuralgia by pudendal nerve entrapment (Nantes criteria). Neurourol Urodyn. 2008;27(4):306–10.
Lawson JO. Pelvic anatomy. I. Pelvic floor muscles. Ann R Coll Surg Engl. 1974;54(5):244–52.
Liao Z, Smith PG. Persistent genital hyperinnervation following progesterone administration to adolescent female rats. Biol Reprod. 2014;91(6):144.
Mahakkanukrauh P, Surin P, Vaidhayakarn P. Anatomical study of the pudendal nerve adjacent to the sacrospinous ligament. Clin Anat. 2005;18(3):200–5.
Maravilla KR, Yang CC. Magnetic resonance imaging and the female sexual response: overview of techniques, results, and future directions. J Sex Med. 2008;5(7):1559–71. doi:10.1111/j.1743-6109.2008.00839.x.
Margulies RU, Hsu Y, Kearney R, Stein T, Umek WH, DeLancey JO. Appearance of the levator ani muscle subdivisions in magnetic resonance images. Obstet Gynecol. 2006;107(5):1064–9.
Masters WH, Johnson VE, Kolodny RC. Masters and Johnson on sex and human loving. Boston: Little Brow; 1986.

Morin M, Bergeron S, Khalife S, et al. Morphometry of the pelvic floor muscles in women with and without provoked vestibulodynia using 4D ultrasound. J Sex Med. 2014;11:776–85.

Murina F, Bianco V, Radici G, et al. Electrodiagnostic functional sensory evaluation of patients with generalized vulvodynia: a pilot study. J Low Genit Tract Dis. 2010;14:221–4.

Netter FH. Atlas of human anatomy. 5th ed. Philadelphia: Saunders-Elsevier; 2010.

O'Connel HE, DeLancey JO. Clitoral anatomy in nulliparous, healthy, premenopausal volunteers using unenhanced magnetic Resonance Imaging. J Urol. 2005;173(6):2060–3.

O'Connel HE, Hutson JM, Anderson CR, et al. Anatomical relationship between urethra and clitoris. J Urol. 1998;159:1892–7.

O'Connell HE, Eizenberg N, Rahman M, Cleeve J. The anatomy of the distal vagina: towards unity. J Sex Med. 2008;5(8):1883–91. doi:10.1111/j.1743-6109.2008.00875.x. Epub 2008 Jun 28.

Oelhafen K, Shayota BJ, Muhleman M, Klaassen Z, Tubbs RS, Loukas M. Benjamin Alcock (1801-?) and his canal. Clin Anat. 2013;26(6):662–6. doi:10.1002/ca.22080. Epub 2012 Apr 9.

Putz R, Pabst R. Sobotta atlas of human anatomy. 14th ed. Munchen: Urban Fischer-Elsevier; 2008.

Ramanah R, Berger MB, Chen L, Riethmuller D, Delancey JO. See it in 3D!: researchers examined structural links between the cardinal and uterosacral ligaments. Am J Obstet Gynecol. 2012;207(5):437.e1–7. doi:10.1016/j.ajog.2012.08.036. Epub 2012 Sep 7.

Ramirez De Knott HM, McCormick TS, Do SO, Goodman W, Ghannoum MA, Cooper KD, et al. Cutaneous hypersensitivity to Candida albicans in idiopathic vulvodynia. Contact Dermatitis. 2005;53:214–8.

Reed BD, Harlow SD, Sen A, et al. Prevalence and demographic characteristics of vulvodynia in a population-based sample. Am J Obstet Gynecol. 2012;206:170e.1–9.

Reed B, Harlow SD, Legocki LJ, Helmuth ME, Haefner HK, Gillespie BW, Sen A. Oral contraceptive use and risk of vulvodynia: a population-based longitudinal study. BJOG. 2013;120:1678–84.

Reed BD, Legocki LJ, Plegue MA, et al. Factors associated with vulvodynia incidence. Obstet Gynecol. 2014;123:225–31.

Regauer S, Eberz B, Beham-Schmid C. Mast cell infiltrates in vulvodynia represent secondary and idiopathic mast cell hyperplasias. APMIS. 2015;123:452–6.

Robert R, Prat-Pradal D, Labat JJ, Bensignor M, Raoul S, Rebai R, Leborgne J. Anatomic basis of chronic perineal pain: role of the pudendal nerve. Surg Radiol Anat. 1998;20(2):93–8.

Schaible HG. Emerging concepts of pain therapy based on neuronal mechanisms. Handb Exp Pharmacol. 2015;227:1–14. doi:10.1007/978-3-662-46450-2-1.

Schober J, Aardsma N, Mayoglou L, Pfaff D, Martín-Alguacil N. Terminal innervation of female genitalia, cutaneous sensory receptors of the epithelium of the labia minora. Clin Anat. 2015;28(3):392–8.

Schraffordt SE, Tjandra JJ, Eizenberg N, Dwyer PL. Surgical anatomy of the pudendal nerve and its terminal branches: a cadaver study. ANZ J Surg. 2004;74(1–2):23–6.

Sommer F, Caspers HP, Esders K, Klotz T, Engelmann U. Measurement of vaginal and minor labial oxygen tension for the evaluation of female sexual function. J Urol. 2001;165(4):1181–4.

Standring S. New focus on anatomy for surgical trainees. ANZ J Surg. 2008;79(3):114–7. doi:10.1111/j.1445-2197.2008.04825.x.

Stein TA, DeLancey JO. Structure of the perineal membrane in female: gross and microscopic anatomy. Obstet Gynecol. 2008;111(3):686–93. doi:10.1097/AOG.0b013e318163a9a5.

Stumpf RM, Wilson BA, Rivera A, Yildirim S, Yeoman CJ, Polk JD, White BA, Leigh SR. The primate vaginal microbiome: comparative context and implications for human health and disease. Am J Phys Anthropol. 2013;152 Suppl 57:119–34. doi:10.1002/ajpa.22395. Epub 2013 Oct 28.

Tagliafico A, Bignotti B, Miguel Perez M, Reni L, Bodner G, Martinoli C. Contribution of ultrasound in the assessment of patients with suspect idiopathic pudendal nerve disease. Clin Neurophysiol. 2014;125(6):1278–84. doi:10.1016/j.clinph.2013.10.053. Epub 2013 Dec 7.

Ting AY, Blacklock AD, Smith PG. Estrogen regulates vaginal sensory and autonomic nerve density in the rat. Biol Reprod. 2004;71:1397–404.

Tommola P, Bützow R, Unkila-Kallio L, et al. Activation of vestibule-associated lymphoid tissue in localized provoked vulvodynia. Am J Obstet Gynecol. 2015;212:4761–8.

Traish AM, Botchevar E, Kim NN. Biochemical factors modulating female genital sexual arousal physiology. J Sex Med. 2010;7(9):2925–46. doi:10.1111/j.1743-6109.2010.01903.x.

Treede RD, Jensen TS, Campbell JN, Cruccu G, Dostrovsky JO, Griffin JW, Hansson P, Hughes R, Nurmikko T, Serra J. Redefinition of neuropathic pain and a grading system for clinical use: consensus statement on clinical and research diagnostic criteria. Neurology. 2008;70:1630–5.

Tunn R, DeLancey JO, Quint EE. Visibility of pelvic organ support system structures in magnetic resonance images without an endovaginal coil. Am J Obstet Gynecol. 2001;184(6):1156–63.

Tunn R, DeLancey JO, Howard D, Ashton-Miller JA, Quint LE. Anatomic variations in the levator ani muscle, endopelvic fascia, and urethra in nulliparous evaluated by magnetic resonance imaging. Am J Obstet Gynecol. 2003;188(1):116–21.

Walker AK, Kavelaars A, Heijnen CJ, Dantzer R. Neuroinflammation and comorbidity of pain and depression. Pharmacol Rev. 2013;66(1):80–101.

Watson JC, Sandroni P. Central neuropathic pain syndromes. Mayo Clin Proc. 2016;91(3):372–85.

Williams PL, Bannister LH. Gray's anatomy of the human body. New York: Churchill Livingstone; 2008.

Xanthos DN, Gaderer S, Drdla R, Nuro E, Abramova A, Ellmeier W, Sandkühler J. Central nervous system mast cells in peripheral inflammatory nociception. Mol Pain. 2011;7:42. doi:10.1186/1744-8069-7-42.

Yang CC, Cold CJ, Yilmaz U, Maravilla KR. Sexually responsive vascular tissue of the vulva. BJU Int. 2006;97(4):766–72.

Yavagal S, de Farias TF, Medina CA, Takacs P. Normal vulvovaginal, perineal, and pelvic anatomy with reconstructive considerations. Semin Plast Surg. 2011;25(2):121–9. doi:10.1055/s-0031-1281481.

Ziouziou I, Bennani H, Zizi M, Karmouni T, Khader KE, Koutani A, Andaloussi AI. Le syndrome du canal d'Alcock ou névralgie pudendale: un diagnostic à ne pas méconnaître. Can Urol Assoc J. 2013;7(7–8):E486–9. doi:10.5489/cuaj.415.

Vulvar Pain in Childhood: A Call for a More Accurate Diagnosis and Care

4

4.1 Introduction

Vulvar pain is an "orphan" symptom in prepubertal children. When a child complains of acute or chronic pain in that area, pediatricians/clinicians refer to "genital pain": certainly a comprehensive, yet not a specific nor a sensitive word.

In this chapter, the focus is on pain precisely referred to the entire vulva or part of it: the clitoris, the labia minora and/or majora, the vestibulum, and the fourchette. The term *vulvar pain* (VP) will be preferred and used here for the sake of clarity, precision, quality of care, detection of vulnerabilities, and prevention of risks to become clinically relevant facts: a must, even more compelling in children and young patients.

Childhood acute vulvar pain is usually found to have a clear biological cause (Clare and Yeh 2011). Accurate national studies have been carried out on unintentional, accidental genital lesions in children, with specific focus on product safety, such as the U.S. Consumer Product Safety Commission (CPSC) National Electronic Injury Surveillance System (NEISS) (Casey et al. 2013; Tasian et al. 2013).

However, systematic studies specifically focused on vulvar pain in children up to the age of puberty are still missing. The literature reports essentially single clinical cases, more focused on acute vulvar pain.

Pain characteristics in this group are similar to adults. The study of the psychological component of vulvar pain is limited due to small numbers of patients available for review. Children who are victims of sexual abuse reported feelings about their genital pain (Sham et al. 2013). Studies on long-term outcome of acute vulvar lesions, and specifically on chronic vulva pain/vulvodynia, are still lacking.

Neglect of childhood vulvar pain may then lead pain to evolve to vestibulodynia/vulvodynia in vulnerable subjects, with a progressive central component in their pain perception.

The goal of this chapter is twofold: first, analyze the existing literature to give a perspective on current issues raised by vulvar pain in children; second, increase the clinical awareness for the need of an early diagnosis and appropriate treatment to avoid the shift to chronic and neuropathic vulvar pain.

A. Graziottin, F. Murina, *Vulvar Pain*, DOI 10.1007/978-3-319-42677-8_4

Table 4.1 Leading etiologies of vulvar pain in children

Traumatic: as a consequence of mechanical injuries on the external genitalia
After a *fall*
Riding toy-related genital injuries (cane bicycle (crossbar)
Play chutes in playground/children garden
On the coccyx, with a later compression of the pudendal nerve at its source at S2,S2,S4 level
After *injuries* while *playing/masturbating* with *foreign objects*
After burns
Sexual abuse, during and after childhood abuse
Ritual, after genital mutilation/cutting/ritual modification
Iatrogenic
When performing invasive maneuvers such as bladder catheterization or vaginal swab, without caring attention
When suturing traumatic unintentional vulvar lesions without proper care
After genital surgery for vulvar cysts (anecdotal case reports)
After chemotherapy and/or radiotherapy, with peripheral neuropathic genital pain
Autoimmune, when lichen sclerosus causes intense itching/pruritus
Neuropathic: vestibulodynia and/or vulvodynia, spontaneous or provoked

4.2 Etiology of Vulvar Pain in Children

Different etiologies may contribute to vulvar pain in prepubertal girls (Table 4.1).

4.2.1 Traumatic Unintentional Accidental Lesions of the Vulva

Traumatic unintentional *accidental lesions of the vulva* in childhood usually cause acute, intense, excruciating vulvar pain, given the extremely rich innervation of the area.

Intensity and duration of vulvar pain depends on:

- *Type of injury*: vulvar cut, hematoma, compression, burn, chemical, iatrogenic, and ritual damages. Injury diagnoses are usually classified as contusion/abrasion, dermatitis, foreign body, hematoma, laceration, strain/sprain, and others (including avulsion, burns, crushing, fracture, hemorrhage, associated internal organ injury, and puncture) (Casey et al. 2013).

  Pediatric external genital trauma because of sports, playground equipment, toys, or furniture does not seem to be uncommon in everyday life. However, the rate of *accidental*, unintentional, *and* nonsexual *pediatric genital injury* is unknown, as most related literature is focused on the association of sexual abuse with genital trauma. Studies focusing on *nonsexual pediatric genital trauma* consist of case reports or small series and focus on either female or male patients exclusively.

  From these studies, it seems that genital injury occurs in 0.4–8 % of reported childhood trauma, and the majority of accidental pediatric genital injury is minor, not requiring surgical or intensive medical treatment.

A retrospective cohort study utilizing the U.S. Consumer Product Safety Commission (CPSC) National Electronic Injury Surveillance System (NEISS) from 1991 to 2010 was performed (Casey et al. 2013) to evaluate pediatric genital injuries.

Pediatric genital injuries represented 0.6 % of all pediatric injuries with *the incidence of injuries rising through the period studied, 1991–2010*. The incidence is raising steadily from 1991 to 2010, in spite of increasing awareness and attention to safety issues for children.

The mean age at injury was 7.1 years and was distributed 56.6 % girls and 43.4 % boys. A total of 43.3 % had lacerations and 42.2 % had contusions/abrasions. The majority of injuries occurred at home (65.9 %), and the majority of patients (94.7 %) were treated and released from the hospital. The most common consumer products associated with pediatric genital trauma were bicycles (14.7 % of all pediatric genital injuries), bathtubs (5.8 %), daywear (5.6 %), monkey bars (5.4 %), and toilets (4.0 %) (Casey et al. 2013).

Another ample study within NEISS indicates that children 4–7 years old were most frequently injured (36.8 % of all injuries), followed by those 8–11 years old (20.6 %). Girls comprised 55 % of the injured children. The most commonly injured organs were female external genitalia (vulva) (37.7 %), penises (21.6 %), and testicles (12 %). Genitourinary injuries were most commonly associated with sporting and exercise equipment (35.7 %), furniture, (15.5 %) and clothing items (11.9 %). Of the patients 91 % were treated at the emergency department and discharged home (Tasian et al. 2013). Bicycle use is responsible for the highest percentage of sport-related genitourinary traumas in children (Bagga et al. 2015).

Blunt perineal injuries that require surgical repair occur predominantly in patients less than 10 years of age who sustain blunt perineal trauma from a variety of causes but rarely motor vehicle crashes. Thus, such patients should undergo aggressive evaluation, including examination under anesthesia (EUA), especially if they present with perineal bleeding, hematoma, or swelling. Furthermore, perineal injuries in children under 4 years should raise the suspicion of abuse (Scheidler et al. 2000).

Lower genitourinary injury may have more serious implication when associated to *pelvic injuries*. Studies indicate that 2.8 % of children with pelvic fractures (6/212) reported bladder and urethral trauma (Tarman et al. 2002). Shared innervation and proximity may increase the vulnerability of the vulvar tissues to short- and long-term consequences. However, this is not specifically reported/quoted in available studies on *genitourinary and pelvic injuries*.

- *Extension, severity, and complexity of vulvar tissue damage*.
- *Involvement of the urethra and/or anal area*.
- *Number of traumatic events*: single versus multiple, for example, repeated fall at the swimming pool or on the cane bicycle.
- *Adequacy of the treatment*, both in terms of quality of primary care, medical and/or surgical, including attention to quality and duration of analgesia and antalgic treatment, while suturing a genital cut, and psychological support to the child and, when indicated, to the family.
- *Quality of the follow-up and pertinent medical/psychosexual intervention and support*.

4.2.2 Sexual Abuse

Every year, about 4–16 % of children are physically abused and one in ten is neglected or psychologically abused. During childhood, between 5 and 10 % of girls and up to 5 % of boys are exposed to penetrative sexual abuse, and up to three times this number are exposed to any type of sexual abuse. However, official rates for substantiated child maltreatment indicate less than a tenth of this burden (Gilbert et al. 2009; Bailhache et al. 2013). Diagnosis can be challenging (Berkoff et al. 2008). Criteria for the clinical diagnosis of children sexual abuse are summarized in Boxes 4.1 and 4.2. A dramatically high percentage of children have increased vulnerabilities to further emotional and physical abuse, neglect, and long-term negative consequences. Severity variables include:

1. *Type of abuse* (nonpenetrative vs. vaginal penetrative sexual abuse): the vestibulum is an extremely vulnerable area for potential long-term consequences in terms of vulvar pain/vestibulodynia, more so as it involves an extremely emotionally charged area such as the vulva.
2. *Number of traumatic events*: single versus multiple, more likely in penetrative abuse when a relative or an acquaintance is the perpetrator (Gilbert et al. 2009; Bailhache et al. 2013).
3. *Associated abuses*: neglect and/or physical abuse.
4. *Vulnerable social context*: poverty, low education, single and/or unemployed mother, and no family/relatives/social support.
5. *Presence of sexually transmitted infections* (STI), such as papillomavirus-induced condylomata (Fig. 4.1). This finding must activate a careful investigation of a potential sexual abuse and the presence of other STI, including gonorrhea and HIV.

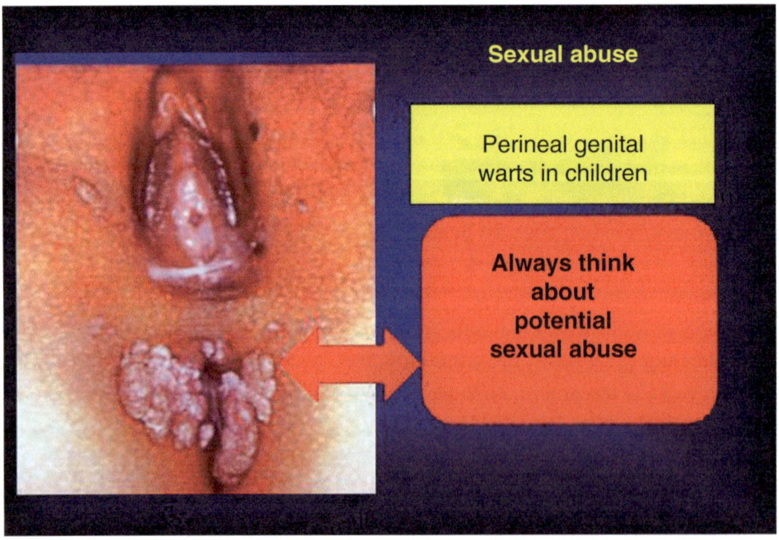

Fig 4.1 Perineal warts in children: healthcare providers must always consider a potential sexual abuse (Picture: courtesy of Metella Dei, MD)

Box 4.1. How to Diagnose a Sexual Penetrative Abuse

Method

The transhymenal diameters and the amount of tissue present between the hymenal edge and vestibule inferiorly at 6 o'clock and laterally at 3 o'clock and 9 o'clock were measured from photographs of 189 prepubertal children with a validated history of digital or penile penetration and 197 children who denied previous sexual abuse. Statistical analyses were conducted to compare the mean values and hymenal symmetry between groups as well as to determine the sensitivity and specificity of various cutoff points.

Results

Comparison of the mean diameters demonstrated *that children with a penetration history had a significantly larger transverse opening than nonabused children when examined in the knee-chest position* (5.6 vs. 4.6 mm). However, there was *extensive overlap in measurements between the 2 groups*. No significant differences were noted between groups in the size of the vertical diameter, the amount of tissue present inferiorly or laterally, or the symmetry of the hymen in either position.

Children with previous penetration were more likely than nonabused children to have a *horizontal opening measuring >6.5 mm in the knee-chest position*, but *the sensitivity and specificity of this test were low* (29 % and 86 %, respectively).

Higher values had better specificity but very low sensitivity. Less than 1.0 mm of hymenal tissue was detected at 6 o'clock only in those with a history of penetration (100 % specificity), but the sensitivity was low (1–2 %) (Berenson et al. 2002).

Conclusion

Most hymenal measurements lack adequate sensitivity or specificity to be used to confirm previous penetration. Less than 1.0 mm of hymenal tissue at 6 o'clock was detected only in victims of penetrative abuse, but the usefulness of this test is limited by the rarity of this finding.

Box 4.2. Classification of Genital Injuries Caused by Sexual Assault*

To ease the clinician's evaluation of the damage and type of intervention, or immediate referral at a tertiary care Pediatric Surgical Unit (Sham et al. 2013):

1. *First-degree tear*: laceration is limited to the fourchette and superficial perineal skin or vaginal mucosa. Perineal body intact.
2. *Second-degree tear*: laceration extends beyond the fourchette, perineal skin, and vaginal mucosa to perineal muscles and fascia, but not the anal sphincter. Perineal body involved.

3. *Third-degree tear*: the fourchette, perineal skin, vaginal mucosa, muscles, and anal sphincter are torn:
   (a) Partial tear of the external anal sphincter involving less than 50 % thickness
   (b) >50 % of external anal sphincter thickness torn
   (c) Internal anal sphincter torn
4. *Fourth-degree tear*: the fourchette, perineal skin, vaginal mucosa, muscles, anal sphincter, and anorectal mucosa are torn.

* It is worth noting that the word "vulva" is not mentioned in spite of the fact that the vulva is frequently, if not always, involved during sexual assaults and that the fourchette is by definition part of the vulva.

Key Learning Points

- Vulvar and genital STI in children should always raise the question of sexual abuse.
- When one infection is diagnosed, screening for other STI with different incubation time and less obvious clinical signs must be done.
- Immediate accurate video recording of the vulvar/genital lesions and audio recording of the child wording (everybody has a mobile phone!) at the very first visit is essential to:
  1. Objectively document the findings
  2. Avoid repeated examination and questioning that may further traumatize the unfortunate child
  3. Prepare a solid, impeccable material for the legal investigation

Figure 4.2 presents a typical case of hymenal damage/change after sexual abuse.

Prospective studies with *careful follow-up* of girls who underwent penetrative abuse focusing on vulvar pain/vestibulodynia and vulvodynia are lacking.

Retrospective studies show conflicting results. Some research groups failed to show an association between sexual abuse and later vulvodynia. The lack of association between sexual abuse and vulvodynia, or vulvar pruritus, was confirmed in more recent studies (Cohen-Sacher et al. 2015).

Other groups, probably because of methodologically more accurate retrospective studies, do instead strongly *support* the association between *sexual abuse and subsequent vulvodynia* (Harlow and Stewart 2005; Khandker et al. 2014).

In 2000–2003, Harlow and Stewart identified 125 women experiencing symptoms of vulvar pain consistent with vulvodynia and 125 age- and community-matched controls from the Boston, Massachusetts, area general population. Telephone-administered questionnaires were used to obtain medical, psychiatric,

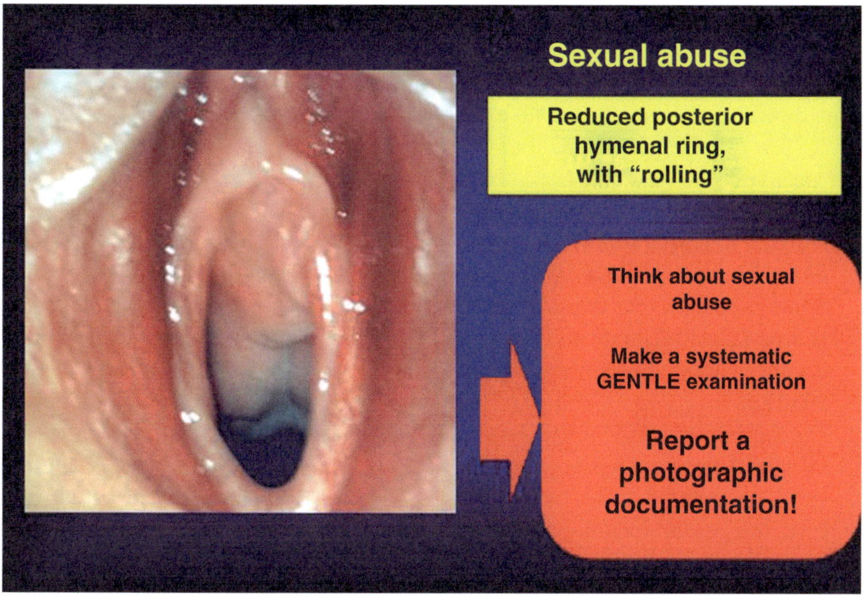

Fig 4.2 Hymen modifications: reduced posterior hymenal ring with "rolling." A potential sexual abuse is to be considered. Gentle and respectful clinical examination is essential. A complete immediate photographic documentation with audio recording of the child wording is mandatory at the very first visit (Picture: courtesy of Metella Dei, MD)

and reproductive histories. Self-administered surveys assessed childhood exposure (age <12 years) to physical and sexual abuse and too poor family support. After authors' adjustment for socioeconomic position, *women with vulvar pain versus controls were 2.6 times more likely to report never/rarely receiving childhood family support*, such as comfort, encouragement, and love [95 % confidence interval (CI): 1.3, 5.1].

Adult-onset vulvodynia was *strongly associated with abuse as a child* more than a few times physically [odds ratio (OR) = 4.1, 95 % CI: 1.7, 10.0] or sexually (OR = 6.5, 95 % CI: 1.2, 35.1). When abused women were compared with those with no history of abuse, the association was largely confined to those harmed by a primary family member (OR = 3.6, 95 % CI: 1.6, 8.0 for physical abuse; OR = 4.4, 95 % CI: 0.9, 22.9 for sexual abuse). The association is impressive and alarming.

Khandker et al. (2014) found that, among women with a history of severe childhood abuse, *those with vulvodynia had three times the odds of living in fear of any abuse* compared to women without vulvodynia (95 % CI: 1.0, 11.0), after adjustment for childhood poverty. Among women with no history of childhood abuse, those with vulvodynia had over six times the odds of antecedent mood disorder compared to women without vulvodynia (95 % CI: 1.9,19.6) (Khandker et al. 2014).

Additional population-based studies of clinically confirmed cases of vulvodynia are needed to replicate this association.

4.2.3 Vestibulodynia/Vulvodynia in Childhood

Vestibulodynia/vulvodynia in childhood is scarcely reported: in the medical perception, the vulva seems to begin "to exist" only after puberty.

A few studies look at the *vulvodynia issue and childhood* with two perspectives:

1. How do *negative experiences such as stress, neglect, and physical or sexual abuse become "predisposing factors"* to the later development of *vulvodynia*? Some authors show that a former childhood stress and/or abuse is a predisposing factor (Harlow and Stewart 2005; Khandker et al. 2014), while others do not support the etiological role of childhood abuse (Cohen-Sacher et al. 2015).
2. *Do children develop vestibulodynia/vulvodynia* during the childhood/prepubertal age? A few case report (Reed and Cantor 2008, focusing on prepubertal girls, and Clare and Yeh 2011, who focus on early postpubertal/adolescent girls) indicates that vestibulodynia/vulvodynia is complained of even in prepubertal girls but is usually *underdiagnosed and undertreated.* The symptom responds usually well to treatment for neuropathic pain, the sooner the better. Vestibulodynia/vulvodynia should be considered in the differential diagnosis when vulvar discomfort/burning pain/chronic or remitting pain is referred to the vulvar region in children, regardless of age (Reed and Cantor 2008).

4.2.4 Ritual Vulvar Damage, After Female Genital Mutilation/Cutting

Female genital mutilation/cutting (FGM/C) is defined by the World Health Organization (WHO) as "all procedures that involve partial or total removal of the external female genitalia or other injury to the female genital organs for non-medical reasons" (WHO 2006, 2008). FGM/C is typically carried out, with or without anesthesia, by a traditional circumciser using a knife or razor. The age of the girls who undergo this procedure varies from weeks after birth to puberty (UNICEF 2013).

Common early complications of FGM/C include uncontrolled bleeding, fever, wound infection, sepsis, and death (Nour 2004). FGM/C is also reported to cause psychological consequences, such as anxiety, horror, posttraumatic stress disorders, and depression.

Long-term complications include dysmenorrhea, dyspareunia, recurrent vaginal and urinary tract infections, infertility cysts, abscesses, keloid formation, obstetric complications, difficulty with childbirth, and sexual dysfunction (WHO 2006). *Vulvar pain is not mentioned in Nour paper, nor in WHO 2006,* in spite of the fact that acute vulvar and genital pain is the most likely symptom when excision is performed in an area like the vulva, with a precise name, and so richly innervated with sensory nerve fibers. *Clitoral cysts are an underdiagnosed late complication* (Rouzi 2010; Rouzi and Alturki 2015).

Excellent reviews of available literature have been recently carried out: 5109 papers were considered, of which 185 studies (3.17 million women surveyed) were of good quality (Berg et al. 2014). Authors have carefully described the long-term gynecologic and obstetric outcomes of FGM/C.

Results indicate significantly increased risks such as urinary tract infections [unadjusted risk ratio (RR) = 3.01], bacterial vaginosis [adjusted OR (AOR) = 1.68], dyspareunia (RR = 1.53), prolonged labor (AOR = 1.49), caesarean section (AOR = 1.60), and difficult delivery (AOR = 1.88). In spite of the huge set of data, vulvar pain is not mentioned in this review, nor in the otherwise very accurate Canadian guidelines (Perron et al. 2013), focused most on *how to manage* appropriate obstetric and gynecological care on FGC, including FGC-related complications.

A recent excellent paper analyzed current limits in research (Abdulcadir et al. 2015).

Only a few recently published clinical cases report epidermoid inclusion cysts, with inguinal (Birge et al. 2015) and/or acute *vulvar pain* (Gudu 2014). Specifically, the first case of *neuropathic pain with sensory neuropathy* has been published in June 2015 (Hadid and Dahan 2015).

Intensity of vulvar pain in childhood and vulnerability to long-term consequences in terms of vulvar pain and other comorbidities (such as urinary recurrent infections, difficulties in urination) and their long-term impact on vulvar health and sexuality depend on a number of variables:

- *Modality/instruments* used to perform cutting, as the damage is more serious when genital mutilation is carried out with primitive objects with complex type of injury (compression, cutting, hematoma, traction/ripping lesions) and more likely subsequent infections, persistent inflammation, and potential neuropathic damage.
- *Site and extension.*
- *Acute and long–term complications* (see Chap. 5).
- *Quality of physical and emotional/affective care after FGC has been performed.*

The goal of this concise paragraph on FGC is to sensitize pediatricians and other healthcare providers to focus on the possibility of *vulvar pain*, and associated comorbidities, every time they consult a child or an adolescent who has undergone FGC. Immigration to European and North American countries makes more likely the possibility to meet patients who have undergone the practice and present with different symptoms we do not even have the proper wording for. Indications on how to appropriately manage FGC and care women after FGC are discussed in the recent excellent Canadian guidelines (Perron et al. 2013) that can help every physician to get more familiar with the cultural, emotional, physical, medical, and technical challenges FGM may imply when symptoms are complained of in the short- and long-term after FGC. "Hot" questions on vulvar pain after FGM are summarized in Box 4.3.

Box 4.3. Vulvar Pain After FMG/C: An "Orphan" Symptom in Childhood

Focusing on children, one sixth to one fifth of those 125 million girls and women are prepubertal, which translates into around 20 million children who recently underwent genital cutting. What are their current symptoms? Is vulvar pain an issue? In which percentage does acute vulvar pain, subsequent to cutting, shift into chronic vulvar pain/vulvodynia? Is there just a "naming/wording" issue? Is the asexual vision of children leading to prefer the "genital pain" wording, instead of "vulvar pain," perhaps because it is perceived as a more "sexually charged" word?

Whatever the reason, vulvar pain/vulvodynia is not mentioned at all in the available literature, and no word/research is spent on vulvar pain in children who underwent FGM/C. Does acute and chronic vulvar pain exist after FMG/C? Or is this issue invisible? That is, is it still under the threshold of clinical perception?

Without attention to this specific symptom, no identification is possible of the subset of children at higher risk of vulvar pain/vulvodynia/dyspareunia, and no early intervention can therefore be offered. Unfortunately, no specific answers to those questions have been found in the pertinent literature. Specific research on acute and chronic vulvar pain in prepubertal children undergoing genital cutting is urgently needed.

4.2.5 Iatrogenic Vulvar Pain

During clinical consultation with the authors (AG and FM), 5.3 % of women with vestibulodynia/vulvodynia reported their pain started after a number of *medical events/interventions during childhood*. More frequent etiologies reported are mentioned here to raise attention to those neglected causes of long-term vulvar pain pediatrician and other healthcare providers could be completely unaware of, in absence of long-term follow-up.

Iatrogenic childhood causes of later vulvar pain include:

- *Invasive maneuvers* such as bladder catheterization and urethral or vaginal swabs, without using two protective attentions:
  - Asking the child to push "as if she wants to urinate" to relax the pelvic floor and allow a less painful introduction of the catheter or the swab.
  - Wetting the swab in physiologic solution, to ease the passage without altering the quality of the sample.
- *Suturing traumatic unintentional vulvar lesions without proper care* (adequate analgesia, tenderness, reassurance, and respect in the clinical approach).
- *After genital surgery for vulvar cysts* (anecdotal case reports).
- *After chemotherapy or radiotherapy*, with peripheral neuropathic genital pain.

As prevention is key, attention to these aspects is of the highest importance, given the high percentage of girls who require medical attention for diagnostic urinary or vaginal exams or suturing of unintentional vulvar/genital trauma (Graziottin et al. 2015).

4.2.6 Autoimmune: Lichen Sclerosus

Childhood *lichen sclerosus* (LS) is a rare and often misdiagnosed inflammatory dermatitis with an unpredictable course. The leading symptom is pruritus/itching, more severe at night. *Itching is considered a subtype of pain* (Papoiu et al. 2013), as many neuronal pathways between itching and pain do partially overlap. It is therefore appropriate to include lichens sclerosus among the etiological conditions responsible for vulvar pain, even during childhood. In brain research, active scratching was accompanied by a higher pleasurability and induced a more pronounced deactivation of the anterior cingulate cortex and insula, in comparison with passive scratching. A significant involvement of the reward system including the ventral tegmentum of the midbrain, coupled with a mechanism deactivating the periaqueductal gray matter (PAG), suggests that itch modulation operates in reverse to the mechanism known to suppress pain. The findings not only confirm a role for the central networks processing reward in the pleasurable aspects of scratching but also suggest they play a role in mediating itch relief (Papoiu et al. 2013).

Besides itching/vulvar pain, the leading complications of LS are:

- *Architectural changes of the vulva*, consequent to the chronic tissue inflammation.
- *Progressive full-thickness involution of the cytoarchitecture of the vulva* (Fig. 4.3). This leads to thinning of the vulvar skin that becomes pale/white; areas of hyper keratinization can be present; the submucosa becomes thinner as well, and vessels, nerves, and smooth muscle cells and fibers undergo the same involutive changes. The involution affects as well the clitoral/cavernosal bodies, the specialized vessels that mediate vulvar/genital arousal.
- The inflammatory infiltrate with mast cells is typical of the acute phases. It tends to disappear when the destruction of the tissue cytoarchitecture is substituted by the collagenous rigid scarring.
- Pain on defecation presenting as constipation and bowel symptoms (24 %), dysuria (24 %), and local bleeding (26 %) is seen significantly more frequently in girls than in women (Cooper et al. 2004).
- *Sexual long-term consequences*, when the child enters adolescence and tries to have the first intercourse:
  - *Introital coital pain* (dyspareunia) is typical when the labia involution leads to the progressive narrowing of the vaginal introitus.
  - *Genital sexual arousal difficulties*, with *vaginal dryness*, and *orgasmic difficulties* up to a frank impossibility to achieve clitoral orgasm in the most severe cases are the clinical consequences of the cavernosal bodies involution.
  - *Acquired avoidance of sexual intercourse becomes a protective attempt against pain*.
  - *Acquired loss of desire* may be the final negative sexual consequence, when LS is not diagnosed and appropriately treated at its onset.
- LS may improve symptomatically, but usually does not entirely resolve at puberty. A retrospective study of 21 postpubertal girls with LS presenting prepubertally revealed that the disorder appeared less active in most cases, but

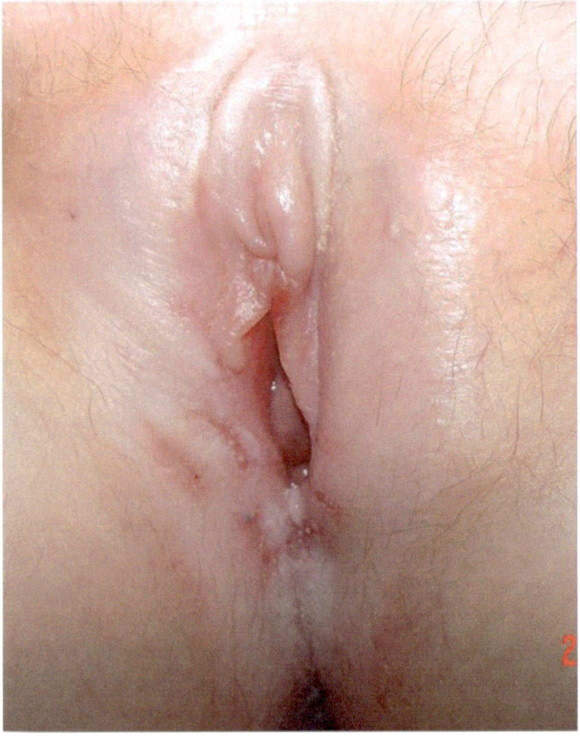

Fig 4.3 Vulvar lichen sclerosus in childhood, with scratching lesions and partial conglutination of labia minora and clitoris

definite physical symptoms and signs persisted in 76 %. A prospective follow-up of 12 children with LS showed that 25 % achieved complete remission prior to menarche. Seventy-five percent of the girls had active LS at puberty and required maintenance therapy after menarche. Fifty percent had a significant disturbance of vulvar architecture (Powell and Wojnarowska 2002; Smith and Fischer 2009).

- *Malignant transformation is possible later in life, in average 5 % of case.* Twenty-one percent of progression of symptomatic LS to squamous vulvar cell carcinoma (SVCC) id reported in the very accurately documented series of adult cases studied by Carlson et al. (1998). Vulvar lichen sclerosus (LS) is an inflammatory dermatosis characterized by clinicopathologic persistence and hypocellular fibrosis (sclerosis). A subset of vulvar SVCCs is significantly associated with the presence of LS and diffusely express the p53 gene product. Keratinocytes affected by LS show a proliferative phenotype and can exhibit markers of neoplastic progression such as increased p53 expression and DNA aneuploidy. As a chronic scarring inflammatory dermatosis, vulvar LS could act as both "initiator and promoter" of carcinogenesis, explaining the frequent coexistence of these diseases. Because keratinocytes of LS significantly express tumor suppressor gene p53 protein, the p53 gene may be involved early in this proposed pathway of carcinogenesis.

Only a minority of lichen sclerosus cases are associated with squamous cell carcinoma. However, the therapeutic implications of a squamous cell carcinoma diagnosis are severe.

Clinically, we lack an understanding of how to separate indolent lichen sclerosus cases from those in danger of progression to squamous cell carcinoma later in life. Several protein markers show promise for further delineating the pathobiology of lichen sclerosus and the potential malignant transformation into squamous cell carcinoma (Carlson et al. 2013).

Early-onset LS tend to progress to vulvar cancer at an earlier age. Early accurate diagnosis, treatment, and follow-up of childhood lichen sclerosus are therefore mandatory, both to relieve the child from an invalidating and often misdiagnosed symptom like vulvar itch/pain (see the clinical case) and to prevent a potential neoplastic evolution.

- *Leading comorbidities include autoimmune disorders, Turner's syndrome, and kidney diseases*. A registry study identified 44 children with LS treated at Tampere University Hospital, Tampere, Finland, from 1982 to 2010. A questionnaire was sent to the identified patients and 15 responded. The clinical depiction of LS varied significantly. LS was diagnosed in only 16% of the patients at the referring unit. Autoimmune disorders were observed in 6 of the 44 patients. High prevalences of Turner's syndrome (2/44) and kidney disease (2/44) were noted. The majority of the patients were treated with topical corticosteroids. Eight developed architectural changes of the vulva. The questionnaire revealed that three of six patients who were asymptomatic at the end of the registry study follow-up experienced a recurrence of symptoms. None of them were undergoing follow-up. Nine of the 15 patients reported reduced quality of life. Childhood LS is a heterogeneous disease with a remarkable effect on quality of life. The misdiagnosis of childhood LS is common. The association between LS and autoimmune diseases should be noted. The high prevalence of Turner's syndrome raises questions regarding the influence of low estrogen levels on the development of LS. The prognosis cannot be predicted, so long-term follow-up is recommended. New tools for diagnosis and surveillance are needed (Lagerstedt et al. 2013).

4.2.7 Neuropathic Vulvar Pain

The lack of neuropathic pain reported in childhood is surprising, given the *high frequency of traumatic nonintentional and intentional vulvar lesions*. This could be the consequence of a real very low frequency due to possible protective factors, such as the lack of fluctuating levels of estrogens, so important in triggering mast cell degranulation in postpubertal fertile women, or to a diagnostic neglect. It is difficult to provide an appropriate diagnosis, if there is no mentioning of a problem and/or if pain is generally labeled as "genital" instead of "vulvar" when the vulva is specifically affected.

Lack of adequate follow-up after traumatic nonintentional and intentional vulvar lesions is one of the leading contributors of missed diagnosis. Pediatricians should be involved in long-term follow-up of vulvar acute pain and lesions of any etiology, to diagnose earlier and better the subset of children at higher risk of chronic vulvar pain in the years after the vulvar trauma.

Key Learning Points

- When acute or chronic pain is reported/referred to the vulvar area, the word "vulvar pain," instead of "genital pain," should be used.
- Childhood vulvar pain is usually found to have an objective biological (genital) cause.
- Careful listening, competent and gentle clinical examination (see the clinical case, Box 4.4), and specific exams when indicated are essential for a timely etiologic diagnosis of childhood vulvar pain.
- Contextual video and audio recording (mandatory after sexual abuse) must be done during the first visit, to avoid multiple repeated examinations and questioning, that further increase the child's distress and the risk of a post-traumatic stress disorder.
- Neglect of a timely diagnosis may facilitate the progression to chronic vulvar pain with a gradual shift to an increase of CNS-driven neuropathic component.
- Long-term follow-up of childhood acute vulvar pain of any etiology is recommended, with special attention after sexual abuse, FGC, lichen sclerosus, and neuropathic pain.

Box 4.4. Clinical Case: The Child Who Was Diagnosed with "Compulsory Masturbation" and "a Nymphomanic Trait"

Linda is a 7-year-old girl, only child of a nice couple with a serene marriage. Both parents adore the child, who "besides this horrible problem" is a most loving and tender little girl. She gets in hesitant in the consulting room, hand in hand with the mom who gets in first. Concerned and hopeful at the same time. Dad waits nervously outside. She looks very thin and tall, with blond hair, big frightened eyes and eyeglasses. Sweet and shy.

Her vulvar symptoms started at the age of four, with progressively intense vulvar itching. The symptom was initially more frequent at night, then became very disturbing and bothersome during the day. It was reported to be more intense when she was distressed, mostly at the kinder garden.

The first pediatrician consulted diagnosed an "impending early puberty" (in spite of the absence of any Tanner sign, pubic, axillary, or mammary) and suggested child psychotherapy. The family agreed, but one year after weekly sessions, the symptom was worsening. Meanwhile the school teacher called the mother as "this continuous genital touching" was considered "very inappropriate" for the age and "sure symptom of serious psychological problems."

A second pediatrician was consulted. She excluded any bowel worm parasitic infection and recommended a different psychotherapeutic approach. A behavioral treatment was then started. Meanwhile the child entered the first year of the elementary school. She was put on the first row, so that the teacher could immediately interrupt and stigmatize the inappropriate behavior. Schoolmates were immediately signaling to the teacher when the child was "beginning to touch herself again." The increasingly distressed child, because of the undiagnosed persistent troublesome itching and the aggressive and emotionally abusive attitude she was the target of, started to have new symptoms: bowel pain (irritable bowel syndrome, IBS) and headache.

A third medical consultation was then requested, with a neuropsychiatrist specialized in children psychopathology with a certificate in sexual medicine. The diagnosis was even more frightening for the parents – "compulsory masturbation with nymphomanic trait" – and recommended low-dose amitriptyline treatment.

Three years had gone since the first symptoms and the condition seemed helplessness and hopeless. Fortunately, while desperately searching on the web, the mother came across a paper of one of the authors (AG) from a lay magazine. She immediately called for an emergency visit: the symptoms the child had been complaining for years where matching exactly the description of LS. Maybe there was new hope.

Questions were very simple, after a gentle general conversation to ease the atmosphere: "Linda, when is itching more intense for you: during the day or at night?". "At night doctor!". "Do you feel that the skin down there is like, say, dry?". "Yes, doctor". "And, Linda, do you feel a sense of relief, say, you feel much better, when you can scratch yourself because of the itching?". "Yes doctor, but I feel also very bad because everybody tells me that I must not touch myself for any reason!". "Ok Linda, I think I have very good news for you! I bet we can perfectly cure this problem!". The child smiles, uncertain. A little thought gets across her eyes "May I trust this doctor or not?". "Linda, may I examine you? I promise I will be very gentle and your mom will stay close to you, hand in hand. May I?". The child nods. The gentle nurse stands behind. The diagnosis is so obvious at first sight that it is almost embarrassing to name it. A serious lichen sclerosus, involving labia majora and minora, almost completely fused with the majora, lichenification of the skin, and signs of recent scratching. "The reason of your itching is very clear Linda. This is great news!!! You can dress yourself". "Besides, your mom is very smart, Linda. I sincerely congratulate her! She found the doctor with the right experience to help you". Linda smiles, with a glimpse of pride, looking up at her mom. "The skin of your genitals is very very dry, as you correctly said before, and this causes the itching. That will disappear in 30 days, Linda, only thirty days, and maybe less, and you will be much better and happy. Let's tell the good news to dad as well!". Treatment was immediately started with clobetasol cream once a day for two weeks and then every other day for two months. Vitamin E spray, twice a day, was added. Vitamin E-based cleansing cream was suggested only once a day.

After 6 weeks, Linda comes in with her mom, both with a radiant smile: "Fantastic Linda, I guess from your beautiful smile that you feel much better! Am I right?". She nods: "Doctor I have a gift for you!". "Really?! How kind of you Linda!". The child hands over a drawing paper: the examining room, Linda, Mom, and the doctor with the white coat. From the lamp hanging from the ceiling, strong yellow rays enlighten the room, and mostly the physician head! The diagnostic lamp was finally turned on (must have thought the smart child).

In fact, symptoms have almost completely disappeared. The skin was much better, so the biopsy for histology was considered not necessary.

Maintenance treatment, with clobesol twice a week, was planned for three months and then reduced to once a week, as symptom improvement was consistent and very reassuring over time. At three-year follow-up, symptom relief is consistent with clobesol once weekly. Unfortunately the conglutination of labia minora is irreversible by now (maybe after puberty topical testosterone of vegetal origin may help to improve the local trophism – AG medical opinion based on other clinical cases).

Headache and IBS, investigated by a competent colleagues, showed to be triggered by gluten. A diagnosis of "gluten sensitivity" was maid (criteria for celiac disease were not fulfilled). A gluten-free diet reduced significantly both symptoms, for Linda' joy.

Key Learning Points

- Lichen sclerosus is an autoimmune-based disease.
- It may affect children; prevalence increases with increasing age.
- In childhood, it is underdiagnosed and undertreated.
- Comorbidity with other autoimmune and/or inflammatory conditions (allergies, food intolerances, IBS, headache, pelvic pain) is frequent.
- Itching, more intense at night, is the most bothersome and typical symptom (cases with the sign of LS, but without itching, are rare).
- Differential diagnosis with worm/parasitic bowel infection (which typically causes itching at night as well) is mandatory.
- Clinical examination of the vulva shows progressive full-thickness involution of the cytoarchitecture of the vulva, with thinning of the vulvar skin that becomes pale/white; area of hyperkeratinizations and fusion of the labia minora with majora become prominent when the disease course progresses undiagnosed.
- Biopsy, with appropriate topical analgesia, should be limited only to cases when vulvar intraepithelial neoplasia, comorbid with LS, is suspected.
- Clobesol cream remains the gold standard for topical treatment.

- Long-term follow-up is recommended because:
  - LS is a chronic progressive autoimmune condition.
  - Autoimmune comorbidities deserve early diagnosis as well.
  - Risk of malignant progression to squamous vulvar cell carcinoma is reported around 5 %.

Conclusions

Vulvar pain is still an orphan concept during childhood. Pediatrician, family physicians, and emergency healthcare professionals should become familiar with the "vulvar" name and use it appropriately when pain referred to the vulvar region is complained of. Long-term follow-up of childhood acute vulvar pain of any etiology is recommended.

Specific training of pediatricians in the area of vulvar pain, of different etiology, is mandatory.

References

Abdulcadir J, Rodriguez MI, Say L. Research gaps in the care of women with female genital mutilation: an analysis. BJOG. 2015;122(3):294–303.

Bagga HS, Fisher PB, Tasian GE, Blaschko SD, McCulloch CE, McAninch JW, Breyer BN. Sports-related genitourinary injuries presenting to United States emergency departments. Urology. 2015;85(1):239–44. doi:10.1016/j.urology.2014.07.075.

Bailhache M, Leroy V, Pillet P, Salmi LR. Is early detection of abused children possible? A systematic review of the diagnostic accuracy of the identification of abused children. BMC Pediatr. 2013;13:202–2010.

Berenson AB, Chacko MR, Wiemann CM, Mishaw CO, Friedrich WN, Grady JJ. Use of hymenal measurements in the diagnosis of previous penetration. Pediatrics. 2002;109(2):228–35.

Berg RC, Underland V, Odgaard-Jensen J, Fretheim A, Vist GE. Effects of female genital cutting on physical health outcomes: a systematic review and meta-analysis. BMJ Open. 2014;4(11):e006316. doi:10.1136/bmjopen-2014-006316.

Berkoff MC, Zolotor AJ, Makoroff KL, Thackeray JD, Shapiro RA, Runyan DK. Has this prepubertal girl been sexually abused? JAMA. 2008;13(23):2779–92.

Birge O, Ozbey EG, Arslan D, Erkan MM, Demir F, Akgor U. Vulvar epidermoid cyst and type 2 radical genital mutilation. Case Rep Obstet Gynecol. 2015;2015:520190. doi:10.1155/2015/520190. Epub 2015 Nov 22.

Carlson JA, Ambros R, Malfetano J, Ross J, Grabowski R, Lamb P, Figge H, Mihm Jr MC. Vulvar lichen sclerosus and squamous cell carcinoma: a cohort, case control, and investigational study with historical perspective; implications for chronic inflammation and sclerosis in the development of neoplasia. Hum Pathol. 1998;29(9):932–48.

Carlson BC, Hofer MD, Ballek N, Yang XJ, Meeks JJ, Gonzalez CM. Protein markers of malignant potential in penile and vulvar lichen sclerosus. J Urol. 2013;190(2):399–406.

Casey JT, Bjurlin MA, Cheng EY. Pediatric genital injury: an analysis of the national electronic injury surveillance system. Urology. 2013;82(5):10.1016.

Clare CA, Yeh J. Vulvodynia in adolescence: childhood vulvar pain syndromes (review). J Pediatr Adolesc Gynecol. 2011;24(3):110–5.

Cohen-Sacher B, Haefner HK, Dalton VK, Berger MB. History of abuse in women with vulvar pruritus, vulvodynia, and asymptomatic controls. J Low Genit Tract Dis. 2015;19(3):248–52.

Cooper SM, Gao XH, Powell JJ, Wojnarowska F. Does treatment of vulvar lichen sclerosus influence its prognosis? Arch Dermatol. 2004;140:702–6.

Gilbert R, Widom CS, Browne K, Fergusson D, Webb E, Janson S. Burden and consequences of child maltreatment in high-income countries. Lancet. 2009;13(9657):68–81.

Graziottin A, Gambini D, Bertolasi L. Genital and sexual pain in women. In: Vodusek D, Boller F, editors. Neurology of sexual and bladder disorders, (Handbook of clinical neurology, vol. 130, 3rd Series). Edinburgh: Elsevier, 2015, p. 395–412.

Gudu W. Acute vulvar pain in a lady with post circumcision inclusion cyst of the vulva containing stones: a case report. BMC Womens Health. 2014;14:2. doi:10.1186/1472-6874-14-2.

Hadid V, Dahan MH. A case of chronic abdominal neuropathic pain and burning after female genital cutting. Case Rep Obstet Gynecol. 2015;2015:906309. doi:10.1155/2015/906309. Epub 2015 Jun 2.

Harlow BL, Stewart EG. Adult-onset vulvodynia in relation to childhood violence victimization. Am J Epidemiol. 2005;161(9):871–80.

Khandker M, Brady SS, Elizabeth G, Stewart EG, Harlow BL. Is chronic stress during childhood associated with adult-onset vulvodynia? J Womens Health (Larchmt). 2014;23(8):649–56.

Lagerstedt M, Karvinen K, Joki-Erkkilä M, Huotari-Orava R, Snellman E, Laasanen SL. Childhood lichen sclerosus – a challenge for clinicians. Pediatr Dermatol. 2013;30(4):444–50. doi:10.1111/pde.12109. Epub 2013 Feb 26.

Nour NM. Female genital cutting: clinical and cultural guidelines. Obstet Gynecol Surv. 2004;59(4):272–9.

Papoiu AD, Nattkemper LA, Sanders KM, Kraft RA, Chan YH, Coghill RC, Yosipovitch G. Brain's reward circuits mediate itch relief: a functional MRI study of active scratching. PLoS One. 2013;8(12):e82389. doi:10.1371/journal.pone.0082389. eCollection 2013.

Perron L, Senikas V, Burnett M, Davis V, Society of Obstetricians and Gynaecologists of Canada. Female genital cutting. J Obstet Gynaecol Can. 2013;35(11):1028–45.

Powell J, Wojnarowska F. Childhood vulvar lichen sclerosus: the course after puberty. J Reprod Med. 2002;47:706–9.

Reed BD, Cantor LE. Vulvodynia in preadolescent girls. J Low Genit Tract Dis. 2008;12(4):257–61.

Rouzi AA. Epidermal clitoral inclusion cysts: not a rare complication of female genital mutilation. Hum Reprod. 2010;25(7):1672–4. doi:10.1093/humrep/deq126. Epub 2010 May 22.

Rouzi AA, Alturki F. Female genital mutilation/cutting: an update. Clin Exp Obstet Gynecol. 2015;42(3):300–3.

Scheidler MG, Schultz BL, Schall L, Ford HR. Mechanisms of blunt perineal injury in female pediatric patients. J Pediatr Surg. 2000;35:1317–9.

Sham M, Singh D, Wankhede U, Wadate A. Management of child victims of acute sexual assault: surgical repair and beyond. J Indian Assoc Pediatr Surg. 2013;18(3):105–11.

Smith SD, Fischer G. Childhood onset vulvar lichen sclerosus does not resolve at puberty: a prospective case series. Pediatr Dermatol. 2009;26(6):725–9. doi:10.1111/j.1525-1470.2009.01022.x.

Tarman GJ, Kaplan GW, Lerman SL, McAleer IM, Losasso BE. Lower genitourinary injury and pelvic fractures in pediatric patients. Urology. 2002;59(1):123–6. discussion 126.

Tasian GE, Bagga HS, Fisher PB, McCulloch CE, Cinman NM, McAninch JW, Breyer BN. Pediatric genitourinary injuries in the United States from 2002 to 2010. J Urol. 2013;189(1):288–93.

UNICEF. Female genital mutilation/cutting: a statistical overview and exploration of the dynamics of change. New York: UNICEF; 2013.

World Health Organization. Eliminating female genital mutilation: an inter-agency statement. Geneva: WHO, OHCHR, UNAIDS, UNDP, UNECA, UNESCO, UNFPA, UNHCR, UNICEF, UNIFEM, WHO; 2008.

World Health Organization study group on female genital mutilation and obstetric outcome, Banks E, Meirik O, et al. Female genital mutilation and obstetric outcome: WHO collaborative prospective study in six African countries. Lancet. 2006;367(9525):1835–41.

Female Genital Mutilations and the Scotomized, Neglected Vulvar Pain: Who Cares?

5

Female genital mutilation/cutting (FGM/C) is defined by the World Health Organization (WHO) as "all procedures that involve partial or total removal of the external female genitalia or other injury to the female genital organs for non-medical reasons" (WHO 2008). It is typically carried out, with or without anesthesia, by a traditional circumciser using a knife or razor. The age of the girls who undergo this procedure varies from weeks after birth to puberty (UNICEF 2013). Different types of FMG/C can be performed (Table 5.1), with different severity of vulvar/genital damage and risk of long-term consequences.

Worldwide, an estimated 125–140 million girls and women live with FGM/C.

Common early complications of FGM/C include uncontrolled bleeding, fever, wound infection, sepsis, and death (Nour 2004). *Vulvar pain, the most obvious consequence, is not mentioned in Nour's and other's papers, although acute vulvar and genital pain is the most likely symptom when excision is performed in an area so richly innervated with sensory nerve fibers*. FGM/C is also reported to cause psychological consequences, such as anxiety, horror, posttraumatic stress disorders, and depression.

Long-term complications include *dysmenorrhea, dyspareunia, recurrent vaginal and urinary tract infections, infertility cysts, abscesses, keloid formation, obstetric complications, difficulty with childbirth, and sexual dysfunctions* (WHO 2006). *Diagnosis requires dedicated medical skills with a nonjudgmental approach* (Hearst and Molnar 2013).

Unfortunately, there is *no mention of vulvar pain* in the WHO 2006's paper as well.

Excellent reviews of available literature have been carried out: 5109 papers were considered, of which 185 studies (3.17 million women surveyed) were of good quality (Berg et al. 2014). Authors have carefully described the long-term gynecologic and obstetric outcomes of FGM/C. Results indicate significantly increased risks such as:

- *Urinary tract infections* (unadjusted RR = 3.01)
- *Bacterial vaginosis* (adjusted OR (AOR) = 1.68)

A. Graziottin, F. Murina, *Vulvar Pain*, DOI 10.1007/978-3-319-42677-8_5

- *Dyspareunia* (RR = 1.53)
- *Prolonged labor* (AOR = 1.49)
- *Caesarean section* (AOR = 1.60)
- *Difficult delivery* (AOR = 1.88)

Vulvar pain is not mentioned as well in this review, nor in the otherwise very accurate Canadian guidelines (Perron et al. 2013), focused most on *how to manage women who underwent FGM/C*, i.e., to indicate the most appropriate obstetric and gynecological care on FGC, including FGC-related complications.

Only a few recently published clinical cases report vulvar epidermoid inclusion cysts, with inguinal (Birge et al. 2015) and/or acute *vulvar pain* (Gudu 2014). Specifically, the first case of *neuropathic pain with sensory neuropathy* has been published in June 2015 (Hadid and Dahan 2015).

Key question: is this case of neuropathic vulvar pain the first ever or is this the first time when neuropathic sensory vulvar pain after FGC receives the proper descriptive name of "vulvar pain"?

Coital pain/introital dyspareunia (CP/ID) is a frequently reported symptom. Its first etiology is the biomechanical narrowing of the vaginal entrance, more frequent in type III FGM/C. CP/ID is a symptom complained of when sexual maturity is achieved and when sexual intercourse is attempted/initiated.

What's behind dyspareunia after FGM/C? Is spontaneous vulvar pain an issue? Is provoked vestibulodynia a leading etiology of CP/ID after FGM/C? Or is coital pain "only" the consequence of the biomechanical narrowing of the vaginal entrance due to cutting and scarring per se, without the specific pathognomonic features of

Table 5.1 The World Health Organization classification of female genital mutilation

Complete typology with subdivisions:
Type I – partial or total removal of the clitoris and/or the prepuce (clitoridectomy)
When it is important to distinguish between the major variations of type I mutilation, the following subdivisions are proposed: type Ia, removal of the clitoral hood or prepuce only, and type Ib, removal of the clitoris with the prepuce
Type II – partial or total removal of the clitoris and the labia minora, with or without excision of the labia majora (excision)
When it is important to distinguish between the major variations that have been documented, the following subdivisions are proposed: type IIa, removal of the labia minora only; type IIb, partial or total removal of the clitoris and the labia minora; and type IIc, partial or total removal of the clitoris, the labia minora, and the labia majora
Note also that, in French, the term "excision" is often used as a general term covering all types of female genital mutilation
Type III – narrowing of the vaginal orifice with creation of a covering seal by cutting and appositioning the labia minora and/or the labia majora, with or without excision of the clitoris (infibulation)
Type IIIa, removal and apposition of the labia minora; type IIIb, removal and apposition of the labia majora
Type IV – all other harmful procedures to the female genitalia for nonmedical purposes, e.g., pricking, piercing, incising, scraping, and cauterization

World Health Organization (2008)

vulvar vestibulitis/provoked vestibulodynia (inflammation, with significant increase of (1) mast cells in the vestibular tissue; (2) degranulated mast cells, indicating a very active release of inflammatory molecules in the vestibular tissue; (3) mast cells closer to the pain nerve fibers)?

"Genital pain" wording is comprehensive, yet not enough accurate. In the available literature on FGM/C (with the abovementioned exception of a few case reports), no mentioning of vulvar pain, either spontaneous or provoked, is usually reported, in spite of the fact that the vulva is the organ more severely cut and wounded.

Even the most recent and accurate papers on research gaps (Abdulcadir et al. 2015a) and on clinical inadequacies in treatment and follow-up (Rouzi and Alturki 2015) do not mention the issue of vulvar pain/vulvodynia after FGM/C. Abdulcadir quotes the "clitoral reconstruction" to relieve clitoral pain in 40 % of women treated by Thabet and Foldès. However, vulvar pain is not mentioned at all in this paper. Only a brief sentence on the improvement of "vulvar appearance" and body image after deinfibulation is reported.

Abdulcadir does mention vulvar pain in two cases of clitoral reconstruction (Abdulcadir et al. 2015b). The current literature seems therefore quote pain only when the clitoris is involved. However, it is very likely that pain is perceived as well in the introitus, given the high percentage of apareunia and introital dyspareunia after FGM/C.

Clitoral reconstruction seems very promising in restoring a better sexual function after FGM/C (Vital et al. 2016).

Case reports on "*clitoral neuromas*" after FGM/C indicate that neurologic complications are present. Fernández-Aguilar and Noël (2003) published the very first clinical case indicating that vulvar pain caused by a neuroma of the clitoris is a serious complications of FGM/C. One more case has been described (Abdulcadir et al. 2012), but a systematic research has not yet been published. Complications leading to vulvar pain are therefore very likely to be underreported.

Specific investigations on acute and chronic vulvar pain after FGM/C should be carried out, with focus on characteristics and vulnerabilities that could predict an evolution toward vestibulodynia, clitorodynia, vulvodynia, and introital dyspareunia. Attention should be paid at the first medical evaluation when a child who underwent FGM/C undergoes pediatric clinical evaluation for whatever reason.

5.1 Vulvar Pain After Female Genital Mutilation/Cutting: A Lifespan Perspective

5.1.1 Children

One sixth to one fifth of those 125 million girls and women are prepubertal, which translates into around 20 million children who recently underwent genital cutting. What are their current symptoms? Is vulvar pain an issue? In which percentage does acute vulvar pain, subsequent to cutting, shift into chronic vulvar pain/vulvodynia? Unfortunately, vulvar pain/vulvodynia is almost not mentioned at all in the available literature, and no word/research is spent on vulvar pain in children who underwent FGM/C. Does acute and chronic vulvar pain exist after FMG/C? Or is this issue invisible? That is, is it still under the threshold of clinical perception?

When clinician/pediatricians talk about "genital pain" after FGM/C, do they include vulvar pain? If yes, why not using a most appropriate wording? If not, why is there such a scotomization of the pain that is most likely to be elicited, given that the cutting acts exactly on that organ called vulva (the clitoris is indeed an anatomic part of it) and primitive suturing involves the labia minora?

Without attention to this specific symptom, with the appropriate wording/naming, no identification is possible of the subset of children at higher risk of long-term vulvar pain/vulvodynia/dyspareunia, and no early intervention can therefore be offered. Specific research on acute and chronic vulvar pain in prepubertal children undergoing genital cutting is urgently needed.

5.1.2 Adolescents

Three million girls in Africa are estimated to be at risk of FGM/C annually. A survey on 258 girls and women who had undergone FGM, most between 10 and 14 years of age, was carried out in Sierra Leone (Bjälkander et al., 2012). Complications were reported by 218 respondents (84.5 %), the most common ones being *excessive bleeding, delay in or incomplete healing, and tenderness.*

Fever was significantly more often reported by girls who had undergone FGM before 10 years of age compared with those who had undergone the procedure later. Out of those who reported complications, 187 (85.8 %) sought treatment, with 89 of them visiting a traditional healer, 75 a Sowei (traditional circumciser), and 16 a health professional. In spite of this very high rate of complications, no mention of acute or chronic vulvar pain is reported.

5.1.3 Adult, Premenopausal Women

FGM/C, according to the extension of the cutting, does remove the glands of the clitoris and part of the clitoral shaft. FGM/C usually does not remove the deeper part of the cavernosal bodies, currently defined as the "bulbs of the clitoris" (O'Connel and De Lancey 2005; O'Connell et al. 2008), and formerly called "bulbocavernosal bodies" deep under the labia minora, unless a very radical and dramatic mutilation is performed. Usually, the crura of the clitoris deep along the crural bones bilaterally and the part of the cavernosal bodies that surround the lower third of the urethra (considered to be the smaller size equivalent of the male corpus spongiosum of the urethra) are not removed.

Data on sexual outcomes and specifically vulvar pain in women who underwent FGM/C are conflicting. Catania et al. (2007) investigated 137 adult women affected by different types of FGM/C: 58 young FGM/C ladies living in the West; 57 infibulated women; 15 infibulated women after the operation of defibulation were studied, with semistructured interviews and the Female Sexual Function Index. Surveyed women affected by different types of FGM/C reported orgasm almost always 86 %, always 69.23 %; 58 mutilated young women reported orgasm in 91.43 %, always 8.57 %; after defibulation 14 out of 15 infibulated women reported orgasm.

The group of 57 infibulated women investigated with the FSFI questionnaire showed significant differences between study group and an equivalent group of control in desire, arousal, orgasm, and satisfaction *with mean scores higher in the group of mutilated women.* No significant differences were observed between the two groups in lubrication and pain (Catania et al. 2007). The maintenance of a consistent part of the cavernosal unit, in spite of the brutal cutting, may explain why the majority of women who underwent FGM/C may experience orgasm, according to this research. The very recent study of Abdulcadir et al. (2016) on anatomy and sexual function after FGM/C was carried out on 15 women with FGM/C and 15 controls using magnetic resonance imaging and validated questionnaires.

Women with FGM did not have significantly decreased clitoral glans width and body length but did have significantly smaller volume of the clitoris plus bulbs. They scored significantly lower on sexual function and desire than women without FGM. They did not score lower on Female Sexual Function Index sub-scores for orgasm, desire, and satisfaction and on the Questionnaire d'Image Corporelle, but did report significantly more dyspareunia. A larger total volume of clitoris and bulbs did not correlate with higher Female Sexual Function Index and Sexual Desire Inventory scores in women with FGM compared with uncut women who had larger total volume that correlated with higher scores. The conclusion was that women with FGM have sexual erectile tissues for sexual arousal, orgasm, and pleasure. Women with sexual dysfunction should be appropriately counseled and treated.

However, the extension of the anatomic vulvar and clitoral damage and the potential neurogenic pain secondary to inflammation, infection, and scarring are expected to cause some long-term consequences in terms of clitorodynia, vulvar pain, vestibulodynia, or vulvodynia, not reported in these studies in spite of the high rate of dyspareunia.

Other researches carried out on larger series indicate a very high risk of *recurrent urinary tract infections* (r-UTI) (unadjusted RR = 3.01) and *dyspareunia* (RR = 1.53). In the existing literature and in the clinical practice, the association between r-UTI and specifically recurrent cystitis and provoked vestibulodynia/introital dyspareunia is as high as 60 % (Salonia et al. 2013). It is therefore surprising that with such a high RR of r-UTI after FGM/C, no risk or association of vestibulodynia/vulvar pain is reported. Moreover, it is surprising that given the higher risk of dyspareunia (RR = 1.53) after FGM/C, at least in the large review of Casey et al. 2013, again *no mentioning of vestibulodynia/vulvodynia/vulvar pain is reported.*

Epidermal clitoral inclusion cysts are not a rare complication of female genital mutilation. *In a series of 28 cases, the subjects underwent surgical excision, and one underwent incision and drainage of a clitoral abscess. No short- or long-term complications occurred* (Rouzi 2010). *No complaints of clitoral pain before or after surgery nor of vulvodynia were reported* (Rouzi 2010).

5.2 Treatments to Improve Women's Sexuality

5.2.1 Defibulation: Treatment Outcomes

Defibulation seems to offer excellent outcomes to women with FGC and their partners (Figs. 5.1 and 5.2). Nour et al. (2006) carried out a retrospective study examining the medical records of 40 consecutive women with a history of type III female genital cutting who underwent defibulation between 1995 and 2003. Telephone surveys were conducted between 6 months and 2 years post procedure to evaluate the long-term health and sexual satisfaction outcomes. Of 40 women identified as having undergone defibulation, 95 % were Somali, 65 % were married, and 73 % were between the ages of 19 and 30. Primary indications for defibulation were being

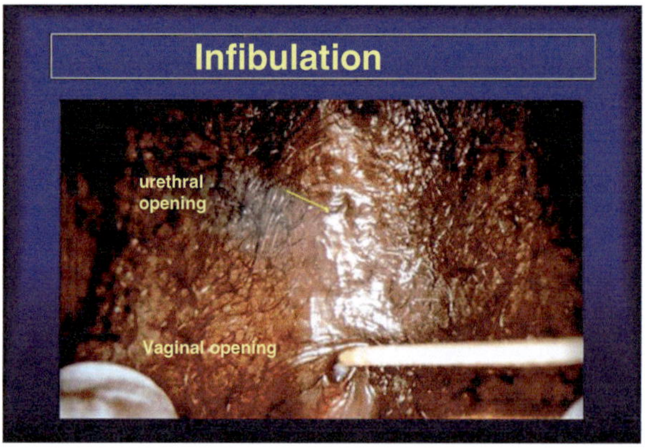

Fig. 5.1 The picture exemplifies the consequences of female genital mutilation/cutting (FGM/C). Labia minora have been cut and sutured along the median line. The urethral opening is surrounded by the skin; the vestibulum is covered by labia's skin. The vaginal opening is narrowed and reduced to a very small passage just for the menstrual blood (Courtesy of Dr. L. Catania and Dr. Omar Abdulcadir, 2015)

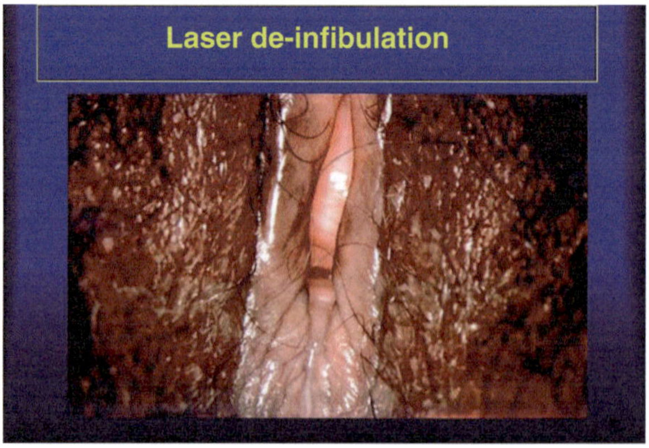

Fig. 5.2 The vulva after laser deinfibulation along the median fusion line of labia minora. The picture well shows the vestibulum and the vagina underneath the line of laser's opening (Courtesy of Dr. L. Catania and Dr. Omar Abdulcadir, 2015)

pregnant (30 %), dysmenorrhea (30 %), apareunia (20 %), and dyspareunia (15 %). Secondary indications were difficulty urinating (12.5 %), apareunia (20 %), and dyspareunia (10 %). 30 % had therefore significant coital difficulties; 65 % had a subcuticular repair; 48 % had an intact clitoris buried beneath the scar. None had intraoperative or postoperative complications. Of the 32 patients reached by telephone, 94 % stated they would highly recommend it to others. 100 % of patients and their husbands were satisfied with the results, felt their appearance had improved, and were sexually satisfied. However, vulvar pain is not mentioned when discussing women's symptoms for the 20 % who could not have intercourse or the 10 % who had severe introital pain.

The persistence of the G spot, usually not lesioned by FGM/C as it is deeper in the anterior vaginal wall (Thabet 2009), helps to understand why women may have a satisfying intercourse with coital orgasm after deinfibulation post FGM/C. However, women with larger mutilations (types II and III) do report a significant sexual impairment, based first on the anatomical and functional damage (Thabet and Thabet 2003).

Figures 5.1 and 5.2 give an immediate perception of the extension of the cutting and median suturing. If the deinfibulation would not have been done, how excruciating, repeated, and prolonged would the vulvar pain have been during the attempts to "naturally" open the suturing (scar defloration)?

5.2.2 Clitoral Reconstruction

Clitoral reconstruction seems a very promising technique to improve women's sexuality and reduce clitoral pain (Foldès et al. 2012; Abdulcadir et al. 2015a, b; Vital et al. 2016). The huge series of Foldès et al., with 2938 women operated of clitoral reconstruction after FGM/C, is impressive. Outcomes seem to be very positive: women had a mean age of 29.2 (SD 7.77 years; age at excision 6.1, SD 3.5 years). Mali, Senegal, and Ivory Coast were the main countries of origin, but 564 patients had undergone female genital mutilation in France. Expectations before surgery were identity recovery for 2933 patients (99 %), improved sex life for 2378 patients (81 %), and pain reduction for 847 patients (29 %).

At 1-year follow-up, 363 women (42 %) had a hoodless glans, 239 (28 %) had a normal clitoris, 210 (24 %) had a visible projection, 51 (6 %) had a palpable projection, and three (0.4 %) had no change. Most patients reported an improvement, or at least no worsening, in pain (821 of 840 patients) and clitoral pleasure (815 of 834 patients). At 1 year, 430 (51 %) of 841 women experienced orgasms. Immediate complications after surgery (hematoma, suture failure, moderate fever) were noted in 155 (5 %) of the 2938 patients, and 108 (4 %) were briefly readmitted to hospital. Foldès et al. conclude that *reconstructive surgery after female genital mutilation seems to be associated with reduced pain and restored pleasure*. Unfortunately, the 1-year follow-up visit was attended only by 866 patients (29 %). This limits the appreciation of the real outcomes: women lost at follow-up could be the least satisfied or have had complications including pain.

5.3 Obstetric Outcomes

Divergent study results have called into question whether FGM/C is associated with obstetric consequences. Berg and Underland (2013) conducted a systematic review of the scientific literature and quantitative meta-analyses of the obstetric consequences of FGM/C. Authors included 44 primary studies, of which 28 were comparative, involving almost 3 million participants. The methodological study quality was generally low, but several studies reported the same outcome and were sufficiently similar to warrant pooling of effect sizes in meta-analyses. The meta-analyses results showed that *prolonged labor, obstetric lacerations, instrumental delivery, obstetric hemorrhage, and difficult delivery are markedly associated with FGM/C*, indicating that FGM/C is a factor in their occurrence and significantly increases the risk of delivery complications. There was no significant difference in risk with respect to cesarean section and episiotomy.

Defibulation seems to facilitate labor and reduce significantly obstetric complications. Wuest et al. (2009) studied 122 pregnant women perinatally: 6 % of patients wished to have their FGM defibulated antenatally; 43 % requested a defibulation during labor; 34 % desired a defibulation during labor only if considered necessary, by the medical staff; and 17 % were unable to express their expectations. There were no differences for FGM patients and controls regarding fetal outcome, maternal blood loss, or duration of delivery. FGM patients had significantly more often an emergency caesarean section and third-degree vaginal tears and significantly less first-degree and second-degree tears. Vulvar pain is never mentioned in the paper.

A recent retrospective study carried out at the University of Geneva (Abdulcadir et al. 2015c) on 129 women who attended a specialized clinic in FGC care indicates that obstetric outcomes were similar to average outcomes for women without FGM presenting at the same department and in Switzerland generally. Specifically, 20 women had a cesarean delivery. An assisted delivery was performed for 18 patients; among these, only eight had experienced obstructed labor. No statistically significant differences were found for the outcome measures when women with FGM type III were compared to FGM type I and II. Routine obstetric follow-up combined with specialized care for women with FGM, including defibulation, can avoid inappropriate obstetric practices and reduce obstetric complications known to be associated with FGM (Abdulcadir et al. 2015c).

Conclusion

FGM/C causes excruciating acute genital pain. Acute vulvar pain during and after the excision is not mentioned in the vast majority of papers, in spite of the cutting being focused on the vulva, an extremely innervated and sensitive organ. Only a few case reports describe vulvar pain in case of neuroma of the clitoris, abscesses, or inclusion cysts.

120–140,000,000 women have undergone FMG/C worldwide, often in dramatic primitive conditions, with scissors, no asepsis, and no accurate wound care.

It is therefore very likely that vulvar, acute, chronic, and, in a subset of women, neuropathic pain is hugely underreported, underinvestigated, and undertreated.

At least 20 % of women have apareunia and 10 % introital dyspareunia. Yet, almost no case of vestibulodynia, vulvodynia, and vulvar pain is reported, with the exception of a few anecdotal recent cases.

This chapter is a call for awareness, research, and action, to understand if *vulvar pain* is *not existing* after FGM/C, in the short and long term. This seems unbelievable. Or if it is an *orphan concept* just waiting to be properly adopted to get the full attention, it deserves with the goal of improving the quality of care, prevention, and follow-up after FGM/C.

With a whish: to hopefully reduce the number of children and girls who have to undergo an excruciating vulvar cutting with cruel pain and persisting dramatic symptoms and comorbidities.

References

Abdulcadir J, Pusztaszeri M, Vilarino R, Dubuisson JB, Vlastos AT. Clitoral neuroma after female genital mutilation/cutting: a rare but possible event. J Sex Med. 2012;9(4):1220–5.

Abdulcadir J, Rodriguez MI, Say L. Research gaps in the care of women with female genital mutilation: an analysis. BJOG. 2015a;122(3):294–303.

Abdulcadir J, Rodriguez MI, Petignat P, Say L. Clitoral reconstruction after female genital mutilation/cutting: case studies. J Sex Med. 2015b;12(1):274–81. doi:10.1111/jsm.12737. Epub 2014 Nov 25.

Abdulcadir J, Dugerdil A, Yaron M, Irion O, Boulvain M. Obstetric care of women with female genital mutilation attending a specialized clinic in a tertiary center. Int J Gynaecol Obstet. 2015c;9.

Abdulcadir J, Botsikas D, Bolmont M, Bilancioni A, Djema DA, Bianchi Demicheli F, Yaron M, Petignat P. Sexual anatomy and function in women with and without genital mutilation: a cross-sectional study. J Sex Med. 2016;13(2):226–37.

Berg RC, Underland V. The obstetric consequences of female genital mutilation/cutting: a systematic review and meta-analysis. Obstet Gynecol Int. 2013;2013:496564. doi:10.1155/2013/496564. Epub 2013 Jun 26.

Berg RC, Underland V, Odgaard-Jensen J, Fretheim A, Vist GE. Effects of female genital cutting on physical health outcomes: a systematic review and meta-analysis. BMJ Open. 2014;4(11): e006316.

Birge O, Ozbey EG, Arslan D, Erkan MM, Demir F, Akgor U. Vulvar epidermoid cyst and type 2 radical genital mutilation. Case Rep Obstet Gynecol. 2015;2015:520190.

Bjälkander O, Bangura L, Leigh B, Berggren V, Bergström S, Almroth L. Health complications of female genital mutilation in Sierra Leone. Int J Womens Health. 2012;4:321–31.

Casey JT, Bjurlin MA, Cheng EY. Pediatric genital injury: an analysis of the national electronic injury surveillance system. Urology. 2013;82(5):10.1016.

Catania L, Abdulcadir O, Puppo V, Baldaro Verde J, Abdulcadir J, Abdulcadir D. Pleasure and orgasm in women with female genital mutilation/cutting (FGM/C). J Sex Med. 2007;4(6): 1666–78.

Fernández-Aguilar S, Noël JC. Neuroma of the clitoris after female genital cutting. Obstet Gynecol. 2003;101(5 Pt 2):1053–4.

Foldès P, Cuzin B, Andro A. Reconstructive surgery after female genital mutilation: a prospective cohort study. Lancet. 2012;380(9837):134–41.

Gudu W. Acute vulvar pain in a lady with post circumcision inclusion cyst of the vulva containing stones: a case report. BMC Womens Health. 2014;14:2. doi:10.1186/1472-6874-14-2.

Hadid V, Dahan MH. A case of chronic abdominal neuropathic pain and burning after female genital cutting. Case Rep Obstet Gynecol. 2015;2015:906309. doi:10.1155/2015/906309. Epub 2015 Jun 2.

Hearst AA, Molnar AM. Female genital cutting: an evidence-based approach to clinical management for the primary care physician. Mayo Clin Proc. 2013;88(6):618–29. doi:10.1016/j.mayocp.2013.04.004.

Nour NM. Female genital cutting: clinical and cultural guidelines. Obstet Gynecol Surv. 2004;59(4):272–9.

Nour NM, Michels KB, Bryant AE. Defibulation to treat female genital cutting: effect on symptoms and sexual function. Obstet Gynecol. 2006;108(1):55–60.

O'Connel HE, De Lancey JOL. Clitoral anatomy in nulliparous, healthy, premenopausal volunteers using unenhanced magnetic Resonance Imaging. J Urol. 2005;173:2060–3.

O'Connell HE, Eizenberg N, Rahman M, et al. The anatomy of the distal vagina: towards unity. J Sex Med. 2008;5:1883–91.

Perron L, Senikas V, Burnett M, Davis V, Society of Obstetricians and Gynaecologists of Canada. Female genital cutting. J Obstet Gynaecol Can. 2013;35(11):1028–45.

Rouzi AA. Epidermal clitoral inclusion cysts: not a rare complication of female genital mutilation. Hum Reprod. 2010;25(7):1672–4.

Rouzi AA, Alturki F. Female genital mutilation/cutting: an update. Clin Exp Obstet Gynecol. 2015;42(3):300–3.

Salonia A, Clementi MC, Graziottin A, Nappi RE, Castiglione F, Ferrari M, Capitanio U, Damiano R, Montorsi F. Secondary provoked vestibulodynia in sexually-active women with recurrent uncomplicated urinary tract infections. J Sex Med. 2013;10(9):2265–73.

Thabet SM. Reality of the G-spot and its relation to female circumcision and vaginal surgery. J Obstet Gynaecol Res. 2009;35(5):967–73.

Thabet SM, Thabet AS. Defective sexuality and female circumcision: the cause and the possible management. J Obstet Gynaecol Res. 2003;29(1):12–9.

UNICEF. Female genital mutilation/cutting: a statistical overview and exploration of the dynamics of change. 2013. UNICEF.

Vital M, de Visme S, Hanf M, Philippe HJ, Winer N, Wylomanski S. Using the Female Sexual Function Index (FSFI) to evaluate sexual function in women with genital mutilation undergoing surgical reconstruction: a pilot prospective study. Eur J Obstet Gynecol Reprod Biol. 2016;202:71–4. Epub 2016 Apr 30.

World Health Organization. Eliminating female genital mutilation: an inter-agency statement. Geneva: WHO, OHCHR, UNAIDS, UNDP, UNECA, UNESCO, UNFPA, UNHCR, UNICEF, UNIFEM, WHO; 2008.

World Health Organization study group on female genital mutilation and obstetric outcome. Banks E, Meirik O, et al. Female genital mutilation and obstetric outcome: WHO collaborative prospective study in six African countries. Lancet. 2006;367(9525):1835–41.

Wuest S, Raio L, Wyssmueller D, Mueller MD, Stadlmayr W, Surbek DV, Kuhn A. Effects of female genital mutilation on birth outcomes in Switzerland. BJOG. 2009;116(9):1204–9.

Vulvar Pain in Adolescents

6

Adolescence is the life period when vulvar pain of various etiologies, and specifically vestibulodynia/vulvodynia, begins to be diagnosed, investigated, and treated (Bachmann et al. 2006; Clare and Yeh 2011; Graziottin and Murina 2011; Reed et al. 2014).

The focus of this chapter will be the analysis of different types of vulvar pain in *nulliparous adolescents* (please see Chap. 7).

Vulvar pain and its different etiologies will be presented with a pathophysiologic reading, carefully based on adolescents' wording, listened to and questioned during almost four decades of clinical practice by one of the authors (AG) ("practice-based evidence") and continuously and dynamically analyzed with the ongoing scientific evidence ("evidence-based medicine").

Vestibulodynia/clitorodynia/vulvodynia are subsets of the vulvar pain. The International Society for the Study of Vulvar Diseases defines vulvodynia as *a chronic pain or discomfort involving the vulva for more than 3 months and for which no obvious etiology can be found* (Haefner 2007). Vulvodynia descriptors are summarized in Box 6.1.

If the etiology is evident (e.g., lichen sclerosus can affect adolescence as well), then the woman has chronic vulvar pain secondary to lichen sclerosus, if this is the only finding (Sadownik 2014). Thus, vulvodynia is a diagnosis of exclusion. However, the woman could also have both conditions, lichen sclerosus *and* vestibulodynia that should be carefully evaluated.

Box 6.1. Vulvodynia Descriptors

- Women *and* adolescents with vestibulodynia/vulvodynia do not usually use the word "pain" to describe their discomfort.
- They use words such as *itching*, *burning*, *stinging*, *irritation*, *stabbing*, *and/or rawness.*

A. Graziottin, F. Murina, *Vulvar Pain*, DOI 10.1007/978-3-319-42677-8_6

- The classification of vulvodynia is currently based on a description of the pain:
  - The adolescent's symptoms may be:
    - *Generalized* to the whole vulva (generalized vulvodynia)
    - *Localized* to a specific area such as the clitoris (clitorodynia) or the vestibule of the vagina (vestibulodynia)
  - The pain may be:
    - *Provoked* (caused by direct touch, inserting a tampon, or sexual touch)
  - *Unprovoked* (spontaneous, i.e., present without touch)
  - *Mixed* (Haefner 2007)

Unfortunately, many healthcare providers (HCPs) consider the "dynia" group the paradigm, the unique essence of vulvar pain, which is not. Therefore, a careful listening to and reporting in the medical record of the precise adolescent's wording may help to exactly qualify her vulvar complaint.

Of note, many predisposing, precipitating, and perpetuating factors are not usually described in the population study on vulvodynia. They will be discussed here because also a few clinical cases may inspire a more comprehensive reading of the complex pathophysiology of vulvar pain. Predictors and vulnerabilities will be briefly considered as well. Preventive strategies with a few key points on treatment principles will be finally summarized (for the detailed discussion, see Chap. 11) (Graziottin and Murina 2011; Frasson et al. 2009; Graziottin 2014; Graziottin et al. 2015; Graziottin and Gambini 2016).

6.1 Epidemiology

Adolescents are *the age cohort more vulnerable to vulvar pain*. A recent study on 1786 women, assessed for onset of vulvodynia, suggests that the incidence rate was 4.2 cases per 100 person-years, and rates per 100 person-years were greater in women who were younger (7.6 cases per 100 person-years at age 20, compared with 3.3 cases per 100 person-years at age 60), Hispanic (9.5), and married or living as married (4.9); had reported symptoms of vulvar pain but did not meet vulvodynia criteria on the initial survey (11.5); and had reported past symptoms suggesting a history of vulvodynia (7.5). Increased risk of new onset vulvodynia also included *baseline sleep disturbance*, *chronic pain in general*, *specific comorbid pain disorders*, and specific comorbid psychological disorders (Reed et al. 2014). Previous studies suggest an overall prevalence of vulvodynia in the general US population of 8.3 % (Reed et al. 2012a). Chronic vulvar pain may affect up to 16 % of the population, according to other studies (Sadownik 2014). Overall, a prevalence of 7–10 % is the most consistent across studies in the USA (Iglesias-Rios et al. 2015).

6.2 The Narrative of Vulvar Pain in Childhood and Adolescence

Vulvar pain may stem in *childhood vulvar lesions*:

- Traumatic:
  - Intentional, after sexual abuse, or after female genital mutilation/cutting (FGM/C) (see Chap. 5)
  - Unintentional
- Infective (herpes)
- Chemical
- Iatrogenic (see Chaps. 4 and 9)

Vulvar pain is not described nor usually considered in childhood. Pediatricians/clinicians usually refer to "genital pain" when symptoms are referred to the vulvar area in prepubertal girls (Casey et al. 2013), with few exceptions (Clare and Yeh 2011). No follow-up prospective studies of children genital pain/vulvar pain have been found in the available literature, with an important wording/naming and research omission.

When intentional vestibular/vulvar trauma (i.e., sexual abuse) is considered, retrospective studies show conflicting results. Some research groups failed to show any specific association between sexual and physical abuse in childhood and later onset vulvodynia (Cohen-Sacher et al. 2015), while others did well indicate how childhood may be the high-risk age for later chronic vulvar pain, up to specific vulvodynia/vestibulodynia in abused children (Harlow and Stewart 2005; Khandker et al. 2014). Among women with a history of severe childhood abuse, those with vulvodynia had three times the odds of living in fear of any abuse compared to women without vulvodynia (95 % confidence interval: 1.0, 11.0), after adjustment for childhood poverty (Khandker et al. 2014).

Lifelong vestibular/vulvar pain since childhood is a still underinvestigated issue in a subset of adolescents complaining of vestibular/vulvar pain. When specifically questioned, many of them recall that vestibular burning symptoms, with or without bladder symptoms, were present well before puberty, but were not listened to by their family and/or by their pediatrician. Attention to comorbidities is mandatory (Reed et al. 2012b).

Key Point
Listening to and gently asking about vestibular/vulvar pain in childhood is of the highest clinical attention as central components of pain, characterized by a progressive neuroinflammation, may become prominent over the years and make the clinical pain picture much more difficult to be effectively treated in the consulting adolescent.

The sad fact is that vulvar pain in childhood is almost totally neglected worldwide. The inflammation that stimulates pain keeps therefore on being active in the shadow of physicians' diagnostic omission. When finally the consulted gynecologist diagnoses *vestibular and/or vulvar pain since puberty*, quite a long period of childhood chronic vulvar pain may have gone undetected.

In other case, vestibular/vulvar pain may be complained of after the very first(s) intercourses: it is defined as *lifelong vestibular/vulvar pain since adolescence*. In these cases it can be a new symptom in a girl otherwise healthy from the general, genital, and vulvar point of view until the symptom was first complained of.

Key Point
When conflicting results are reported, the authors of this book focus on the pathophysiology of vulvar pain and vestibulodynia/vulvodynia to give meaning to those results, with the aim of distilling useful infos for the clinicians in their daily practice first and researchers second.

6.3 Vulvar Pain: The New Entry in Adolescents' Diagnostic Scenario

Why is there such a change in the diagnostic/naming attitude of physicians, who finally call *vulvar pain* the formerly defined "genital pain," or "female genital pain"?

Reasons include, but are not limited to:

- Habit, as the literature tends to be quite conservative in the diagnostic labeling, unless major discussion arises worldwide.
- Different training and diagnostic attitudes between gynecologists, trained to call the vulva with this name, whatever the age of the patient, and pediatricians, trained to generally call the vulva "genital." However, pediatricians correctly call differently the glans, the penis, and the scrotum of little boys, without encompassing them all in the term "genitals," as they do for girls (Casey et al. 2013).
- The tendency to talk about vulvar pain in adolescents and young women in reproductive age, when genital pain is associated with sexual intercourse or early tampon use (Clare and Yeh 2011).
- The *sexual reading of the vulva*, so that the name is (unconsciously?) considered appropriate for the organ *only after puberty*.

6.4 Risk Factors for Vulvar Pain in Adolescence

Risk factors can be clustered under three major headings: *predisposing*, *precipitating, and perpetuating factors*, for the sake of clarity. The goal is to facilitate a more structured learning, hopefully useful in the clinical practice.

In real life risk factors for vulvar pain in adolescence may partly overlap. This is specifically true for the *sexual factor*, a major player in the game of predisposing, precipitating, and perpetuating factors.

The skilled physician should try to make the more comprehensive diagnosis with a careful evaluation of the different factors more relevant in the individual case (Box 6.2).

Box 6.2. The Pain Movie

The diagnosis is a photogram in the movie, i.e., in the film of a disorder or a disease. The skilled clinician should look at the photogram of the vestibular/vulvar pain complaint (or any other pain) with an investigative and pathophysiologically oriented mind. He/she should look for the protagonist(s) of the pain movie, for the co-protagonists, and for the passing-by actors reading carefully (within) the plot. From the medical point of view, predisposing, precipitating, and perpetuating factors/actors should be recognized.

The skilled clinician knows that the photogram of the first diagnosis identifies a critical crossroad. According to the adequacy and quality of the diagnosis and consequent multimodal treatment decisions, the pain movie can continue with different narrative plots, until a:

- *Dramatic end*: a neuropathic persistent devastating pain when it is neglected, banalized, undiagnosed, and untreated
- *Disappointing end*, when the diagnosis is inadequate and/or incomplete and when treatment is minimalistic, partial, short-living, or inappropriately surgically aggressive
- *Very rewarding happy end*, when predisposing, precipitating, and perpetuating factors are diagnosed and treated and when the pharmacologic treatment is successful in addressing the central neuroinflammatory component of the pain process

6.5 Predisposing Factors

6.5.1 Traumas

Unintentional sportive and other types of accidental vulvar traumas may cause vulvar pain in adolescents, similar to what happens during childhood (Smith et al. 2013).

Genitofemoral neuralgia is often the consequence of such traumas, in adolescent and, as well, in adult women (Verstraelen et al. 2015). Pain may be perceived and complained of immediately after the trauma (acute vulvar pain) and then resolved. It may reappear and/or worsen months and years after the primary insult.

Vulvar pain may also be the result of a *pudendal neuralgia of posttraumatic origin*, for example, after a traumatic fall over the coccygis years before the clinical complaint of vulvar pain (Graziottin et al. 2015).

Intentional traumas, such as sexual abuse, are discussed below under the heading of precipitating sexual factors (please see also Chap. 4).

Female genital mutilation/cutting (FMG/C) is a traumatic and potentially devastating cause of vulvar pain when performed during the childhood and, probably even more, after puberty. The many issues involved are discussed in detail in the pertinent chapter (please see the Chap. 5).

Key Point

Vulvar and pelvic traumas should be actively questioned in every adolescent complaining of vulvar pain. The girl should be encouraged to recall childhood traumas, if present, and to ask the mother about this event even at a very small age, particularly when a coccygeal trauma and a pudendal neuralgia appear as potential contributors.

6.5.2 Herpes Virus 1 and 2 (HSV1, HSV2)

Herpes virus type 2 vulvitis is more prevalent than thought. A recent study shows that in Germany HSV-2 prevalence increases from ~3 % in children aged 10–15 years to 7 % among 16–18-year-olds and to 14 % among adults. It causes *acute vulvar pain, itching, and burning*; in a subset of cases, it may cause intermittent recurrent infections (see the excellent review of Sauerbrei 2016).

HSV-1 and HSV-2 may cause peripheral neuropathy. In rare cases this may evolve to chronic neuropathic vulvar pain.

6.5.3 Papillomavirus

The role of papillomavirus-induced vulvar lesions as potential triggers of vulvar pain is still under debate (Graziottin and Serafini 2012).

The most credited reading is that not the HPV infections per se but the outcome of treatments (laser, thermocoagulation, thermic) may be responsible for the subset of vulvar pain complained of after an HPV infection (Graziottin and Serafini 2012).

6.5.4 Vulvar Lichen Sclerosus

Vulvar lichen sclerosus (VLS) is *an autoimmune disease of genital/vulvar and extragenital skin* (Fistarol and Itin 2013). It causes *chronic inflammation* of the vulvar tissue, with progressive full-thickness tissue destruction of the vulvar cytoarchitecture and function. Labia involution, thinning, and clitoral conglutination of the hood may result. It may affect children (please see the clinical case described in Chap. 4) and adolescents, with prevalence increasing with age. The main symptom is vulvar itching, more disturbing and intense at night. *Itching is a subtype of pain.* When people feel itching, MRI indicates that brain pain areas are activated. When people scratch the itching area, brain pain areas are silenced and pleasure/reward mediating areas are activated. Other symptoms include pain, dysuria, and restriction of micturition.

In the long term, if left untreated, VLS causes the full-thickness tissue involution which progresses to involve as well the corpora cavernosa. A progressive reduction of the sexual response may then be complained of, in parallel to the worsening itching, unless appropriate treatment is adequately prescribed in the long term. Treatment includes topical cortisone, topical testosterone (of vegetal origin or propionate), and vitamin E cream. They are usually adequate to control both symptoms and the progression of the disease. VLS deserves periodic clinical monitoring, as 5 % may evolve to vulvar cancer (Fistarol and Itin 2013). The probability is higher in cases with early onset.

When VLS causes progressive stenosis of the vestibular area and of the vaginal entrance, *it may cause severe introital dyspareunia and progressive sexual dysfunction in women* (Fistarol and Itin 2013): this is usually a late complication, but it may be an unexpected contributing factor to introital pain also in young women. Treatment of lichen sclerosus in the adolescence requires a very careful and competent approach (Gurumurthy et al. 2012; Simonetta et al. 2015).

6.5.5 Sexual Factor

The *sexual factor* is a major protagonist in the narrative of vestibular pain in adolescents. It may behave as:

- *Predisposing factor*, when it causes the *first inflammatory trauma* of the vestibular mucosa, which was normal and healthy until that very moment.
- *Precipitating factor*, when it *exacerbates the role of other predisposing factors* such as a hyperactive pelvic floor and/or a recurrent *Candida* vaginitis or of vaginal dryness associated with hypothalamic amenorrhea or hormonal contraceptive use.
- *Perpetuating factor*, when *the adolescent continues to accept the intercourse*, with the consequent repeated mechanical trauma of the introital mucosa, in spite of a worsening pain, for fear of being abandoned, or in the vain hope that insisting on having intercourse will "cure" the problem, or because she is forced to accept intercourse by an abusive partner. A dramatic *iatrogenic component* is in play when some physicians recommend the use of an *anesthetic cream* "to allow the intercourse with less pain." In the short term, this *antitherapeutic suggestion* may seem to reduce pain during intercourse, but it will perpetuate a worsening trauma of the vestibular mucosa. Which physician would recommend the use of an anesthetic to allow the walking on a broken leg? Why should he/she recommend the anesthetic to allow the partner to "use" a wounded, inflamed vestibule and vagina?

The focused listening to adolescents reporting their experiences "in their own words" across many decades of clinical practice leads one of the authors (AG) to identify different pain experiences contributing to different types of vulvar and vestibular pain and to understand why the sexual factor plays a major role in the etiology of vestibular and vulvar pain and associated comorbidities.

Different types of vestibular/vulvar pain will be described in a polarized structured approach for the sake of clarity. In real life intermediate pathophysiologic mechanisms can be in play. This description is aimed at giving clinical meaning to adolescents' wording and to ease the diagnostic and therapeutic work of clinicians who are committed to help their young patients in their daily work.

The scenario of *vulvar pain triggered by sexual intercourse* presents with different leading features:

1. *Acute transient nociceptive vestibular pain and acute introital dyspareunia*
2. *Chronic/intermittent vestibular pain and recurrent introital dyspareunia*
3. *Lifelong (primary) neuropathic vestibular pain and lifelong introital dyspareunia*
4. *Acquired (secondary) vestibular pain and acquired introital dyspareunia, either acute/nociceptive or, later, chronic and then neuropathic*

The descriptions focus first on desired, accepted first experiences, to analyze the biological mechanisms that are in play in the perception of sexually triggered vestibular pain.

Unwanted sex, sexual harassment, and sexual assault may further complicate the vulvar pain scenario according to the adolescent's (or child's!) age, the identity of the perpetrator (relative, acquaintance, or unknown), the severity of the physical trauma and other associated lesions, emotional and psychosexual impact of the sexual trauma, frequency of sexual abuse, the emotional context, quality of family support (or neglect), and quality of medical and psychological support.

Key Point

The precise gentle questioning about the presence of vestibular/vulvar (and/or bladder) pain *during childhood* is a vital part of the medical history. Causes of childhood vulvar pain should be quoted with the adolescent's words. Specific traumatic events, including sexual abuse but also painful diagnostic genital/vulvar maneuvers during childhood (such as suturing of labia's unintentional trauma without analgesia/anesthesia, repeated urethral catheterization for whatever reason, and so on), should be investigated and recorded. In the author's (AG) experience, in 5.3% of later vulvar pain, the only recalled childhood trauma was linked to medical invasive exams, such as urethroscopy, tampon swab, vaginal swab, "urethral dilatation," suturing of unintentional traumas without analgesia, and so on.

The four different types of *vulvar pain triggered by sexual intercourse* will be briefly discussed, trying to identify critical passages and pathophysiologically relevant events contributing to the shift from acute to chronic to neuropathic pain.

6.5.5.1 Acute Transient Nociceptive Vestibular Pain and Acute Introital Dyspareunia

Almost every adolescent girl can experience *short-living*, *transient acute vestibular pain and introital dyspareunia* of variable intensity, from very mild/negligible to severe, at first desired sexual intercourse or a few more, when the *hymen is broken* during the first penetration(s).

This pain is triggered by *hymenal sexual abrasions/lacerations/lesions*; it has a "*microtraumatic*" *etiology*; it is "*nociceptive*," i.e., it indicates a tissue damage that should be repaired by the physiologic inflammatory process. It indicates therefore the presence of a transient hymenal mucosal damage that normally will be rapidly repaired by *an inflammatory process of limited intensity and duration*, finalized to restore the normal anatomic and physiologic conditions ("resolving inflammation") (Fig. 6.1).

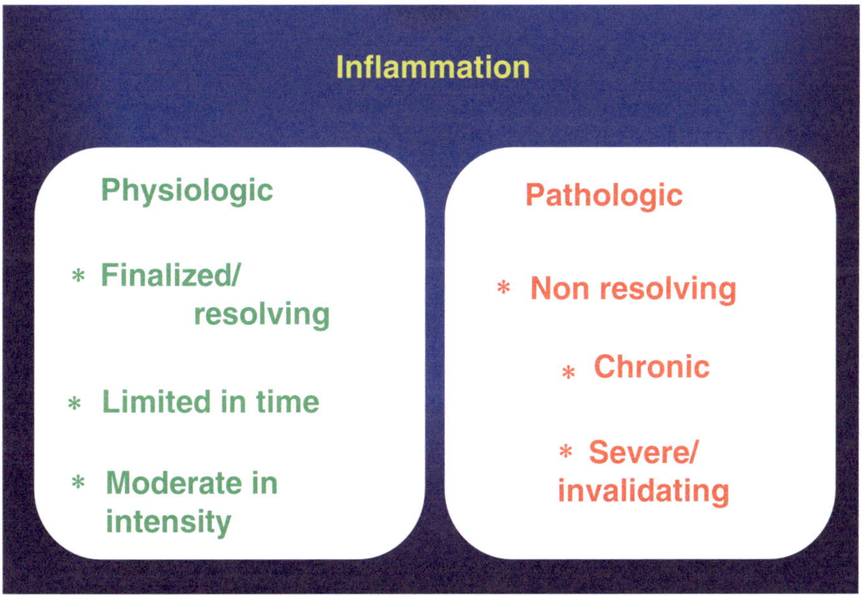

Fig. 6.1 Inflammation's key features are summarized here. The figure highlights the fact that inflammation is a physiologic process necessary to maintain health when it is "resolving," i.e., when it is *finalized* to restore the normal cytoarchitecture and function of a tissue, after an infection or a trauma. Typical examples of physiologic, periodic inflammation include ovulation, menstruation, or delivery, just to mention three typical events in women's health. When inflammation is physiologic, it is also, by definition, of *limited duration*, sufficient to restore the normal tissue well-being, and of *limited intensity. Inflammation* becomes progressively *pathologic* when it is *non-resolving* and *chronic* and when it becomes more and more *severe and invalidating* (Graziottin 2015b)

Vestibular pain can be *repeated and more prolonged* when a tightened, fibrous, rigid hymen is present. After a few more attempts, if there are no other cofactors, if the desire and arousal of the girl remain intense, and if the sense of intimacy and love is emotionally rewarding, then the hymen is gradually dilated and a normal, painless intercourse can be finally enjoyed.

6.5.5.2 Chronic/Intermittent Vestibular Pain and Recurrent Introital Dyspareunia

Vestibular pain triggered by sexual intercourse *persists beyond 36 months* when:

- The *hymen is cribrous, or very thick.*
- A *hyperactive pelvic floor is present.*
- *Fear of pain (up to a frank vaginismus) blocks the genital arousal*, leading to vaginal dryness, and further triggers a defensive contraction of the levator ani.
- *Sexual pain (introital dyspareunia) inhibits sexual desire* and *central and peripheral arousal* (Graziottin 2015a).

Penetration can therefore become extremely painful or impossible. If the partner insists in his attempts, an *inflammatory* repeated *trauma* of variable intensity, *of the vestibular area, and of the external part of the hymen is in play.* Mast cells are a critical factor in the activation and persistence of inflammation progressively moving from the genitals to the brain (Graziottin et al. 2013, 2014; Skaper et al. 2014).

This *vestibular/hymenal inflammation* can:

- Finally *resolve* ("*resolving inflammation*," a physiologic process), when the penetration is accomplished, the girl manages to relax the pelvic floor, and the residual hymenal remnants gradually heal with a nonpainful residual scar
- Be maintained and become a "*chronic vestibular inflammation*" of the vestibular area, with *continuous or intermittent sexual pain at intercourse*

Vaginismus with myogenic hyperactivity of the levator ani may be so biologically driven to require pharmacologic treatment with botulinum toxin. Otherwise it will perpetuate as persistent predisposing factor to introital trauma and chronic vestibular inflammation. A botulinum toxin treatment (Bertolasi et al. 2009) may be necessary both in primary and secondary vaginismus when the myogenic component is nonresponsive to conventional psycho-behavioral and physiotherapic treatments. Central components of vaginismus should be assessed as well (Frasson et al. 2009).

6.5.5.3 Lifelong (Primary) Neuropathic Vestibular Pain and Lifelong Introital Dyspareunia

When the microtraumatic abrasions of the introital mucosa are repeated, *the inflammatory process further changes its characteristics within the vestibular mucosa*:

- From "resolving," finalized at restoring the normal cytoarchitecture and integrity of the vestibular mucosa, with a limited duration and intensity, the inflammatory process gradually shifts into a *lifelong vulvar vestibulitis since adolescence.*

- *Mast cell involvement* (Graziottin 2009; Graziottin et al. 2013, 2014) significantly increases, with increased production and release within the vestibular mucosa of many cytokines, of *nerve growth factor (NGF), and of other neurotrophins*. Local proliferation of nerve pain fibers is the histologic correlate of the *hyperalgesia*, i.e., the amplification of the intensity of the stimulus perceived by the woman. Mast cells produce as well tryptase and heparanase, lytic enzymes responsible for the creation of tunnels across the basal membrane.
- Pain fibers penetrate along these microscopic tunnels and superficialize across the cells of the vestibular mucosa. This process is responsible for another typical pain feature: *pain perception shifts from a tactile stimulus into "burning pain,"* "as if I were burned with a hot iron," as many young women frequently say to the listening physician. This shifting is defined as *allodynia* and is typically found when the physician gently touches ("tactile stimulus") at 5 and 7 o'clock of the vestibular introitus, looking at it as a clock face, and the woman perceives a burning pain. The tactile stimulus is then "read" by the brain as a painful one.
- *Lifelong "provoked vestibulodynia"* is the current definition of this specific pain experience that is the leading etiology of *lifelong introital dyspareunia, i.e., persistently painful intercourse* in adolescents.
- The very same type of *vestibular burning pain* is experienced *during and after intercourse.*
- *Pelvic symptoms and comorbidities* are increasingly reported, when the vestibular *inflammation mechanically induced* by the intercourse persists and is reactivated at every penetration. The inflammatory process tends to involve the neighboring organs, the *urethra and the bladder* first. This involvement is more likely when a hyperactive pelvic floor, either lifelong and/or acquired in response to pain, is in play (Graziottin 2014, 2015a; Graziottin and Gambini 2015; Graziottin et al. 2016).
- *Recurrent cystitis* and *provoked vestibulodynia* are reported by 60% of women when accurately investigated (Salonia et al. 2013). Postcoital cystitis, usually complained of 24–72 h after intercourse, and *a pain bladder syndrome* (Peters et al. 2007) are frequently reported in the natural history of *lifelong vulvar vestibulitis/provoked vestibulodynia and introital dyspareunia since adolescence.*

Neuroinflammation becomes a prominent feature when the inflammatory process becomes non-resolving, i.e., unable to restore the return to normal anatomic and physiologic conditions, either because the precipitating traumatic factor (intercourse) is repeated or because other contributing factors (see below) remain undiagnosed/unaddressed (Xanthos et al. 2011; Walker et al. 2013; Ru-Rong et al. 2014; Xanthos and Sandkühler 2014).

When the *hyperactivated mast cells* keep on producing and releasing in the tissue inflammatory molecules such as cytokines, tumor necrosis factor alpha, and others, a progressive *neuroinflammation* takes place. Neuroinflammation is characterized by infiltration of immune cells, activation of glial cells, and production of inflammatory mediators in the peripheral and central nervous system (Ru-Rong et al. 2014). It has an important role in the induction and maintenance of chronic pain.

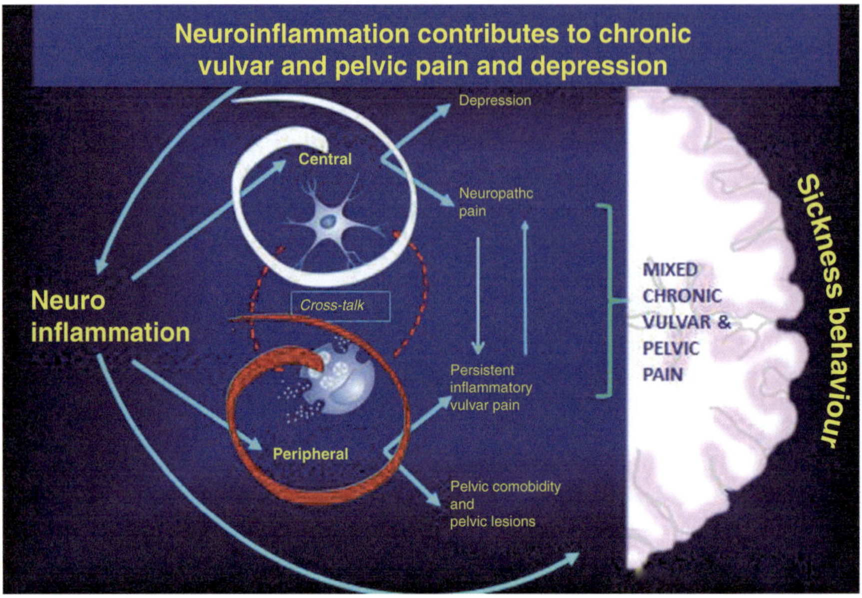

Fig. 6.2 Neuroinflammation is characterized by infiltration of immune cells, activation of glial cells, and production of inflammatory mediators in the peripheral and central nervous system. It has an important role in the induction and maintenance of chronic pain. Specifically, it contributes to the *neurogenic* maintenance of chronic vulvar and pelvic pain, to maladaptive sickness behavior and depression, to central sensitization, and to the progressive shift of pain from nociceptive to chronic and neuropathic, a real disease of the pain system per se (Graziottin 2014)

Inflammatory molecules can either pass across the brain barrier and/or be produced within the brain by the hyperactivated microglia (Xanthos et al. 2011; Walker et al. 2013; Ru-Rong et al. 2014; Xanthos and Sandkühler 2014).

When *neuroinflammation becomes chronic and prominent*, *pain* gradually shifts from *nociceptive*, a "friendly" pain signal, to *neuropathic*, *i.e.*, *a disease of the pain system* per se. The *brain takes the lead* in the inflammatory process with four major interacting and reciprocally potentiating consequences (Fig. 6.2):

- *A neurogenic peripheral inflammation*, when nerve fibers can trigger mast cell degranulation in the vestibular (or bladder) tissue
- *A neurogenic neuroinflammation*, when the inflammation is maintained *within the brain* by the hyperactivated glial cells
- *A central sensitization*, with a progressive lowering of the pain threshold
- *Depression caused by neuroinflammation*, besides psychosexual factors

Mood changes, a maladaptive sickness behavior, and depression may be multifactorial and stem from:

- Progressive neuroinflammation (Xanthos et al. 2011; Walker et al. 2013; Graziottin et al. 2013, 2014, 2016)

- The persistent frustrating experience of coital pain, with many consequences for the couple dynamics
- The "mysterious" invalidating vestibular burning pain, causing anxiety and further coping difficulties

Menstrual flares of vestibular pain further worsen pain perception. Menstrual worsening is reported by the subset of adolescents more sensible to the degranulating effect that the menstrual fall of estradiol and progesterone may have on the mast cells and, likely, on the microglia. Shortening the menstrual period (Graziottin 2015b), or reducing the number of periods per year, can etiologically reduce this contributing factor to vestibular pain.

This pathophysiologic reading of the narrative of vulvar/vestibular pain distilled from women's wording is substantiated by scientific evidence. The sexual factor is indeed of special relevance in adolescents. An interesting survey on women affected with *bladder pain syndrome/interstitial cystitis* (BPS/IC) and controls (Peters et al. 2007) will indicate that affected women are significantly more likely to have suffered from *lifelong vaginismus*, *lifelong fear of pain at intercourse,* and *lifelong introital dyspareunia* than controls.

This supports the hypothesis that a *lifelong hyperactive pelvic floor*, associated with vaginismus and/or lifelong dyspareunia, can be a *"biomechanical" predisposing factor to recurrent postcoital cystitis* (which are complained of 24–72 h after intercourse), contributing to a *bladder pain syndrome* and *comorbidity with vestibular pain*, in line with the pathophysiologic reading of vestibular and bladder comorbidities described above (Graziottin 2014, 2015a; Graziottin and Gambini 2015; Graziottin et al. 2016; Xanthos and Sandkühler 2014).

When unaddressed, the persistent bladder inflammation caused by the intercourse and associated pathogenic biofilms of *Escherichia coli* (or other pathogens) contributes to BPS (Graziottin 2014; Graziottin and Zanello 2015). If unaddressed, it can become as well a perpetuating factor for both the bladder and vestibular symptoms. This contributes to maintain the pelvic chronic inflammation while increasing the neuroinflammation and the shifting of pain from nociceptive to neuropathic, a real disease per se (Xanthos et al. 2011; Walker et al. 2013; Graziottin et al. 2013, 2014; Graziottin 2015a).

Low desire, inadequate central and peripheral arousal with vaginal dryness reduces both the vaginal lubrication and the congestion of the vessel and cavernosal body around the lower third of the urethra (equivalent to part of the male corpus spongiosum), thus depriving the urethra of a vasocongestive "airbag" against the potential trauma of the intercourse. The traumatic potential is higher if the entrance of the vagina is reduced by the contraction of the surrounding elevator ani muscle, contributing to introital dyspareunia and PVD. In a series of 60 women with r-UTIs, Salonia et al. (2013) recently proved that secondary/acquired PVD was reported by 36 (60%) out of the 60 patients. Women with PVD had a higher prevalence of UTIs over the last 12 months (χ^2, 4.54; $p=0.03$) and more frequently suffered from UPEC-related r-UTIs (χ^2, 5.92; $p=0.01$) compared to those without PVD. Moreover, women with PVD showed significantly lower scores for the Female Sexual Function Index domains (all

$p \leq 0.01$) as compared with PVD negative individuals. Uropathogenic EC-related r-UTIs (OR, 3.1; $p=0.01$), a number of UTIs ≥6 (OR, 2.8; $p=0.01$) over the last 12 months, and having being treated with ≥3 antibiotics throughout the same period (OR, 2.1; $p=0.04$) emerged as independent predictors of PVD (Salonia et al. 2013).

Sexual factors can contribute in parallel to both r-UTI and PVD, as common denominators of the tissue's traumas activating a chronic process of local inflammation, with specific characteristics according to the organ tissue (vulvar vestibule or urethra/bladder) involved.

When vestibular pain turns into the characteristics of *provoked vestibulodynia*, interesting changes are in play also from the histologic point of view between lifelong (*primary*) *provoked vestibulodynia and* acquired (*secondary*) *provoked vestibulodynia*. Primary and secondary vestibulodynia may have distinct histopathologic pathways. Both subtypes show increased chronic inflammation with *mast cell recruitment*. However, primary type presents with significant *neural hypertrophy and hyperplasia*.

6.5.5.4 Acquired (Secondary) Vestibular Pain and Acquired Introital Dyspareunia, Either Acute/Nociceptive or, Later, Chronic and Then Neuropathic

Adolescents may experience months and years of serene, painless, joyful sexual activity. Then something suddenly or progressively changes the sexual experience for the worse.

Precipitating infectious diseases, causing *recurrent vaginitis and cystitis*, may induce vulvar/vestibular pain of different severity and duration.

Contributing factors include:

- An *hyperactive pelvic floor* triggered or further stimulated by the recurrent inflammation and pain induced by recurrent vulvovaginal and/or bladder inflammation
- A *metabolic factor*, when an excessive sugar intake, an inadequate peripheral use of insulin, and/or diabetes increases glycemia and the vulnerability to recurrent vulvovaginal and bladder infections
- *Hormonal factors*, such as hypothalamic amenorrhea, and the use of hormonal contraception

6.5.6 Recurrent Vaginitis

Candida infections: this microorganism is leading the infectious etiology of *acquired vestibular and vulvar pain* (Graziottin and Murina 2011; Murina et al. 2011; Farmer et al. 2011; Reed et al. 2014). More than 70 % of vulvodynia patients report the occurrence of prior chronic *Candida* infections, which is accompanied by localized inflammation fibroblast-mediated and fibroblast-elevated production of proinflammatory/pain-associated interleukin 6 (IL-6) and prostaglandin E2 (PGE2), with a higher activation of fibroblasts (Falsetta et al. 2015).

The classic *acute Candida vaginitis* causes acute, short-living vulvar pain, characterized by reddening and swelling of the vulvar skin and vestibular mucosa, increasing local temperature, burning pain, itching, and acute introital pain at attempts of intercourse. The symptoms are limited to the duration of the acute inflammatory phase: this is a typical example of "resolving" inflammation, finalized at restoring the tissue integrity and function, therefore with a physiologic reparative inflammatory process of limited intensity and limited duration.

In *recurrent Candida*, when the infection is repeated, the pathophysiology of the tissue response does change dramatically over time. The *inflammation* gradually becomes "*non-resolving*" and *chronic*, somehow no more finalized to restore the mucosal tissue's integrity. When intercourse happens in conditions of hyperactive, tightened pelvic floor and/or with poor/absent lubrication and/or when the penis diameter is above the norm, it may cause microabrasions of the delicate introital mucosa. Mast cells and other defense cells get in contact with the *Candida* antigens, even when the number of this normal component of the vaginal microbiota is within or slightly above the normal (Graziottin and Zanello 2015; Jayaram et al. 2014).

In subjects with an allergic genetic background, this dangerous meeting may lead to a disregulated immune response with hyperergic local reactions (Graziottin and Murina 2011).

Histologic findings with immunostaining of the vestibular mucosa support this reading, showing the triad typical of an upregulated inflammatory response in the bioptic specimen:

1. Significant increase of mast cells
2. Significant increase of degranulated mast cells
3. Significant increase of mast cells in close proximity with pain nerve fibers (Graziottin et al. 2013, 2014; Chatterjea and Martinov 2015)

Correctly Chatterjea and Martinov define mast cells as "the versatile gatekeeper of pain." This and other studies strongly support the role of inflammation in the first pathophysiologic steps of vestibulodynia. The wording "vulvar vestibulitis" maintains its appropriate descriptive values, as these authors have always supported. The vestibular inflammation is certainly the first step of a "biochemical fire" causing genital pain and progressive brain involvement, with neuroinflammation.

Symptoms gradually shift to an increasingly severe burning pain of the vestibular mucosa. *Acquired provoked vestibular burning pain* is elicited at the contact with the examining gloved finger and/or with a swab, mimicking the type of pain the woman perceives at and, above all, after intercourse. When the inflammation induced by the immuno-hyperergic reaction to the *Candida* antigen persists inadequately diagnosed and treated, *the acquired burning pain becomes intermittent or continuous* and independent from the precipitating triggering factor of the intercourse.

A progressive involvement of the brain is in play, with *neuroinflammation* contributing to sickness behavior and depression (Graziottin et al. 2013, 2014; Xanthos et al. 2011; Walker et al. 2013). Further steps of this perverted, pathologic inflammatory shift mirror what has been described for the lifelong vestibular pain:

1. The "*neurogenic peripheral inflammation*" contributes to maintain the inflammation in the peripheral tissues.
2. The "*neurogenic neuroinflammation*" maintains it within the brain.

3. This will induce acquired *central sensitization*, with reduced central pain threshold.
4. Neuroinflammation will as well contribute to *maladaptive sickness behavior and depression*.

The final *pathophysiology leading to "vestibulodynia/vulvodynia" is completed.* The relationship between repeated *Candida* vaginitis and VVS/PVD has been proven in an animal model (Farmer et al. 2011).

6.5.7 Immunoallergic Factors

Clinical histories of adolescents strongly support the increased vulnerability to vestibular pain and vulvodynia stemming in the form of *allergic-hyperergic reactions* to acute *Candida* infections in women with *self-reported allergies*.

Harlow et al. (2009) showed that the association indeed increases the risk. Women with *self-reported hives* prior to first report of vulvar pain were *2.5 times more likely to develop vulvodynia* (95 % CI 1.7–4.4). Those reporting a history of allergic reactions to insect bites were 2.1 times more likely (95 % CI 1.1–4.0), and those reporting a history *of seasonal allergies were 2.0 times* (95 % CI 1.3–3.2) *more likely to develop vulvodynia*. Findings were similar in a restricted subset of clinically confirmed cases and matched controls.

6.5.8 Repeated Antibiotics

Candida infections are often triggered by *antibiotic courses* for whatever reason. In women, antibiotics used to treat cystitis devastate the intestinal and vaginal microbiota (Graziottin 2014; Graziottin and Zanello 2015).

Together with a hyperactive pelvic floor, they constitute the leading etiology of the comorbidity between recurrent cystitis and vulvar vestibulitis/provoked vestibulodynia (VVS/PVD) that can be as high as 60 % (Salonia et al. 2013). Listening carefully to *women's wording* increases the ability to recognize *critical factors predisposing, precipitating, and maintaining recurrences of VVS/PVD and/or r-UTIs* and specifically of postcoital cystitis so frequent in the clinical history of women with VVS/PVD. To understand the shared pathophysiology behind this frequent comorbidity is useful in planning a strategic and effective treatment.

Key Point

The precise questioning about former antibiotic treatment(s) is mandatory in women complaining of recurrent *Candida* infections and should be carefully reported in the clinical record. A pharmacologic treatment of intestinal *Candida* is part of an effective treatment of VVS/PVD (please see Chap. 11).

6.5.9 The Recurrent Bladder Factor: Cystitis

The bladder factor: the urothelium is coated by glycosaminoglycans (GAGs) and proteoglycans. This functional a-cellular layer, referred to as "bladder coating," is the first line of defense at the bladder's luminal surface (Anand et al. 2012). It ensures the impermeability of the bladder surface to urine's ions and bacteria, neutralizes toxic compounds, inhibits the passage of small molecules, and inhibits the adhesion of UPEC and the formation of microcrystals. A defective bladder coating may lead to the passage of urine's constituents and bacteria across the urothelial barriers, till it reaches the interstitial space.

Mast cell activation and its consequent proinflammatory cascade of events may follow to bladder's barrier violation (Graziottin 2009; Graziottin et al. 2013, 2014). A *mast cell-mediated neurogenic inflammation, both peripheral and central*, can give rise to *neurogenic pain*, as it happens in the bladder pain/painful bladder syndrome and in the interstitial cystitis. The GAG layer is dynamically altered during the course of UTI. This bladder originated inflammation and pain may contribute to increase the flow of the systemic "*river of pain*," thus worsening pain perception in both the bladder and the vestibular area.

The urethral factor: the urethral mucosal, submucosal, and muscular layers should ensure a good "sealing effect" of the urethral lumen, thus preventing ascending infections during intercourse. This protective mechanism is partially estrogen and partially androgen dependent and may become defective in prolonged acquired amenorrhea of the adolescent. The amenorrhea may be caused by binge eating disorders, acute/chronic physical or emotional stress, or breastfeeding.

Key Point
Comorbidity between vestibular/vulvar pain and bladder symptoms is frequent (up to 60 % of cases). It should be actively investigated with appropriate listening and questioning. When comorbidity is present, common predisposing, precipitating, and maintaining factors should be investigated and addressed.

6.5.10 The Pelvic Floor Factor

Pelvic floor muscles:

- *Are critical "biomechanical" factors* in the etiology of traumatic inflammation of the vulvar vestibule and/or of the urethral tissues.
- Can be *lifelong hyperactive*: typical childhood symptoms include lifelong obstructive constipation and/or urgency and frequency.
- May as well *react to tissue inflammation* becoming dysfunctional and tense. The either lifelong or acquired hyperactive elevator ani contributes to the mechanical trauma of the urethra when intercourse is accepted without adequate lubrication and genital congestion. The latter is associated with inadequate congestion of the

periurethral equivalent of the male corpus spongiosum of the urethra, with loss of its "airbag-like" protective role vs. the intercourse-induced mechanical trauma of the urethra (Graziottin 2014, 2015a; Graziottin and Gambini 2015; Graziottin et al. 2016).

A defensive hyperactive pelvic floor is in play also when *fear of intercourse* is prominent, as is typically seen in women affected by *vaginismus*. Recurrent cystitis and dyspareunia since adolescence are significantly associated with bladder pain syndrome and interstitial cystitis (Peters et al. 2007; Graziottin 2006, 2015a).

Last but not least, the risk of pelvic floor dysfunction, with dyspareunia and bladder symptoms, doubles (OR = 2.4) after sexual abuse (Postma et al. 2013).

Key Point

A hyperactive pelvic floor, either lifelong or acquired, is a frequent predisposing factor to vestibular/vulvar pain and introital dyspareunia. This powerful contributor must be investigated, diagnosed when present, and accurately treated.

6.5.11 The Metabolic Factor

Adolescents with type 1 diabetes have an increased risk of recurrent *Candida* vaginitis and UPEC cystitis. On a general note, *insulin-treated diabetes* is a powerful predisposing factor for r-UTIs (with OR ranging from 2.0 to 3.4, across different studies) (Donders 2002; Jackson et al. 2004; Gorter et al. 2010). Relapses and reinfections were reported in 7.1 and 15.9 % of women with diabetes versus 2.0 and 4.1 % of women without diabetes. There was an independent higher risk of recurrent UTI in women with diabetes compared with women without diabetes (OR 2.0; 95 % CI 1.4–2.9). Women taking oral blood glucose-lowering medication (OR 2.1; 95 % CI 1.2–3.5) or insulin (OR 3.0; 95 % CI 1.7–5.1), or who had had diabetes for ≥5 years (OR 2.9; 95 % CI 1.9–4.4), or who had retinopathy (OR 4.1; 95 % CI 1.9–9.1), were at risk of recurrent UTI (Gorter et al. 2010).

More recent researches confirm that obesity and diabetes increase the risk of r-UTIs (Saliba et al. 2012) and that women with r-UTIs have a cluster of risk factors, diabetes first (Yoon et al. 2013). Authors' clinical experience indicates that family history of diabetes increases the vulnerability to recurrent vaginitis and cystitis also in adolescents, more so if their diet is rich in sugars such as glucose, long before the woman develops diabetes herself. Overweight/obesity further contributes to worsen this important – and underevaluated – predisposing factor.

6.5.12 The Hormonal Factor

In adolescents two leading hormonal factors may contribute to vestibular/vulvar pain, with a controversial evidence:

1. *Hypothalamic amenorrhea*
2. *Oral contraceptives (OC)/hormonal contraception (HC), in selected cases*

Estrogens maintain the lactobacilli-dominated healthy vaginal ecosystem and a low vaginal pH. Recent data suggest that in the fertile age, female genital tract secretions are bactericidal for *Escherichia coli* ex vivo. The bactericidal activity and concentration of immune mediators in cervicovaginal lavage (CVL) reduced the number of *E. coli* colonies by 68 %. CVL were active against laboratory and clinical isolates of *E. coli*, but were inactive against *Lactobacillus* species (Kalyoussef et al. 2012). The role of vaginal ecosystem, estrogen dependent, further supports the preventing role of estrogens in the strategy of maintenance of a better vulvovaginal trophism, vaginal ecosystem and protective microbiota, and vaginal low pH, contributing to prevent vestibular pain at intercourse and r-UTIs.

6.5.12.1 Hypothalamic Amenorrhea

Acquired persistent hypothalamic amenorrhea may predispose to *acquired VVS/PVD* through vaginal hypoestrogenism, with the associated changes in the vaginal microbiota, loss of lactobacilli, and increase of pathogenic biofilms with enterobacteria (Graziottin and Zanello 2015), increased vaginal dryness, and genital arousal difficulties.

A hyperactive pelvic floor is often copresent. This facilitates the microabrasions of the vestibular mucosa during intercourse and contributes to *acquired introital dyspareunia*.

6.5.12.2 Oral Contraceptives

OCs (but hormonal contraception, HC, would be more appropriate if contraceptive patches and rings, or even implants or IUD, are included) are credited to contribute to increased vulnerability to VVS/PVD with a number of mechanisms:

- *Reduced sexual desire and reduced arousability* because of the reduction of ovarian production of testosterone associated with HC; this sexual consequence is complained of by about 20–26 % of women on HC.
- *Vaginal dryness*, due to relative vaginal hypoestrogenism induced by some pills and/or reduced vaginal response to the low estrogenic levels of pills containing 15 or 20 mcg of ethinyl estradiol.
- *Changes in vaginal microbiota*, with increased pathogenic biofilms (Graziottin and Zanello 2015).
- *Increased vulnerability to Candida vaginitis.*
- *Acquired introital dyspareunia.*

Harlow et al. (2008) conducted a population-based study of 177 women experiencing vulvar pain consistent with clinical criteria for vulvodynia and community-matched controls. Analyses were repeated and validated in clinically confirmed clinic-based and population-based cases and matched controls. In their analyses of population-based cases and controls, oral contraceptive use was associated with a nonsignificant, 30 % increase in the risk of vulvodynia (95 % CI 0.7–2.3) and was highest among women whose first use occurred before age 18 (OR = 2.5, 95 % CI 1.1–5.8). These findings were similar when restricted to clinically confirmed cases (Harlow et al. 2008). He showed that women who use HC are significantly more likely to have a hyperactive pelvic floor and significantly more difficulties in tampon use than controls. This suggests that probably HC acts as precipitating cofactor of a stronger predisposing factor such as the hyperactive pelvic floor.

Reed et al. (2013) did not find as well that OCs increase the risk of vulvodynia.

The author's (AG) clinical experience suggests that adolescents who choose hormonal contraception *before* the first intercourse are particularly motivated to self-control and self-protection, that is, very good, but are more likely to have a hyperactive pelvic floor, a lower genital arousability, and a higher vulnerability to vestibular pain and introital dyspareunia.

However, no specific studies have been carried out so far on the psychosexual attitude of young women who ask for contraception before having the first intercourse, in the author's knowledge.

Key Point
Hormonal factors should be explored, carefully evaluated, and treated. This does not imply necessarily to give up the HC but to diagnose concomitant factors (such as a hyperactive pelvic floor) to address it.

6.5.13 The Vaginal pH and Ecosystem

Estrogens are essential in maintaining the normal vaginal ecosystem, with the prominent lactobacilli, which is mirrored by a vaginal pH of 4.0–4.5. A vaginal pH of 5 or more is associated with bacterial vaginosis, vaginitis, and cystitis.

Key Point
The vaginal pH should be always evaluated and recorded. It immediately gives a comprehensive evidence of:

- Levels of vaginal estrogenization, even during hormonal contraception
- Prominent microorganisms living in the vaginal microbiota
- The likely presence of pathogens and pathogenic biofilms

Normalizing vaginal pH is part of a comprehensive treatment of factors predisposing to vestibular pain.

6.5.14 The Intestinal Factor

The *gut* is the most important immunitary organ of the human body.

The *intestinal microbiota* may be dramatically altered by gastroenteritis, antibiotic treatments, celiac disease, food allergies, and intolerances, such as gluten sensitivity or lactose intolerance. This may lead to the overgrowth of enterobacteria, the causative agents of the majority of r-UTIs, of which UPEC is the most frequently involved, and pathogenic vaginal biofilms and to comorbidity with VVS/PVD (Graziottin and Zanello 2015).

The *irritable bowel syndrome* (IBS) with the associated hyperactive mast cells in the intestinal mucosa and the increased passage ("translocation") of intestinal germs through the intestinal cells (barrier violation) is a key predisposing factor to r-UTIs (Donskey 2004; Stanghellini et al. 2010; Rescigno 2011). It is frequently comorbid with VVS/PVD.

Obstructive constipation, often associated with a hyperactive pelvic floor, is another contributing factor to vestibular pain.

Key Point

The gut can be a powerful and yet inadequately evaluated contributor of VVS/PVD and r-UTI. When symptoms suggestive of gut disorders are present, their treatment should be included in collaboration with a skilled gastroenterologist.

6.5.15 The Diet Factor

A diet rich in sugar (glucose) and yeast-containing food may alter the intestinal microbiota, contribute to the overgrowth of *Candida* and pathogenic biofilm, and increase the vulnerability to irritable bowel syndrome (IBS) and to recurrent *Candida* vaginitis.

Gluten sensitivity may further contribute to IBS and the leaky gut syndrome, say the increased gut's vulnerability to the passage of allergens and pathogens in the blood and increased vulnerability to recurrent vaginitis and cystitis, predisposing factors to VVS/PVD.

Alcohol use, with its high sugar and yeast content, is to be firmly discouraged in adolescents, both for its negative direct and indirect effect on the intestinal microbiota and its neurotoxic effect, definitely stronger on the adolescent brain.

Iron deficiency anemia (*IDA*) is highly prevalent in women worldwide (30–50 % of women are affected). Low iron increases the sensitivity to pain by lowering the central threshold, almost doubles the vulnerability to depression, and significantly increases fatigue. Diagnosing the etiology of IDA (low iron intake with the diet, increase gastrointestinal or menstrual losses, reduced intestinal absorption, increased need, such as in adolescence and pregnancy), and curing it, is still an underappreciated contributor to improving the coping ability of the young woman and the likelihood of a successful treatment outcome of VVS/PVD. Shortening the duration and the intensity of the menstrual bleeding, while using a pill which offers continuous/constant plasmatic levels of estradiol, improves IDA and reduces the degranulation of mast cells, with consequent dramatic reduction of the menstrual flares of vestibular pain (Graziottin 2015b).

6.5.16 The Physical Exercise Factor

Inadequate/absent physical exercise may:

- *Predispose to overweight/obesity*, contributing to a progressively elevated production of inflammatory cytokine with increasing weight. They contribute to increase the systemic "river of inflammation" increasing the vulnerability to neuroinflammation, central sensitization, and depression.
- *Reduce the peripheral use of insulin*, contributing to increase the plasmatic levels of glucose, with increased vulnerability to pathogenic biofilms, recurrent vaginal *Candida* infections, r-UTI, and VVS/PVD.
- *Reduce the ability to express the negative emotions* through the relieving pathway of the physical exercise. This translates into a higher vulnerability to anxiety and depression and reduced ability to cope with vestibular pain and to be adherent to the treatment plan.

6.5.17 The Sleep Factor

Chronic sleep shortage, so frequent among adolescents, is a powerful biological stressful factor as it activates the *corticotrophin-releasing pathway* (CRP). This translates into increased vulnerability to depression, anxiety, irritability, catastrophism, and loss of sexual desire and reduced ability to cope with the distressing challenge of vestibular and vulvar pain. It increases as well neuroinflammation, thus contributing to the neurogenic neuroinflammation and peripheral inflammation, with neurogenically induced increased degranulation of mast cells in the inflamed tissue and reduction of the central threshold of pain.

Reduced quality of sleep is reported as a significant contributor of vulvodynia in Reed et al.'s survey (2014). The reduced quality could be either a predisposing factor or a consequence of neuroinflammation, sickness behavior, depression, and anxiety.

Ideally every adolescent should sleep *8 h per night*, i.e., 1 h sleep for 2 h of wake.

Key Point
Attention to lifestyles, and recommendation to adhere to a more healthy lifestyle profile, is one of the most critical and neglected factors of reducing direct and indirect predisposing contributors to VVS/PVD.

6.5.18 Psychosocial and Contextual Factors

Psychosocial factors may predispose to *vestibular/vulvar pain* with multiple mechanisms (Bergeron et al. 2014; Graziottin et al. 2016):

- *Restrictive/repressive education on sexuality*, more present in young women suffering of vaginismus and/or lifelong dyspareunia

- *Passive models*, poor self-esteem, low assertiveness reducing the ability to say "no," or "please stop" to sexual intercourse when introital dyspareunia is experienced
- *Catastrophism* as a leading coping attitude
- *Emotional neglect/physical abuse* activating depression and/or a posttraumatic stress disorder
- *Physical and emotional distress*

Depression and posttraumatic stress disorder may specifically affect the pain experience of women with vulvodynia (Iglesias-Rios et al. 2015). According to her study, women who screened positive for depression had a 53 % higher prevalence of having vulvodynia (PR = 1.53; 95 % CI: 1.12, 2.10) compared with women who screened negative for depression. Women who screened positive for PTSD had more than a twofold increase in the prevalence of having vulvodynia (PR = 2.37; 95 % CI: 1.07, 5.25) compared with women who screened negative for PTSD. The increased prevalence of vulvodynia among those screening positive for depression or PTSD suggests that these disorders may contribute to the likelihood of reporting vulvodynia. Alternatively, and very likely, the neuroinflammation caused by vulvodynia may contribute to depression. PTSD may stem from previous or current contextual negative factors and further contribute to neuroinflammation. Therefore, they could have a common pathophysiological and risk profile (Iglesias-Rios et al. 2015).

Key Point
Psychosocial factors should be investigated. Psychosexual support/therapy may prove extremely useful for a subset of women where psychosocial factors are leading contributors. It should be considered carefully in the treatment plan.

6.6 Precipitating Factors

Intercourse may precipitate:

- *VVS/PVD*, more likely so when one or more predisposing factors such as a hyperactive pelvic floor, vaginal dryness, and/or a *Candida* vaginitis are already in play. A comprehensive evaluation of all the potentially interacting factors should be carefully carried out.
- *R-UTI*, highly comorbid with VVS/PVD (Salonia et al. 2013). On average, 60 % of r-UTIs are postcoital. The risk of symptomatic UTI has a three- to fourfold increase on the second day after sexual intercourse. In multivariate analysis, frequency of sexual intercourse is the strongest risk factor for recurrence (Sen 2008). This vulnerability increases in women reporting introital dyspareunia, either lifelong (Peters et al. 2007) or acquired (Graziottin and Murina 2011; Gardella et al. 2011; Salonia et al. 2013).

Antibiotic courses may precipitate a *Candida* vaginitis a few days after an antibiotic course.

Acute stress may precipitate or worsen VVS/PVD through a neurogenic peripheral inflammation when a neuropathic vulvar pain is already in play.

6.7 Perpetuating Factors

Sexual intercourse maintained in spite of the vestibular inflammation and introital pain: often the adolescent continues to accept the intercourse, with the consequent repeated mechanical trauma of the introital mucosa, in spite of a worsening pain, for fear of being abandoned, or in the vain hope that insisting on having intercourse will "cure" the problem, or because she is forced to accept intercourse by an abusive partner, as mentioned above.

A dramatic *iatrogenic component* is in play when some physicians recommend the use of an *anesthetic cream* "to allow the intercourse with less pain." In the short term, this *antitherapeutic* suggestion may seem to reduce pain during intercourse, but it will perpetuate a worsening trauma of the vestibular mucosa.

The *diagnostic omission* of the complex pathophysiology of VVS/PVD is the most important predictor of further recurrences.

Inadequate treatment strategies contribute to recurrences, when predisposing, precipitating, and perpetuating factors are not comprehensively addressed.

Poor adherence to healthy lifestyle and treatment protocol may further contribute to VVS/PVD and associated comorbidities, r-UTI first.

Conclusions

The sexual debut is particularly vulnerable to the onset of vestibular and vulvar pain. The caring physician should not be minimalistic but devote adequate consulting time to the listening and questioning about the many contributing factors potentially in play in the consulting young woman.

Women are not "walking vulvas." The vestibular/vulvar health is not isolated, but it is the tip of the iceberg of multiple systemic vulnerabilities that should be addressed if an effective treatment is to be designed and pursued.

Unfortunately the hyperspecialistic approach to the vulvar organ, as if it were "separated" by the rest of the body, leads to minimalistic treatment, the most shortsighted of all being vestibulectomy. No peripheral surgery will ever cure the neuroinflammation typical of the neuropathic pain, for the very same reason why amputating the hand will not resolve the problem of neuropathic hand pain. Long-term follow-up has proven that this aggressive attitude is not and cannot be the first answer to vestibular and vulvar pain.

This is the leading reason why this chapter has been carefully devoted to analyze all the potential systemic and local factor contributing to vestibular/vulvar vulnerabilities up to burning neuropathic pain and introital dyspareunia.

References

Anand M, Wang C, French J, Isaacson-Schmid M, Wall LL, Mysorekar IU. Estrogen affects the glycosaminoglycan layer of the murine bladder. Female Pelvic Med Reconstr Surg. 2012;18(3):148–52. doi:10.1097/SPV.0b013e31824b76bd.

Bachmann G, Rosen R, Pinn V, Utian W, Ayers C, Basson R, Binik Y, Brown C, Foster D, Gibbons J, Goldstein I, Graziottin A, Haefner H, Harlow B, Kellogg Spadt S, Leiblum S, Masheb R, Reed B, Sobel J, Veasley C, Wesselmann U, Witkin S. Vulvodynia: a state-of-the-art consensus on definitions, diagnosis and management. J Reprod Med. 2006;51(6):447–56.

Bergeron S, Likes WM, Steben M. Psychosexual aspects of vulvovaginal pain. Best Pract Res Clin Obstet Gynaecol. 2014;28:991–9.

Bertolasi L, Frasson E, Cappelletti JY, Vicentini S, Bordignon M, Graziottin A. Botulinum neurotoxin Type A injections for vaginismus secondary to vulvar vestibulitis syndrome. Obstet Gynecol. 2009;114(5):1008–16.

Casey JT, Bjurlin MA, Cheng EY. Pediatric genital injury: an analysis of the national electronic injury surveillance system. Urology. 2013;82(5):10.1016.

Chatterjea D, Martinov T. Mast cells: versatile gatekeepers of pain. Mol Immunol. 2015;63(1):38–44.

Clare CA, Yeh J. Vulvodynia in adolescence: childhood vulvar pain syndromes (review). J Pediatr Adolesc Gynecol. 2011;24(3):110–5.

Cohen-Sacher B, Haefner HK, Dalton VK, Berger MB. History of abuse in women with vulvar pruritus, vulvodynia, and asymptomatic controls. J Low Genit Tract Dis. 2015;19(3):248–52.

Donders GG. Lower genital tract infections in diabetic women. Curr Infect Dis Rep. 2002;4(6):536–9.

Donskey CJ. The role of the intestinal tract as a reservoir and source for transmission of nosocomial pathogens. Clin Infect Dis. 2004;39(2):219–26.

Falsetta ML, Foster DC, Woeller CF, Pollock SJ, Bonham AD, Haidaris CG, Stodgell CJ, Phipps RP. Identification of novel mechanisms involved in generating localized vulvodynia pain. Am J Obstet Gynecol. 2015;213(1):38e.1–12. doi:10.1016/j.ajog.2015.02.002. Epub 2015 Feb 12.

Farmer MA, Taylor AM, Bailey AL, Tuttle AH, MacIntyre LC, Milagrosa ZE, et al. Repeated vulvovaginal fungal infections cause persistent pain in a mouse model of vulvodynia. Sci Transl Med. 2011;3:101ra91.

Fistarol SK, Itin PH. Diagnosis and treatment of lichen sclerosus: an update. Am J Clin Dermatol. 2013;14(1):27–47.

Frasson E, Graziottin A, Priori A, Dall'Ora E, Didonè G, Garbin EL, Vicentini S, Bertolasi L. Central nervous system abnormalities in vaginismus. Clin Neurophysiol. 2009;120(1):117–22.

Gardella B, Porru D, Nappi RE, Daccò MD, Chiesa A, Spinillo A. Interstitial cystitis is associated with vulvodynia and sexual dysfunction – a case-control study. J Sex Med. 2011;8(6):1726–34. Epub 2011 Apr 7.

Gorter KJ, Hak E, Zuithoff NP, Hoepelman AI, Rutten GE. Risk of recurrent acute lower urinary tract infections and prescription pattern of antibiotics in women with and without diabetes in primary care. Fam Pract. 2010;27(4):379–85. Epub 2010 May 12.

Graziottin A. Sexual pain disorders: dyspareunia and vaginismus. In: Porst H, Buvat J, editors. ISSM (International Society of Sexual Medicine) standard committee book, standard practice in sexual medicine. Oxford, UK: Blackwell; 2006. p. 342–50.

Graziottin A. Mast cells and their role in sexual pain disorders. In: Goldstein A, Pukall C, Goldstein I, editors. Female sexual pain disorders: evaluation and management. Chichester: Blackwell Publishing; 2009. p. 176–9.

Graziottin A. Recurrent cystitis after intercourse: why the gynaecologist has a say. In: Studd J, Seang LT, Chervenak FA, editors. Current progress in obstetrics and gynaecology, vol. 2. Mumbai: Suketu P. Kothari – TreeLife Media; 2014. p. 319–36.

Graziottin A. Female sexual dysfunction: assessment. In: Bø K, Berghmans B, Mørkved S, Van Kampen M, editors. Evidence-based physical therapy for the pelvic floor – bridging science and clinical practice. 2nd ed. Oxford, UK: Elsevier; 2015a. p. 243–57.

Graziottin A. "The shorter, the better": a review of the evidence for a shorter contraception hormone-free interval. Eur J Contracept Reprod Health Care. 2015b;20:1–13.

Graziottin A, Gambini D. Female sexual dysfunction: treatment. In: Bø K, Berghmans B, Mørkved S, Van Kampen M, editors. Evidence-based physical therapy for the pelvic floor – bridging science and clinical practice. 2nd ed. Oxford, UK: Elsevier; 2015. p. 258–70.

Graziottin A, Murina F. Clinical management of vulvodynia. Milano: Springer Verlag Italia; 2011.

Graziottin A, Serafini A. HPV infection in women: psychosexual impact of genital warts and intraepithelial lesions. In: Takac I, editor. Recent advances in cervical cancer. Kerala: Transworld Research Network; 2012. p. 69–85.

Graziottin A, Zanello PP. Pathogenic biofilms: their role in recurrent cystitis and vaginitis (with focus on D-mannose as a new prophylactic strategy). In: Studd J, Seang LT, Chervenak FA, editors. Current progress in obstetrics and gynaecology, vol. 3. 2nd ed. Mumbai: Kothari Medical; 2015. p. 218–38.

Graziottin A, Skaper S, Fusco M. Inflammation and chronic pelvic pain: a biological trigger for depression in women? J Depress Anxiety. 2013;3:142–50.

Graziottin A, Skaper S, Fusco M. Mast cells in chronic inflammation, pelvic pain and depression in women. Gynecol Endocrinol. 2014;30(7):472–7.

Graziottin A, Gambini D, Bertolasi L. Genital and sexual pain in women. In: Vodusek D, Boller F, editors, Neurology of sexual and bladder disorders (Handbook of clinical neurology, vol. 130, 3rd series). Edinburgh: Elsevier; 2015. p. 395–412.

Graziottin A, Gambini D. Evaluation of genito-pelvic pain penetration disorder. In: Waguih WI, editor. The textbook of sexual medicine. Springer; 2017 (in press).

Gurumurthy M, Morah N, Gioffre G, Cruickshank ME. The surgical management of complications of vulval lichen sclerosus. Eur J Obstet Gynecol Reprod Biol. 2012;162(1):79–82.

Haefner HK. Report of the International Society for the Study of Vulvovaginal Disease: terminology and classification of vulvodynia. J Low Genit Tract Dis. 2007;11:48–9.

Harlow BL, Stewart EG. Adult-onset vulvodynia in relation to childhood violence victimization. Am J Epidemiol. 2005;161(9):871–80.

Harlow BL, Vitonis AF, Stewart EG. Influence of oral contraceptive use on the risk of adult-onset vulvodynia. J Reprod Med. 2008;53(2):102–10.

Harlow BL, He W, Nguyen RH. Allergic reactions and risk of vulvodynia. Ann Epidemiol. 2009;19(11):771–7. doi:10.1016/j.annepidem.2009.06.006.

Iglesias-Rios L, Harlow SD, Reed BD. Depression and posttraumatic stress disorder among women with vulvodynia: evidence from the population-based woman to woman health study. J Womens Health (Larchmt). 2015;24(7):557–62.

Jackson SL, Boyko EJ, Scholes D, Abraham L, Gupta K, Fihn SD. Predictors of urinary tract infection after menopause: a prospective study. Am J Med. 2004;117(12):903–11.

Jayaram A, Witkin SS, Zhou X, Brown CJ, Rey GE, Linhares IM, Ledger WJ, Forney LJ. The bacterial microbiome in paired vaginal and vestibular samples from women with vulvar vestibulitis syndrome. Pathog Dis. 2014;72(3):161–6. doi:10.1111/2049-632X.12197. Epub 2014 Jul 10.

Kalyoussef S, Nieves E, Dinerman E, et al. Lactobacillus proteins are associated with the bactericidal activity against E. coli of female genital tract secretions. PLoS One. 2012;7(11):e49506. doi:10.1371/journal.pone.0049506. Epub 2012 Nov 19.

Khandker M, Brady SS, Elizabeth G, Stewart EG, Harlow BL. Is chronic stress during childhood associated with adult-onset vulvodynia? J Womens Health (Larchmt). 2014;23(8):649–56.

Murina F, Graziottin A, Felice R, Radici GL, Di Francesco S. The recurrent vulvovaginal candidiasis: proposal of a personalized therapeutic protocol. ISRN Obstet Gynecol. 2011;2011: Article ID 806065, 4 pages

Peters KM, Killinger KA, Carrico DJ, Ibrahim IA, Diokno AC, Graziottin A. Sexual function and sexual distress in women with interstitial cystitis: a case control study. Urology. 2007;70(3): 543–7.

Postma R, Bicanic I, van der Vaart H, Laan E. Pelvic floor muscle problems mediate sexual problems in young adult rape victims. J Sex Med. 2013;10(8):1978–87. doi:10.1111/jsm.12196. Epub 2013 May 16.

Reed BD, Harlow SD, Sen A, Legocki LJ, Edwards RM, Arato N, Haefner HK. Prevalence and demographic characteristics of vulvodynia in a population-based sample. Am J Obstet Gynecol. 2012a;206(2):170.e1–9.

Reed BD, Harlow SD, Sen A, Edwards RM, Chen D, Haefner HK. Relationship between vulvodynia and chronic comorbid pain conditions. Obstet Gynecol. 2012b;120:145–51.

Reed BD, Harlow SD, Legocki LJ, Helmuth ME, Haefner HK, Gillespie BW, Sen A. Oral contraceptive use and risk of vulvodynia: a population-based longitudinal study. BJOG. 2013;120(13):1678–84.

Reed BD, Legocki LJ, Plegue MA, Sen A, Haefner HK, Harlow SD. Factors associated with vulvodynia incidence. Obstet Gynecol. 2014;123(2 Pt 1):225–31.

Rescigno M. The intestinal epithelial barrier in the control of homeostasis and immunity. Trends Immunol. 2011;32(6):256–64. doi:10.1016/j.it.2011.04.003. Epub 2011 May 11. Review.

Ru-Rong JI, Zhen-Zhong XU, Gao YJ. Emerging targets in neuroinflammation-driven chronic pain. Nat Rev Drug Discov. 2014;13(7):533–48.

Sadownik LA. Etiology, diagnosis, and clinical management of vulvodynia. Int J Womens Health. 2014;6:437–49.

Saliba W, Barnett-Griness O, Rennert G. The association between obesity and urinary tract infection. Eur J Intern Med. 2012;29 [Epub ahead of print].

Salonia A, Clementi MC, Graziottin A, Nappi RE, Castiglione F, Ferrari M, Capitanio U, Damiano R, Montorsi F. Secondary provoked vestibulodynia in sexually-active women with recurrent uncomplicated urinary tract infections. J Sex Med. 2013;10(9):2265–73.

Sauerbrei A. Optimal management of genital herpes: current perspectives. Infect Drug Resist. 2016; 9:129–41.

Sen R. Recurrent cystitis in non-pregnant women. BMJ Clin Evid (online). 2008;208:0801.

Simonetta C, Burns EK, Guo MA. Vulvar dermatoses: a review and update. Mo Med. 2015;112(4):301–7.

Skaper SD, Facci L, Giusti P. Mast cells, glia and neuroinflammation: partners in crime? Immunology. 2014;141(3):314–27. doi:10.1111/imm.12170.

Smith LA, Price N, Simonite V, Burns EE. Incidence of and risk factors for perineal trauma: a prospective observational study. BMC Pregnancy Childbirth. 2013;13:59.

Stanghellini V, Barbara G, Cremon C, et al. Gut microbiota and related diseases: clinical features. Int Emerg Med. 2010;5 Supp 1:57–63.

Verstraelen H, De Zutter E, De Muynck M. Genitofemoral neuralgia: adding to the burden of chronic vulvar pain. J Pain Res. 2015;8:845–9. Published online 2015 November 30.

Walker AK, Kavelaars A, Heijnen CJ, Dantzer R. Neuroinflammation and comorbidity of pain and depression. Pharmacol Rev. 2013;66(1):80–101.

Xanthos DN, Sandkühler J. Neurogenic neuroinflammation: inflammatory CNS reactions in response to neuronal activity. Nat Rev Neurosci. 2014;15(1):43–53. doi:10.1038/nrn3617. Epub 2013 Nov 27.

Xanthos DN, Gaderer S, Drdla R, Nuro E, Abramova A, Ellmeier W, Sandkühler J. Central nervous system mast cells in peripheral inflammatory nociception. Mol Pain. 2011;7:42. doi:10.1186/1744-8069-7-42.

Yoon BI, Kim SW, Ha US, Sohn DW, Cho YH. Risk factors for recurrent cystitis following acute cystitis in female patients. J Infect Chemother. 2013;19(4):727–31.

Vulvar Pain During Pregnancy and After Childbirth

7

Pregnancy is a special period in a woman's life. The childbirth involves significant physical, hormonal, psychological, social, and cultural changes that may influence her own sexuality as well as the health of the couple's sexual relationship.

Vulvar pain is often sadly neglected during pregnancy and particularly after delivery, despite its frequent comorbidity with introital dyspareunia in this vulnerable phase of a woman's life.

Women's sexual dysfunctions are frequently reported after childbirth. Among them, dyspareunia carries the highest risk of long-term systemic, genital, sexual, and relational consequences. Therefore, the twin problem "vulvar pain and dyspareunia" requires a very committed clinical approach, with specific medical/gynecological attention to its biological basis, as well as careful evaluation of the delivery outcome and the condition of the pelvic floor.

This chapter is prominently focused on the biological etiology of vulvar pain and dyspareunia, while psychosexual and contextual factors will be considered when appropriate for a balanced vision of the vulvar pain scenario at pregnancy and after childbirth.

7.1 Vulvovaginal Pain During Pregnancy

Vulvovaginal pain during pregnancy may have three major timing reading, according to the author's clinical experience. It may:

- Be rooted in *previous vulvar vestibulitis/provoked vestibulodynia*, inadequately diagnosed and addressed before pregnancy
- Be the exacerbation of a *vulvar pain caused by a previous delivery* and remained untreated/insufficiently cured
- Have the *first onset during the current pregnancy*

A. Graziottin, F. Murina, *Vulvar Pain*, DOI 10.1007/978-3-319-42677-8_7

Vulvovaginal discomfort usually varies across pregnancy. In the first trimester, higher percentages of this symptom may be attributed to the concerns and anxiety related to the onset of the new pregnancy. In the second trimester, it is usually reported as significantly milder, coherently with the mother's adaptation to pregnancy. Fears of early labor and the emotional alert toward the delivery tend to increase again the perception of it in the third trimester. It was demonstrated that 76–79 % of women enjoyed sexual intercourse before pregnancy (7–21 % not at all), while this decreased to 59 % in the first trimester, 75–84 % in the second trimester, and 40–41 % in the third trimester (Johnson 2011). Moreover, coital frequency tends to decline with advancing gestational age. This trend is further negatively influenced by dyspareunia and decreased orgasmic quality (Leeman and Rogers 2012).

As pregnancy progresses, vaginal discomfort may become more pronounced as a result of changes in vaginal physiology in response to hormonal changes wherein the connective tissue of the vagina decreases and the muscle fibers of the vaginal wall increase in size in preparation for delivery (Erol et al. 2007).

During the third trimester, vaginal contractions are weaker and tonic muscle spasms may occasionally occur, which may influence orgasmic response.

Candida vulvovaginitis (CVV) is a specific and usually neglected contributor of genital discomfort and introital dyspareunia in pregnancy. Frequency of *Candida* infections increases significantly during pregnancy. The vulnerability to CVV is higher in women who were already vulnerable to this germ's infections, who had history of vulvar vestibulitis/provoked vestibulodynia, who are diabetic and/or presented with gestational diabetes, or have family/genetic predisposition to diabetes, and/or who have an excess weight gain in pregnancy (Martins and Kroumpouzos 2016).

In a recent prospective study on 210 pregnant women, aged 10–42, 38.1 % were symptomatic. Symptoms were most prevalent in the second and third trimesters of pregnancy coincident with a major prevalence of microorganisms. In this study, 39.5 % of pregnant women had normal microbial biota, and symptoms of CVV due to noninfectious causes were observed (6.2 %). The occurrence of vulvovaginal candidiasis was 25 %, and *Candida albicans*, with a prevalence of 80.7 %, was the dominant species ($P=0.005$), while non-*Candida albicans* species and other yeast were more common in asymptomatic ones ($P=0.0038$) (Mucci et al. 2016).

Key Points

- CVV *should be considered* in women with vulvar pain and/or vulvovaginal discomfort in pregnancy.
- Attention should increase in women with history of CVV and/or leading risk factors such as diabetes.
- Accurate diet, change of the circadian rhythm of sugar/carbohydrates intake, and control of weight increase are leading preventing strategies to reduce the vulnerability to CVV in pregnancy (Box 7.1).

Box 7.1. Prevention of *Candida* Vulvovaginitis in Pregnancy

- *Control weight gain:* the woman who has a normal body weight at the onset of pregnancy should ideally increase on average of 1000 g per month in the first trimester, 1.200 g/month in the second trimester, and 1.500 g/month in the third trimester, with a total weight gain ranging between 11 and 13 kilograms at term. Overweight/obese women should ideally reduce their body weight *before the onset of a new pregnancy,* to prevent/reduce the risk of fetal and maternal complication, including but not limited to CVV. Combined diet and physical exercise appear to be significantly effective in reducing gestational weight gain (GWG) (Muktabhant et al. 2015).
- *Change the circadian rhythm of source of calories intake.* Human placental lactogen (HPL) is a placenta hormone leading the placental control of maternal glucose homeostasis. Its activity is aimed at maintaining a favorable gradient between the plasmatic levels of glucose in the mother blood (physiologically, between 80 and 90 mg/dL) and that of the child (physiologically, between 50 and 60 mg/dL). Passage of glucose from mom to child is essential to guarantee his/her optimal growth. The night hours of fasting are more likely to reduce the gradient, impairing child nutrition, more so when animal protein intake is preferred in the evening, while higher carbohydrate intake at lunch turns into conversion into glycogen and fat. Authors' clinical wisdom, physiologically based, suggests therefore to prefer moderate sugar/fruit intake at breakfast, protein intake (fish or meat with vegetables) at lunch, and carbohydrates (rice and legumes, cereals, raw pasta) in the evening, to maintain a long-lasting modest increase of plasmatic maternal glucose levels and a persisting favorable gradient during the night hours while preventing hypoglycemic night crisis in the mother. Prevention of glucose daily peaks further reduces the vulnerability of *Candida* shifting from the spora to the active hypha state (Groot et al. 2014; Mending and Brash 2012).
- *Reduce the intake of yeast-containing food* (bread, cakes, biscuits) and prefer fresh vegetables and fruits.
- *Avoid alcohol completely:* to prevent embryo and fetal toxicity, to reduce useless calories intake, and to prevent changes in the colonic microbiota.
- *Enjoy 45 min/1 h of brisk walking every day:* it optimizes the peripheral insulin metabolism, contributes to maintain physiologic glycemic levels, reduces the risk of gestational diabetes and contributes to an optimal weight gain, reduces systemic inflammation associated with overweight, improves mood, contributes to a better pregnancy outcome, and is very democratic as it can be practiced at every income level.

  The preventive impact of daily exercise on onset and progression of gestational diabetes is discussed in the comprehensive work of Angina et al. (2016).

Benefits of physical exercise on diabetic risk are reviewed as well in the meta-analysis of Di Mascio et al. (2016) on 2019 pregnant subjects randomized to aerobic exercise and controls before 23rd week. Women in the exercise group (35–90 min of aerobic exercise 3–4 times a week) had a significantly lower incidence of gestational diabetes mellitus (2.4 % vs. 5.9 %; RR 0.41, 95 % CI 0.24–0.68) and significantly lower incidence of hypertensive disorders (1.9 % vs. 5.1 %; RR 0.36, 95 % CI 0.19–0.69) compared to controls.

7.2 Etiology of Women's Sexual Dysfunctions *After* Childbirth

Vulvar pain and dyspareunia after childbirth are usually rooted in a more complex biological and psychosexual dysfunctional scenario that must be understood and investigated to prevent/avoid minimalistic approaches and therapeutically disappointing outcomes.

The first 6 months after delivery can have a profound impact on a woman's sexual quality of life. Sexual dysfunctions usually recognize *a multifactorial etiology* that should be carefully investigated in the presenting woman and couple (Table 7.1). Vulvar pain and dyspareunia may indeed just be the tip of the iceberg of multiple biological and psychosexual causes, easy to be addressed when appropriately diagnosed. Leading neglected contributors include:

7.2.1 Systemic Factors

- *Hormonal contributors*, prominent in breastfeeding women, where high prolactin causes the "ovarian silence," with minimum levels of estradiol, progesterone, and testosterone. This hormonal milieu leads to consequent silencing of the first endocrine motor of sexual drive and of central and genital arousal, leading to vaginal dryness, and changes in the vaginal microbiota and pH. It was demonstrated that breastfeeding confers an increased odds ratio of 4.4 (95 % CI 2.7–7.7) for dyspareunia at 6 months. It has been shown that at 6 weeks, bottle-feeding women who have an earlier recovery of ovarian function are more likely to return to intercourse and their rates of sexual difficulties fall (Rowland et al. 2005).
- *Iron deficiency anemia* (IDA), highly prevalent after delivery. Iron is key for the dopaminergic system mediating sexual drive, vital energy, mood and physical strength. IDA increases depression and pain perception, an aspect that few physician seem to consider. Early iron supplementation in mothers with postpartum depression (PPD) significantly improves the iron stores and causes a significant improvement in PPD with a 42.8 % improvement rate during 6 weeks (Sheikh et al. 2015).
- *Low mood/depression,* due to *anemia* (which doubles the risk of depression) *and neuroinflammation.* Inflammatory cytokines may increase dramatically during

Table. 7.1 Leading contributors to sexual dysfunction after childbirth

Biological factors
Systemic
Breastfeeding-induced amenorrhea
High prolactin and low levels of estradiol and testosterone
Iron deficiency anemia
Depression
Fatigue
Sleep reduction/insufficient quality
Obesity
Genital
Vulvovaginal tears during delivery
Spontaneous genital tract trauma
Episiotomy discomfort
Inadequate healing of episiorrhaphy
Pelvic floor trauma during operative delivery
Pelvic floor dysfunction
Pudendal nerve trauma
Vaginal bleeding
Vaginal discharge
Urinary stress incontinence
Anal incontinence
Postcoital cystitis
Psychosexual factors
Decreased sense of attractiveness
Reduced sexual drive and central arousal
Decreased lubrication
Vaginal dryness
Dyspareunia
Fear of further genital injuries and pain
Contextual/relational factors
Inadequate transition to parenthood
Marital crisis
Loss of desire in the partner
Concerns about the child's health, in case of baby's perinatal problems
Fear of awakening the baby or not hearing him/her

the immediate postpartum, due to (1) the massive physiologic uterine muscular catabolism (from 1000 to 1500 g at the end of pregnancy of uterine muscle to average 70–80 g of uterine weight in a nonpregnant woman) and (2) the intense adipocyte production, higher in overweight/obese women.

- *Sleep reduction,* due to night breast feeding and/or child's frequent awakenings. Poor quality of sleep is another neglected contributor of depression, fatigue, low vital energy and consequently low sexual drive.
- *Fatigue,* which recognizes biological and psychological contributors.
- *Obesity,* because of systemic and brain inflammation, skins stretches and marks, fatigue, poor body image.

7.2.2 Genital Factors

- *Genital tract trauma during delivery*, either spontaneous or iatrogenic, with episiotomy discomfort and/or inadequate healing of episiorrhaphy.
- *Pelvic floor trauma during spontaneous or operative delivery and Kristeller maneuver*, more practiced than reported in the medical chart, is another neglected factor of lesions of the pubococcigeal component of the levator ani, contributing to loss of vaginal sensitivity and urinary incontinence. Operative deliveries may further contribute to subclinical lesions of the anal sphincter, which are diagnosed with the ecographic probe up to 25–33 % of postpartum women.
- *Pelvic floor dysfunction,* due to functional/anatomic lesions of the levator ani in case of macrosomic babies and/or prolonged second phase of labor or posterior rotation of the baby's head.
- *Pudendal nerve trauma:* is a most concerning complication of delivery. It can be subclinical or overt and can occur more during operative than during spontaneous delivery.
- *Vaginal bleeding* due to prolonged postpartum endometrial involution.
- *Vaginal discharge* due to vaginitis.
- *Urinary stress incontinence:* stress incontinence may specifically affect women during thrusting, while urge incontinence is more reported at orgasm.
- *Anal incontinence* to gas and feces, in more serious cases. Incontinence, either urinary and/or anal, is a threatening consequence of delivery. It is underdiagnosed, underreported and undertreated, therefore persisting as a major neglected contributor to sexual dysfunction long term after delivery. It has both biological and psychosexual consequences as it may affects the sense of self-worth, self-esteem with heavy impairment of the social life, dramatically reduced because of the incontinence (Rezvan et al. 2015).
- *Postcoital cystitis*: reduction of the congestion of periurethral corpus spongiosum (equivalent of part of male's urethral corpus spongiosum) deprives the woman's urethra of a functional protective "airbag" during thrusting, with increased risk of postcoital cystitis, more frequently complained of 24–72 h after intercourse. Hypoestrogenism during breastfeeding changes the vaginal microbiota and pH, further increasing vaginal and urethral vulnerability to microtraumas and pain after delivery.

7.2.3 Psychosexual Factors

- Decreased sense of sexual attractiveness.
- Reduced sexual drive and reduced central arousal with decreased lubrication, because of the abovementioned systemic and genital factors, which are prominent after delivery. They set the biological and psychosexual scenario of an increased psychosexual vulnerability to vulvovaginal discomfort and vaginal dryness after delivery. All these factors potentiate each other in a vicious circle, where negative feedbacks play a prominent role (Fig. 7.1).

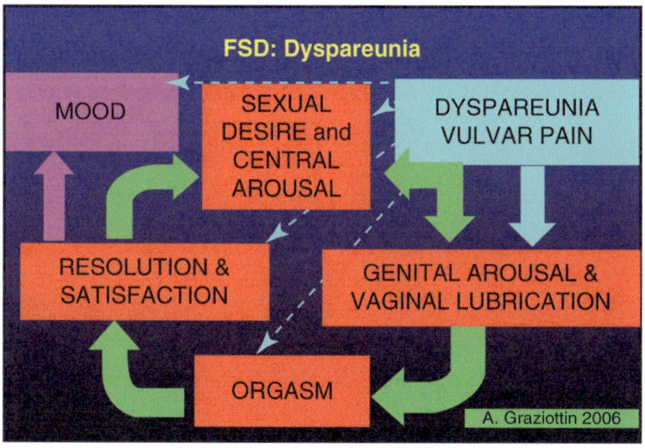

Fig. 7.1 Impact of dyspareunia on women's sexual function. Dyspareunia and vulvar pain directly impair genital arousal and vaginal lubrication. Indirectly they may affect coital orgasm and level of sexual satisfaction, thus modulating both mood and levels of sexual desire and central arousal

- Dyspareunia: introital pain is a powerful reflex inhibitor of genital arousal, worsening vaginal dryness and reducing cavernosal bodies' congestion.
- Fear of further genital injuries and pain may further contribute to sexual dysfunction after delivery.

7.2.4 Contextual/Relational Factors

- *Transition to parenthood* is a major revolution in the couple's affective and sexual relationship. When the transition is difficult or inadequate, it may affect as well partner's sexual drive and motivation to sexual intimacy, impairing the woman's sense of self-worth and self-esteem and further affecting her sexual desire.
- *Marital crisis*, because of an inadequate transition to parenthood or other factors, may increase the physical and emotional distance in a subset of vulnerable couples: vulvar pain may be even "used" or read as the last straw, or the "drop that makes the vase overflow" of a prolonged sexual dissatisfaction. Unaddressed or inadequately treated vulvar pain before pregnancy, further worsened after delivery, may turn into becoming the precipitating factor of a major marital crisis up to divorce (Korja et al. 2016).
- *Loss of desire in the partner*: depression triggered by the baby's birth because of jealousy toward the newborn, sense of inadequacy, and sexual difficulties worsening after a long period of abstinence during pregnancy and/or of economic concerns may further affect the partner's sexual desire in a complex relational interplay of negative factors.
- *Concerns about the child's health*, in case of baby's perinatal problems, premature deliveries, need of intensive care, and risk of long-term consequences, may affect mood and motivation to intimacy in both partners, with mothers usually reporting the more severe negative impact on mood and desire.
- *Fear of awakening the baby or not hearing him/her*.

7.2.4.1 Practical Tips

- All these negative biological, sexual, and contextual factors set the scenario of an increased woman's sexual vulnerability to genital pain after delivery.
- They may differ in their relative weight in the individual woman and couple.
- Vulvar pain may just be the tip of the iceberg of a complex multifactorial etiology that must be investigated and addressed if a successful physical, sexual, and relational outcome is to be pursued.
- Genital factors specific to delivery must be competently diagnosed early on after childbirth, to prevent long-term consequences that may affect the future of the woman's sexuality, the sexual relationship, and the marriage/family itself.

7.3 Vulvar Pain and Dyspareunia After Childbirth

7.3.1 Epidemiology

The prevalence of female sexual dysfunction (FSD) is high after childbirth, in the postpartum and puerperium periods. Data indicate that up to 86 % of women report one or more FSD soon after delivery. The most frequently reported complaint is low libido, which is more prevalent in women who are breastfeeding. High prolactin has a negative impact on the neurobiological basis of sexual drive and central and genital arousal, in addition to inducing amenorrhea. Dyspareunia and vaginal dryness frequently occur after childbirth. They may further independently contribute to a reduction in sexual drive, because of the negative feedback from the genitals.

Dyspareunia is reported by 41–67 % of women within 2–3 months postpartum. At 3 months postpartum, 30 % of women reported persistence of dyspareunia, while about 20 % continued to experience dyspareunia at 6 months postpartum according to Barrett et al. (2000).

In another study problems with intercourse were reported by 569/1075 (53 %) of women in the first 8 weeks after delivery and by 215/435 (49 %) in the subsequent year. Women who reported perineal pain, depression, or tiredness experienced problems related to intercourse more often than those who did not. Women who breastfed their infants were significantly less interested in intercourse than those who bottle-fed, irrespective of tiredness or depression, but this effect did not persist in the long term (Glazener 1997).

In a more recent study (McDonald et al. 2015), long-term negative consequences on sexuality are reported with almost overlapping figures with Glazener's data. The study on 1507 nulliparous women reports that dyspareunia at 3, 6, 12, and 18 months was complained of by 44, 43, 28, and 23 %, respectively. Sad to say, "lack of professional recognition" as Glazener (1997) pertinently said so many years ago persists almost unchanged.

7.3.2 Vulvar Pain After Delivery: Frequently Asked Questions (FAQ) in the Clinical Setting

Physicians and midwives, women, and partners have leading, "hot," questions focused on etiology, classification, prevention, and treatment of vulvar pain during pregnancy and after delivery.

This FAQ section is committed to help healthcare providers in their daily clinical work while easing communication on these issues with their patients. It is distilled from the interplay between authors' clinical experience and scientific evidence.

FAQ 1. What Are the Leading Genital Contributors of Vulvar Pain and Dyspareunia After Childbirth?

Vulnerability to vulvar pain and dyspareunia after childbirth recognizes two major genital contributors, overlapping and exacerbating the role of systemic factors discussed above and summarized in Table. 7.1. In case of vulvar pain complaint after childbirth, healthcare providers should mandatorily investigate, diagnose, and, if present, appropriately treat the specific role of the following factors.

7.3.2.1 Pudendal Nerve Damage

The pudendal nerve is the primary afferent nerve for the perineum, vulva, and clitoris and mediates some of the reflex pathways involved with female sexual function.

Intrapartum pudendal nerve injury may occur from compression of the nerve by the fetal head, resulting in acute nerve dysfunction and ischemic injury, which is similar to the neuropathy that can occur from compartment syndrome.

Compartment syndrome is a condition in which increased tissue pressure within a limited tissue space compromises the circulation and function of the contents of the space. During delivery, and particularly in case of prolonged second stage labor, ischemic damage of the pudendal nerve caused by the fetal head may lead to sensory and/or motor dysfunctions of this nerve causing paresthesias, sense of pins and burning pain, referred pain, dyspareunia, and sexual dysfunction. Stretch injury to the pudendal nerve can also occur with a prolonged second stage of labor, operative delivery, and large fetal birth weight, potentially worsening the ischemic damages to the nerve. The strain in the perineal nerve branch innervating the anal sphincter can reach 33 % (Lien et al. 2005).

7.3.2.2 Vulvo-perineal Trauma

Perineal trauma is defined as any damage to the genitalia during childbirth, either spontaneously or due to an episiotomy, that in its extent can be considered as the equivalent of a spontaneous second-degree perineal tear. Although laceration rates vary based on patient characteristics, birth settings, and obstetric care provider practices, 53–79 % of women will sustain some type of laceration at vaginal delivery (Smith et al. 2013).

Vulvo-perineal trauma (Fig. 7.1) and its scarring effects are associated with postpartum dyspareunia and sexual dysfunctions. Klein et al. (1994) found that women who underwent episiotomy, with or without additional perineal trauma, had higher rates of postpartum dyspareunia when compared with women who delivered with an intact perineum or spontaneous perineal trauma.

Signorello et al. (2001) also found that women who sustain a second-degree laceration had an 80 % increased incidence of dyspareunia at 3 months postpartum compared with women who delivered with an intact perineum.

When a wound complication occurred, a terminal swelling or end bulb can be observed with axonal sprouting occurring. This can lead to formation of a neuroma, a tangled mass that is formed when the axon cannot completely reconnect and/or is partially entrapped in the scar tissue. The neuroma generates abnormal activity that is called "ectopic" because it does not generate from the physiologic stimuli of nerve endings. In more unfortunate cases, after traumatic delivery pudendal nerve neuroma can trigger vulvar pain, limiting sexual function and decreasing the woman's quality of life.

Key Points

- The potential role of pudendal nerve damage and vulvo-perineal trauma must be accurately investigated, documented, and appropriately treated in every woman complaining of vulvar pain after delivery.
- The sooner, the better, to prevent long-term negative genital, sexual, and functional (incontinence!) outcomes.

FAQ 2. How Should the Severity of Perineal Trauma Be Classified?

Classification of perineal trauma's severity into different degrees may be recorded depending on the anatomical structures involved (modified from ACOG 2014):

- *First degree*: injury to perineal skin only
- *Second degree*: injury to perineum involving perineal muscles but not involving the anal sphincter
- *Third degree*: injury to perineum involving anal sphincter complex
  1. 3a: less than 50 % of external anal sphincter thickness torn
  2. 3b: more than 50 % external anal sphincter thickness torn
  3. 3c: both external anal sphincter and internal anal sphincter torn
- *Fourth degree*: injury to perineum involving anal sphincter complex (external anal sphincter and internal anal sphincter) and anal epithelium

During childbirth, women may also sustain other traumas to the perineal area such as labial, anterior vaginal wall and paraurethral tears.

Key Points

- Postpartum perineal pain after a laceration is a common cause of vulvar pain and introital dyspareunia.
- Pain is usually more severe and lasts longer with third-degree or fourth-degree lacerations compared with first-degree or second-degree lacerations, which are limited to perineal skin and the perineal body muscles.
- However, subclinical damages of the pudendal nerve not immediately evident after delivery may occur even in women with first- or second-degree lacerations and must be investigated.
- The complaint of vulvar pain, and not only the severity of perineal tears and injuries, must lead the clinical approach.

FAQ 3. Which Maternal and Fetal Factors Increase the Risk of Perineal Trauma at Birth?

Maternal factors increasing the vulnerability to perineal traumas and vulvar pain include:

- *The first vaginal birth*: which is a significant risk factor for perineal trauma (odds ratio 2.88) and may reflect the relative inelasticity of previously unstretched perineal tissues
- *Advanced maternal age at first child*, as age increases the inelasticity of the pelvic floor muscles further contributing to the vulnerability of the first childbirth
- *Pelvic floor-related and genital factors* such as an hyperactive pelvic floor, an untreated or inadequately treated lifelong vaginismus and scarring outcomes of female genital mutilation
- *Prepregnancy diabetes and gestational diabetes* leading to high birth weight (macrosomic child) and complicated delivery
- *Accelerated second stage labor, with rapid delivery*

(Schmitz et al. 2014)

Fetal factors include:

- *Fetal malposition*: it increases the risk for perineal trauma, probably due to a larger circumference of the presenting vertex and hence greater distension of the perineal tissues, longer second stage of labor, and higher risk of operative deliveries. Indeed, a study of 1481 women found that any fetal position other than occipito-anterior was associated with a significant risk of perineal trauma (odds ratio 1.30).
- *Birth weight > 4000 g* (odds ratio 3.98, 95 % confidence interval 2.12–7.40) and the use of *oxytocic augmentation during labor* (OR 2.0, CI 1.13–2.53) have been shown to be significantly associated with severe perineal trauma (Webb and Sherburn 2014).

Key Points

- Prevention of *maternal factors* increasing the vulnerability to genital traumas during delivery includes:
  - Accurate monitoring of the woman's weight gain
  - Control of diabetes
  - Appropriate counseling to reduce the progression of the gestational diabetes
  - Relaxation of the pelvic floor with hands-on massage, physiotherapy, and midwives promoting preparation of the pelvic floor.
- Prevention of *fetal factors*, high weight at birth first, includes:
  - Diet monitoring
  - Diabetes' care
  - Recommendation of daily physical exercise
  - Early diagnosis of high birth weight (more dangerous in small women) and/or malposition to shift to cesarean section when indicated

FAQ 4. Which Type of Suturing Should Be Recommended After First- and Second-Degree Tears or Episiotomy?

A systematic review of two randomized controlled trials (2603 women) found that leaving the perineal skin unsutured but well apposed (with the vagina and perineal muscles appropriately sutured) may be more effective than conventional repair in reducing dyspareunia and perineal pain in first-degree and second-degree tears and episiotomies (Kettle and Tohill 2011).

Continuous suturing of a second-degree laceration is preferred over interrupted suturing.

Trials that compared continuous versus interrupted absorbable sutures for repair of episiotomy and second-degree perineal tears found that continuous repairs are associated with less pain for up to 10 days postpartum, less analgesia use, and a lower risk of having to have suture material removed postpartum. However, no differences were seen in dyspareunia, long-term pain, or the need for wound resuturing (Kettle et al. 2012).

Key Points

- Leaving the perineal skin unsutured but well apposed (with the vagina and perineal muscles appropriately sutured) may be more effective than conventional repair in reducing dyspareunia and perineal pain in first-degree and second-degree tears and episiotomies.

FAQ 5. What Are the Indications for Episiotomy in Contemporary Obstetric Practice?

Episiotomy is a surgical enlargement of the posterior aspect of the vagina by an incision of the perineum during the last part of the second stage of labor. The more common type of episiotomy performed in the Europe is mediolateral episiotomy;

this starts within 3 mm of the midline in the posterior fourchette and is directed laterally at an angle of at least 60° from the midline toward the ischial tuberosity. In the USA, a midline (also known as median) is more frequently performed, which starts within 3 mm of the midline in the posterior fourchette and extends downward between 0° and 25° of the sagittal plane.

Comparing restrictive episiotomy practices to routine performance, a meta-analysis of eight randomized trials (5541 women) found that *restrictive practices were associated with a lower risk of severe perineal trauma* (RR 0.67), *posterior perineal trauma* (RR 0.88), *need for suture repair of perineal trauma* (RR 0.71), and *healing complications* compared with patients in the routine episiotomy study arm (Carroli and Mignini 2009).

Accurate suturing of the episiotomy/episiorrhaphy is a simple but not insignificant medical procedure. When it is not adequately performed, with no respect for the appropriate reconstruction of different tissues and planes, or when rigorous asepsis is not respected, infection and local abscesses may dramatically increase the risk of a retracting scar, painful introital trigger points, or dyspareunia and vulvodynia.

Key Points

- There are no specific/standard situations in which episiotomy is essential.
- The decision to perform episiotomy should be based on clinical considerations focused on the individual case.
- Restrictive episiotomy use is recommended over routine episiotomy.
- Accurate episiorrhaphy is to be performed to reduce the risk of negative genital outcomes and chronic vulvar pain.

FAQ 6. Which Are the Two Golden Rules to Prevent Vulvar Pain After Childbirth?

A number of different perineal management interventions have been used in the antepartum period or at the time of delivery in an effort to reduce perineal trauma and vulvar pain:

1. *Perineal massage* (antepartum or during the second stage of labor) is intended to decrease perineal muscular tension/resistance and reduce the likelihood of laceration at delivery. In an analysis of four trials that compared antenatal perineal massage to no-massage controls, *digital perineal massage from 30 weeks of gestation onward* was associated with a *reduction in perineal trauma* that required repair with suture and *decreased episiotomy* in women without previous vaginal birth. Moreover, a statistically significant reduction in the incidence of pain at 3 months postpartum was reported (Beckmann and Stock 2013).
2. *Empower the midwives' role in the pelvic floor training and relaxation during pregnancy.*

It is very important for the clinician to trust and empower the role of well-trained midwives.

Midwives are the healthcare providers that are best placed for, and trained in, teaching pregnant women a number of key steps of self-awareness and empowerment:

- Knowledge of the pelvic floor, its muscles, and their functions
- Increasing competence in responding to the command to contract and completely relax the pelvic floor, with appropriate breathing (yoga can help)
- Learning a competent and efficient "pull strategy"

  In the case of a hyperactive pelvic floor (which is more frequently associated with lifelong dyspareunia, vaginismus and/or vulvodynia), it is essential to use "hands-on" *training* to teach the woman to relax the pelvic floor, using more specific physiotherapy techniques such as pelvic floor stretching and perineal work.

  The economic cost of this preventive intervention is hugely compensated by the cost saving in terms of reduction of maternal and fetal damages and related prolonged hospitalization, of pelvic floor integrity preservation, of prevention of urinary and fecal incontinence and further uterovaginal prolapse, of sexual dysfunctions, and of rehabilitative and surgical costs, not to mention the unquantifiable costs in terms of personal suffering and long-term comorbidities of problematic deliveries.

FAQ 7. What Causes the Shift from Acute Nociceptive Postpartum Vulvar Pain to Chronic Neuropathic Vulvar Pain/Vulvodynia?

Factors contributing to the neuropathic shift include (Graziottin et al. 2015):

- Persistence of vulvar inflammation, in infected episiorrhaphies and/or genital abscesses
- Retracted episiorrhaphy scars, with genital cutaneous nerve entrapment syndrome
- Repeated intercourses, in spite of pain (and/or the wrong use of topical anesthetics to reduce it), worsening the introital mucosal damage, increasing the mast cell degranulation and upregulation, proliferation, and superficialization of introital pain nerve fibers, with hyperalgesia and allodynia, systemic and brain inflammation, and neuroinflammation contributing to neurogenic pain (Graziottin 2009; Graziottin et al. 2014)
- Incomplete/inadequate healing of pudendal nerve damage
- Pudendal nerve neuroma

FAQ 8. Which Postnatal Advices Should Be Offered to for Women with Perineal Trauma and/or Episiotomy?

More useful advices include:

- *Check the woman's general health* and well-being first. Leading attention should be devoted to screen for:
  1. *Iron deficiency anemia* (IDA), highly prevalent after delivery particularly in low-income countries and women with low family/personal income;

supplement with iron, folic acid, and possibly lactoferrin and vitamin C should be prescribed for at least 3 months after delivery.
2. *Depression*, as it increases the vulnerability to pain, decreases search of professional help, and reduces adherence to treatment(s).

- *Ensure good perineal hygiene*, keeping the area clean and dry as much as possible and changing sanitary protection regularly.
- *Wash hands regularly*, especially before and after changing sanitary protection, during cleaning of the perineum, and after toileting/cleaning the child genitals.
- *Take a daily bath or shower*, making sure the perineum is washed with gentle soap with acid pH and water only and rinsed with clear water. It is important that the wound is dried as much as possible either by patting gently with a soft, clean towel or using a hairdryer on a "cool" setting.
- Be vigilant for *signs and symptoms of perineal infection*, such as an increase in pain, excessive discharge that has changed in color or offensive smells, swelling, suture breakdown, and hematoma.
- Maintain *a well-balanced diet* with adequate fluid intake to help promote healing and assist with breast milk production if required.
- Undertake regular, gentle *physical activity*, such as progressively active walking outdoor, to enjoy energy comeback and social interactions congratulating the mom with the newborn.
- *Start pelvic floor muscle exercises* within 5–7 days of delivery.

(Modified from Webb and Sherburn 2014)

Key Points

- Early recognition of postpartum dyspareunia, and adequate diagnosis and treatment of the different biological systemic and genital contributory factors, may significantly reduce postpartum vulvar pain and coital pain.
- It may also reduce the number of women whose pain, if persistently unaddressed and untreated, may shift from being nociceptive to becoming neuropathic, contributing to provoked and then spontaneous vulvodynia.

FAQ 9. What Is the Most Effective Treatment Plan to Cure Vulvar Pain After Delivery?

Accurate diagnosis of different factors contributing to vulvar pain is the first step of an effective treatment plan. According to the relevant contributors in the individual woman, leading biological therapeutic strategies include addressing the following factors.

7.3.2.3 Systemic Factors

- Treat iron deficiency anemia and depression, systemic factors that contribute to sexual dysfunction and increase vulnerability to pain.
- Improve the quality of sleep to reduce tiredness and fatigue.

- Improve quality of diet, with reduced yeast food and sugar to reduce the vulnerability to *Candida* infections and recurrences.
- Reduce body weight to reduce systemic inflammation and improve body image and self-esteem.
- Reduce neuropathic vulvar pain with:
  - Alpha-lipoic acid (600 mg/day)
  - Palmitoylethanolamide plus transpolydatin, to reduce neuroinflammation and pain perception (Murina et al. 2013)
  - Daily aerobic exercise (30–60 min) to reduce systemic inflammation and pain, reduce body weight (if indicated), improve peripheral use of insulin, and increase sexual drive, central arousal, and genital responsiveness
- Consider probiotics in case of comorbid irritable bowel syndrome (IBS). Well-selected probiotics appear to modulate the gut-brain axis and vulnerability to depression and further pain.

7.3.2.4 Genital Factors

- Avoid penetrative intercourse until the healing process is completed, to avoid worsening of the clinical picture and pain, and recommend other forms of sexual intimacy to encourage sexual closeness and pleasure.
- Select "hands-on" physiotherapy, stretching, electromyographic biofeedback, and self-massage to treat local inflammation contributing to the painful pelvic floor and retrain the pelvic floor muscles (Graziottin and Gambini 2015).
- Improve vestibular/vaginal trophism, choosing among hyaluronic acid, vitamin E, colostrum gel, D-mannose, and N-acetyl cysteine-based cream, to prevent vaginitis from *Escherichia coli* and associated comorbidities.
- Consider topical estriol during breastfeeding, to improve the genital trophism and reduce vaginal dryness.
- D-mannose and cranberry are orally indicated, twice per day, to reduce the bladder vulnerability to recurrent *Escherichia coli* uropathogenic (UPEC) infections (Graziottin and Zanello 2015; Graziottin 2014).
- Vaginal probiotics may contribute to restore the physiologic vaginal microbiota (Murina et al. 2014).
- Prevent recurrent vulvovaginal *Candida* with a personalized fluconazole protocol (Murina et al. 2011).

7.3.2.5 Psychosexual and Contextual Factors

- A competent psychologist may contribute to address leading psychosexual and contextual factors, interacting with the biological ones, with the goal of reducing vulvar pain.

Conclusions

Vulvar pain during pregnancy may stem from previous vulvar vestibulitis/provoked vestibulodynia, inadequately diagnosed and addressed before pregnancy; exacerbation of vulvar pain caused by a previous delivery and remained untreated/insufficiently cured; or the first onset during the current pregnancy.

Recurrent CVV is a leading contributor of vulvovaginal discomfort/vulvar pain during pregnancy. Accurate diet monitoring with weight gain control, daily exercise, reduction of gestational diabetes onset, and progress may significantly reduce the risk of vulvovaginal discomfort and reduce critical predisposing factors to vulvar pain after delivery.

Vulvar pain after childbirth recognizes predisposing, precipitating, and perpetuating factors. A rigorous medical approach is the golden path to the appropriate diagnosis and treatment of the multifactorial etiology of vulvar pain. Healthcare providers should provide a teamwork both in the preventive and treatment setting during pregnancy and during and after delivery, with balanced attention to biological, psychosexual, and contextual factors.

A well-orchestrated clinical work, inspired by a genuine passion for women's health; a solid medical attention to the biological contributors of vulvar pain, so often neglected after delivery; and a collaborative attitude with the other precious health providers such as midwives, physiotherapists, psychotherapists, and sexual therapists may offer women and couples a very effective way to cope and overcome vulvar pain after childbirth, to fully enjoy their family life with their child.

References

American College of Obstetricians and Gynecologists. Obstetric data definitions [version 1.0]. Washington, DC: American College of Obstetricians and Gynecologists; 2014.

Anjana RM, Sudha V, Lakshmipriya N, Anitha C, Unnikrishnan R, Bhavadharini B, Mahalakshmi MM, Maheswari K, Kayal A, Ram U, Ranjani H, Ninov L, Deepa M, Pradeepa R, Pastakia SD, Malanda B, Belton A, Mohan V. Physical activity patterns and gestational diabetes outcomes – the wings project. Diabetes Res Clin Pract. 2016;116:253–62.2.

Barrett G, Pendry E, Peacock J, Victor C, Thakar R, Manyonda I. Women's sexual health after childbirth. BJOG. 2000;107:186–95.

Beckmann MM, Stock OM. Antenatal perineal massage for reducing perineal trauma. Cochrane Database Syst Rev. 2013;(4):CD005123.

Carroli G, Mignini L. Episiotomy for vaginal birth. Cochrane Database Syst Rev. 2009;(1):CD000081. doi:10.1002/14651858.CD000081. pub2. (Meta-Analysis).

De Groot LJ, Beck-Peccoz P, Chrousos G, Dungan K, Grossman A, Hershman JM, Koch C, McLachlan R,New M, Rebar R, Singer F, Vinik A, Weickert MO, editors. Management of diabetes in pregnancy. MDText.com, Inc.; 2000–2014.

Di Mascio D, Magro-Malosso ER, Saccone G, Marhefka GD, Berghella V. Exercise during pregnancy in normal-weight women and risk of preterm birth: a systematic review and meta-analysis of randomized controlled trials. Am J Obstet Gynecol. 2016.

Erol B, Sanli O, Korkmaz D, Seyhan A, Akman T, Kadioglu A. A cross-sectional study of female sexual function and dysfunction during pregnancy. J Sex Med. 2007;4:1381–7.

Glazener CM. Sexual function after childbirth: women's experiences, persistent morbidity and lack of professional recognition. Br J Obstet Gynaecol. 1997;104(3):330–5.

Graziottin A. Mast cells and their role in sexual pain disorders. In: Goldstein A, Pukall C, Goldstein I, editors. Female sexual pain disorders: evaluation and management. Blackwell Publishing; 2009. p. 176–9.

Graziottin A. Recurrent cystitis after intercourse: why the gynaecologist has a say. In: Studd J, Seang LT, Chervenak FA, editors. Current progress in obstetrics and gynaecology, vol. 2. Mumbai: Suketu P. Kothari – TreeLife Media; 2014. p. 319–36.

Graziottin A, Gambini D. Female sexual dysfunction: treatment. In: Bø K, Berghmans B, Mørkved S, Van Kampen M, editors. Evidence-based physical therapy for the pelvic floor – bridging science and clinical practice. 2nd ed. Oxford, UK: Elsevier; 2015. p. 258–70.

Graziottin A, Gambini D, Bertolasi L. Genital and sexual pain in women. In: Vodusek D, Boller F, editors. Neurology of sexual and bladder disorders (Handbook of clinical neurology, Volume 130, 3rd Series). Elsevier; 2015. p. 395–412.

Graziottin A, Skaper S, Fusco M. Mast cells in chronic inflammation, pelvic pain and depression in women. Gynecol Endocrinol. 2014;30(7):472–7. doi:10.3109/09513590.2014.911280. Epub 2014 May 8.

Graziottin A, Zanello PP. Pathogenic biofilms: their role in recurrent cystitis and vaginitis (with focus on D-mannose as a new prophylactic strategy). In: Studd J, Seang LT, Chervenak FA, editors. Current progress in obstetrics and gynaecology, vol. 3. 2nd ed. Mumbai: Kothari Medical; 2015. p. 218–38.

Johnson CE. Sexual health during pregnancy and the postpartum. J Sex Med. 2011;8:1267–84.

Kettle C, Dowswell T, Ismail KM. Continuous and interrupted suturing techniques for repair of episiotomy or second-degree tears. Cochrane Database Syst Rev. 2012;11:CD000947.

Kettle C, Tohill S. Perineal care. BMJ Clin Evid. 2011;2011:140.

Klein MC, Gauthier RJ, Robbins JM, Kaczorowski J, Jorgensen SH, Franco ED, et al. Relationship of episiotomy to perineal trauma and morbidity, sexual dysfunction, and pelvic floor relaxation. Am J Obstet Gynecol. 1994;171:591–8.

Korja R, Piha J, Otava R, Lavanchy-Scaiola C, Ahlqvist-Björkroth S, Aromaa M, Räihä H, STEPS-study. Mother's marital satisfaction associated with the quality of mother-father-child triadic interaction. Scand J Psychol. 2016;57(4):305–12.

Leeman LM, Rogers RG. Sex after childbirth: postpartum sexual function. Obstet Gynecol. 2012;119(3):647–55.

Lien KC, Morgan DM, Delancey JO, Ashton-Miller JA. Pudendal nerve stretch during vaginal birth: a 3D computer simulation. Am J Obstet Gynecol. 2005;192(5):1669–76.

Martins NR, Kroumpouzos G. Oral and vulvovaginal changes in pregnancy. Clin Dermatol. 2016;34(3):353–8.

McDonald EA, Gartland D, Small R, Brown SJ. Dyspareunia and childbirth: a prospective cohort study. BJOG. 2015;122(5):672–9. doi:10.1111/1471-0528.13263. Epub 2015 Jan 21.

Mendling W, Brasch J. Guideline vulvovaginal candidosis (2010) of the German Society for Gynecology and Obstetrics, the Working Group for Infections and Infectimmunology in Gynecology and Obstetrics, the German Society of Dermatology, the Board of German Dermatologists and the German Speaking Mycological Society. Mycoses. 2012;55 Suppl 3:1–13.

Mucci MJ, Cuestas ML, Cervetto MM, Landaburu MF, Mujica MT. A prospective observational study of vulvovaginitis in pregnant women in Argentina, with special reference to candidiasis. Mycoses. 2016;59(7):429–35.

Muktabhant B, Lawrie TA, Lumbiganon P, Laopaiboon M. Diet or exercise, or both, for preventing excessive weight gain in pregnancy. Cochrane Database Syst Rev. 2015;(6):CD007145.

Murina F, Graziottin A, Felice R, Radici GL, Di Francesco S. The recurrent vulvovaginal candidiasis: proposal of a personalized therapeutic protocol. ISRN Obstet Gynecol. 2011;2011:806065, 4 pages. doi:10.5402/2011/806065.

Murina F, Graziottin A, Felice R, Radici G, Tognocchi C. Vestibulodynia: synergy between palmitoylethanolamide + Transpolydatin and transcutaneous electrical nerve stimulation. J Low Genit Tract Dis. 2013;17(2):111–6.

Murina F, Graziottin A, Vicariotto F, De Seta F. Can Lactobacillus fermentum LF10 and Lactobacillus acidophilus LA02 in a slow-release vaginal product be useful for prevention of recurrent vulvovaginal candidiasis? A clinical study. J Clin Gastroenterol. 2014;48 Suppl 1, Proceedings From The 7th Probiotics, Prebiotics & New Foods Meeting Held In Rome On September 8–10, 2013:S102–105.

Rezvan A, Jakus-Waldman S, Abbas MA, Yazdany T, Nguyen J. Review of the diagnosis, management and treatment of fecal incontinence. Female Pelvic Med Reconstr Surg. 2015;21(1):8–17.
Rowland M, Foxcroft L, Hopman W, Patel R. Breastfeeding and sexuality immediately postpartum. Can Fam Physician. 2005;51:1366–7.
Schmitz T, Alberti C, Andriss B, Moutafoff C, Oury JF, Sibony O. Identification of women at high risk for severe perineal lacerations. Eur J Obstet Gynecol Reprod Biol. 2014;182:11–5.
Sheikh M, Hantoushzadeh S, Shariat M, Farahani Z, Ebrahiminasab O. The efficacy of early iron supplementation on postpartum depression, a randomized double-blind placebo-controlled trial. Eur J Nutr. 2015.
Signorello LB, Harlow BL, Chekos AK, Repke JT. Postpartum sexual functioning and its relationship to perineal trauma: a retrospective cohort study of primiparous women. Am J Obstet Gynecol. 2001;184:881–8.
Smith LA, Price N, Simonite V, Burns EE. Incidence of and risk factors for perineal trauma: a prospective observational study. BMC Pregnancy Childbirth. 2013;13:59.
Webb S, Sherburn M. Managing perineal trauma after childbirth. BMJ. 2014;349:g6829.

Vulvar Pain After the Menopause

8

Women have a much longer life expectancy than men: around 80–85 years of age in the high-income countries. This means 30–35 years after the menopause. This translates into *an incredible gain in life duration* (30 years on average) in comparison to only 100 years ago, when the mean life expectancy for women, in Western Europe for example, was 48 years.

Life expectancy is not enough. Women would love to have a more appealing and longer health expectancy (HE). A longer, and hopefully happy, sexual life is part of the dream. Menopause, ongoing diseases, and a pathologic aging are the first enemies of the pursuit of a longer HE, with specific and rapid negative effects on the sexual function.

8.1 Postmenopausal Genital, Vaginal, Vulvar, Urinary, and Sexual Aging: The "Renaming" Problems

Soon after the menopause *the disappearance of the ovarian sex hormones* threatens the basic roots of genital arousal, dramatically affecting the anatomy and function of women's genital organs, vulvar and vaginal aging leading the list (Graziottin and Gambini 2015; Graziottin 2015a).

Vulvovaginal aging causes tissues' involution, named *vulvovaginal atrophy* (VVA). This causes a constellation of symptoms that include vaginal dryness and dyspareunia, the most frequently reported; vulvar and vaginal irritation; burning and itching (Phillips et al. 2015); soreness; vaginal discharge; postcoital bleeding; and postcoital cystitis (Graziottin 2014; Graziottin and Zanello 2015), just to mention the most bothersome (Graziottin et al. 2015; Graziottin and Lukasiewicz 2016).

All these symptoms are reported after a natural menopause and, with a more invalidating impact, after premature menopause (Graziottin and Lukasiewicz 2015), more so if associated with oncologic surgery and treatments (Graziottin and Lukasiewicz 2016).

A. Graziottin, F. Murina, *Vulvar Pain*, DOI 10.1007/978-3-319-42677-8_8

The term VVA has been recently modified in *Genitourinary Syndrome of the Menopause (GSM)* (Portman and Gass 2014) (Box 8.1), more inclusive of the comorbid urinary symptoms. Women may present with some or all the signs and symptoms. However, most of the published literature is still using the VVA definition (Freedman 2009; Nappi and Kokot-Kierepa 2012; Nappi et al. 2013; Nappi and Palacios 2014; Parish et al. 2013). VVA can be definitely considered the vulvovaginal component of GSM (Genitourinary Syndrome of the Menopause). Therefore both terms will be used here.

Box 8.1. The Genitourinary Syndrome of the Menopause (GSM)
It includes:

- *Genital symptoms*: vulvovaginal atrophy, vulvar burning, vulvar itching, soreness, and vaginal discharge
- *Sexual symptoms*: vaginal dryness, genital arousal difficulties, dyspareunia (painful intercourse), and postcoital bleeding
- *Urinary symptoms*: urgency, frequency, urinary incontinence, and recurrent cystitis

The same classification problems hold true for coital pain. While dyspareunia translates easily into "painful intercourse" in the clinical setting, *classification difficulties make definitions very complex and still under debate*. The same pathophysiology of dyspareunia is discussed. Dyspareunia has been now renamed genito-pelvic pain penetration disorder (GPPPD) in DSM V (2015), with critical aspect in differential diagnosis between vaginismus and dyspareunia still unresolved (Lahaie et al. 2015; Reissing et al. 2014).

For example, in every woman the clinician should assess how much of the coital pain depends on:

- The vulva (and specifically here from the vulvar aging after the menopause)
- The vestibular mucosa changes or frank inflammation (postmenopausal vulvar vestibulitis (VV) or provoked vestibulodynia (PVD)
- The vaginal dryness and aging
- The hyperactive pelvic floor
- An inadequate processing of painful stimuli potentiated by fear in a subset of women

Of note, the neuropathic vulvar pain labeled as "provoked vestibulodynia" and "vulvodynia" is not limited to younger women (although it certainly peaks around the 30 years of age) but can affect as well the postmenopausal women.

A recent very accurate paper of Philips et al. (2015), aimed at describing similarities and differences in symptoms of PVD in pre- and postmenopausal women, indicate that postmenopausal women reported significantly more *vulvar burning* (70.00 % vs 43.42 %, $P = 0.03$), but there were no differences in vulvar itching

(20.00 % vs 22.37 %, $P=0.82$), vulvar stinging (40.00 % vs 36.84 %, $P=0.79$), vulvar aching (50.00 % vs 63.16 %, $P=0.28$), and vulvar stabbing (60.00 % vs 71.06 % $P=0.34$) or in mean number of symptoms (2.40 ± 1.0 vs 2.37 ± 1.4, $P=0.92$). In conclusion, pre- and postmenopausal women with PVD have similar pain scores and with the exception of a higher incidence of burning vulvar pain in postmenopausal women and similar presenting clinical symptoms.

Pain is therefore one of the leading and often neglected symptoms of the menopausal genital, vulvar, and sexual aging. This chapter will focus specifically on *vulvar pain after the menopause* and related genital and sexual symptom, considering VVA a part of GSM. The term dyspareunia or coital pain will be preferred, with the most recent acronym GPPPD used in brackets. Given this complexity, the Authors accept the challenge of trying to give *a systematic perspective* within the limits of a very magmatic classification and the persisting uncertainties from the clinical and pathophysiologic point of view.

Falling estrogen and testosterone levels after the menopause may trigger different types of vulvar pain and introital dyspareunia or genito-pelvic pain penetration disorders (GPPPD), according to different anatomic, functional, and clinical pictures, that can partly overlap. Besides aging:

- *Candida* infections may re-exacerbate PVD, in women who suffered from it in the fertile age.
- Papillomavirus infections may contribute to the oncogenic process leading to vulvar cancer and pain (Alkatout et al. 2015).

Leading etiologies of vulvar pain after the menopause are summarized in Box 8.2, where different potential contributors are "polarized" for the sake of clarity. In the clinical setting, they can be comorbid and need to be carefully diagnosed to be properly addressed.

Box 8.2. Leading Etiologies of Vulvar Pain After the Menopause

Etiologies of vulvar pain include:

1. *The VVA*, with the associated anatomic and functional changes that lead to a progressive increasing thinning of the vestibular mucosa and vulvar skin, reduced lubrication, increased pH, altered vaginal and vulvar microbiota, and increased vulnerability to microabrasions and introital pain (dyspareunia, GPPPD), with secondary reflexive contraction of the levator ani.
2. *The vestibular pain (PVD)*, histologically more similar to the picture demonstrated in the PVD of the younger cohort, with a prominent inflammatory (mast cell dominated) tissue finding. The development of a subtype of menopausal vestibulodynia can explain the number of cases of postmenopausal coital pain. We hypothesize that the vestibule is more sensitive to withdrawal of estrogen during menopause and develops the features of vestibulodynia alongside visual changes of atrophy, at least in a subset of

vulnerable patients. The vagina can also develop marked atrophy but does not become tender to the same degree as the vestibule because it has a different innervation.

3. *The vulvar/vestibular pain* that can be associated with a more prominent vulvar dermatoses, like lichen sclerosus, which contributes to the narrowing of the vaginal introitus and introital dyspareunia.
4. *Vulvar cancer*, HPV or not HPV associated, can cause/contribute to vulvar pain.
5. *Iatrogenic vulvar pain* after vulvar, anal, or bladder surgery and radio/laser therapy.
6. *Post-traumatic vulvar pain, unintentional and intentional* (sexual abuse).

In the real life these pictures can partly overlap.

8.2 Impact of Estrogens' and Androgens' Loss on Genital and Vulvar Trophism

Hot flashes are the most commonly identified hallmark of menopause and aging. However, many women also suffer with *a constellation of vulvovaginal symptoms* as a result of lowered estrogen and androgens (Graziottin and Lukasiewicz 2015). They are the tip of the iceberg of an underlying progressive genital involution leading to *VVA, GSM, and vulvar pain.* Genital menopausal and urinary symptoms become rapidly prominent in the majority of women, because the urogenital epithelium is particularly vulnerable to hormonal changes, unless an appropriate hormonal menopause therapy, at least topical, is performed. The characteristic vulvovaginal changes that occur during and after the menopause are due to the combination of pathophysiologic aging, hypoestrogenism, and hypoandrogenism (Graziottin and Gambini 2015).

Estradiol, the primary form of estrogen produced by a woman's ovary during her reproductive years, plays an essential role in maintaining the elasticity and health of the genital tissues, including *an appropriate vaginal and vulvar microbiota and an adequate low vaginal pH* (Graziottin and Zanello 2015) The genital involution is more rapid and anticipated in women affected by a premature ovarian insufficiency (Graziottin and Lukasiewicz 2015). An iatrogenic menopause after gynecologic cancers may have an even more dramatic impact on anatomy and function of genital organs, when the premature or anticipated menopause is complicated with the side effects of vaginal/pelvic radiotherapy (Lukasiewicz and Graziottin 2015; Graziottin and Lukasiewicz 2016).

Testosterone is responsible for the hormone-dependent involution of the cavernosal bodies (clitoral, bulbocavernous, and part of the equivalent of the male corpus spongiosum, around the urethra), of the androgen-dependent cells of the skin, of the connective tissue (fibroblasts and myocells), and of the androgen-dependent nitrergic nerve fibers, present at vaginal (1/3 nitrergic, 2/3 vipergic) and vulvar level (Graziottin and Gambini 2015).

8.3 Postmenopausal Dyspareunia

Dyspareunia, genital pain associated with sexual intercourse, is a common symptom in postmenopausal sexually active women. It can adversely affect their sexual quality of life or intensify preexisting sexual disorders (Schneidewind-Skibbe et al. 2008):

- Approximately 40 % of postmenopausal women report dyspareunia.
- Fifty-two percent of women 50–79 years of age have been sexually active with a partner in the past year.
- Twenty-two percent of married women, 70–79 years of age, report that they still have sexual intercourse.

8.4 VVA: The Three Enemies of Vulvovaginal Health in the Clinical Setting

Three major problems impair the appropriate diagnosis and treatment of VVA (Graziottin 2015a), including vulvar pain: symptoms caused by VVA are *underreported*, *underdiagnosed*, and *undertreated*.

8.4.1 Underreported

Embarrassment, related to the intimacy of the complaints, holds women back to seek professional advice. However, in the VIVA survey among 3520 postmenopausal women, 53 % of participants said that they would feel comfortable discussing "vaginal" discomfort with their doctor (of note, many women call "vagina" the vulva!), while 37 % would not raise the subject or hesitate to do so (Nappi and Kokot-Kierepa 2012). A third would not even tell their partner (Nappi et al. 2013).

A pervading *collusion of silence* that translates into a substantial diagnostic neglect is preventing effective communication, both in the high- and low-income world. In addition, general ignorance about the condition also plays a major role in the underreporting, with only 4 % of women attributing their symptoms to vulvovaginal atrophy and 63 % failing to recognize vulvovaginal atrophy as a chronic condition that requires ongoing treatment of the underlying cause (Nappi and Kokot-Kierepa 2012).

Few women attributed symptoms to menopause (24 %) or hormonal changes (12 %) (Kingsberg et al. 2013). Many women expect their doctor to start the discussion about postmenopausal vaginal health, but 50 % of the total survey population claimed that their doctor had not raised the subject (Nappi and Kokot-Kierepa 2012). Even less women think that the vulva "could age," because of the menopause. They usually report symptoms only when vulvar itching and scratching (usually associated with lichen sclerosus) become a problem.

8.4.2 Underdiagnosed

Vulvovaginal atrophy is also called *atrophic vaginitis*. This wording is accurate as the increase of inflammatory molecules in the vagina, particularly IL-1 and IL-8, is the leading feature of this organ after menopause, without hormone therapy. It parallels the increase of vaginal pH and the decrease of lactobacilli. It is a chronic, progressive condition that results from the decrease in estrogen levels in the vagina that commonly occurs after the menopause.

The *diagnosis* of VVA is commonly based on a combination of symptoms, gynecological history and clinical findings of vulvovaginal atrophy during examination (atrophy of the introitus and labia, disappearance of the rugae, and a dry, thin, friable mucosa which can be reddened or paled with petechiae), sometimes supported by pH testing (pH>5) and the Vaginal Maturation Index (e.g., <5 % superficial cells) (MacBride et al. 2010). It is a clinical diagnosis, but requires the doctor to have an interest in the vaginal and vulvar health of the patients with 40 % of patients expecting the doctor to initiate the discussion (Kingsberg et al. 2013). It is estimated that between 69 (Gass et al. 2011) and 98 % (Freedman 2009) of postmenopausal women have signs of vulvovaginal atrophy, with worsening features with increasing age after the menopause. More than 70 % of men note that their partner avoided sexual intimacy because of vaginal discomfort (Nappi et al. 2013)

Despite the impact on quality of life and relationships, the fact that 62 % of women complain of moderate or severe symptoms and 55 % had the symptoms for 3 or more years (Nappi and Kokot-Kierepa 2012), vulvar and vaginal atrophy remains an underreported, underdiagnosed, and therefore also an undertreated condition (Parish et al. 2013) for a number of different reasons. The figures are constant worldwide. It is estimated that 10–40 % of postmenopausal women experience discomfort due to a vulvovaginal atrophy (VVA) that requires treatment, but only 25 % of these women seek treatment. Seventy-five percent of postmenopausal women suffer vaginal dryness; 15 % complain of vulvovaginal itching, discharge, and pain (The North American Menopause Society Menopause 2013).

It is important for physicians to have a clinical interest in maintaining the sexual function and erotic value of the vagina and vulva of their patients (even if these do not specifically and clearly ask for help), with a clinically accurate diagnosis and treatment (Nappi et al. 2016).

8.4.3 Undertreated

The underreporting and underdiagnosing of VVA itself lead to undertreatment of the condition. The REVIVE US survey among postmenopausal US women with VVA revealed that only 40 % was using any form of treatment, with those who discussed the condition with their doctor being twice as likely to have treatment than those who did not (Kingsberg et al. 2013).

In the VIVA survey, just under half (49 %) of all women with VVA complaints had tried lubricants and moisturizers, but these do not treat the underlying condition (Nappi and Kokot-Kierepa 2012), and the efficacy on vaginal symptoms is lower than that of topical estrogen therapy in the trials published thus far. Systemic HRT, on the other hand, relieves vaginal atrophy in about 75 % of women, but is usually not recommended in women with vaginal symptoms only (Sturdee and Panay 2010). The mainstay of treatment for VVA has been local vaginal estrogens.

However, in the VIVA survey, 30 % of women said that they would not consider taking local estrogen therapy, even if they knew it to be effective (Nappi and Kokot-Kierepa 2012). In the REVIVE EU survey, less than half (45 %) of the participants were satisfied with their current treatment. For over-the-counter (OTC) products, the concerns were mainly about efficacy, and for local estrogens they were about safety (REVIVE EU 2015). Among those who expressed a preference for treatment administration, 55 % indicated they would prefer an oral product (Kingsberg et al. 2013). Finally, the labels of all local estrogens exclude women with a history of breast cancer and other hormone-dependent cancers, as systemic absorption has been demonstrated for these treatments (Labrie et al. 2009; Del Pup et al. 2012).

Key Point

Vulvovaginal atrophy in postmenopausal women can lead to symptoms, including vulvar and vestibular pain that significantly impact self-esteem, quality of life, and relationships.

There is a dire need to educate such women about the potential for effective treatment. Doctors and other healthcare providers should be willing to open up the conversation about vaginal health to assist in diagnosing and treating all those women who come to seek help.

8.5 Genital Arousal Disorders and Dyspareunia (GPPD) in VVA and GSM

Vaginal dryness is the first and leading symptom of VVA, and therefore of GSM, contributing to genital arousal disorders after the menopause. It may cause coital pain/dyspareunia. It is (still) neglected in the majority of women after the menopause for the abovementioned reasons.

Contributors include *vaginal atrophy*, *vulvar dystrophy*, and *vestibular atrophy with hyperalgesia*, the most neglected contributor to introital dyspareunia in postmenopausal women. In more rare cases, an (advanced) *vulvar cancer* may overlap with the atrophic changes.

Urogenital epithelium is particularly vulnerable to *hormonal changes*.

The characteristic vulvovaginal changes that occur during and after the menopause are due to the combination of physiological aging, hypoestrogenism, and hypoandrogenism. The latter is responsibile for the hormone-dependent involution of the cavernosal bodies (clitoral, bulbocavernous, and part of the equivalent of the male corpus spongiosum, around the urethra), of the androgen-dependent cells of the vulvar skin, of the connective tissue (fibroblasts and myocells), and of the nitrergic nerve fibers contributing to 1/3 of vaginal nerve fibers and the majority of vulvar nerve fibers. Notably, nitrergic fibers recognize testosterone as "permitting factor" potentiating the vascular-mediated genital arousal response in both genders.

8.6 Diagnosis: The Clinical Examination Is Key (also) After the Menopause

The vagina loses elasticity, shortens, narrows, becomes less distensible, and can, therefore, be easily traumatized and irritated. Vaginal secretions may decrease, and evidence of inflammation and small petechiae may be visible.

A watery, scalding discharge may be present and superficial fissuring is not an unusual finding, and lack of estrogen depletes vaginal intracellular glycogen, resulting in reduced lactobacilli bacteria, causing increased vaginal pH that should be recorded. Accurate physical examination is key (Box 8.3).

Box 8.3. Vulvovaginal Anatomic Changes Caused by Decreased Hormone Levels in Menopause (Figs. 8.1 and 8.2)

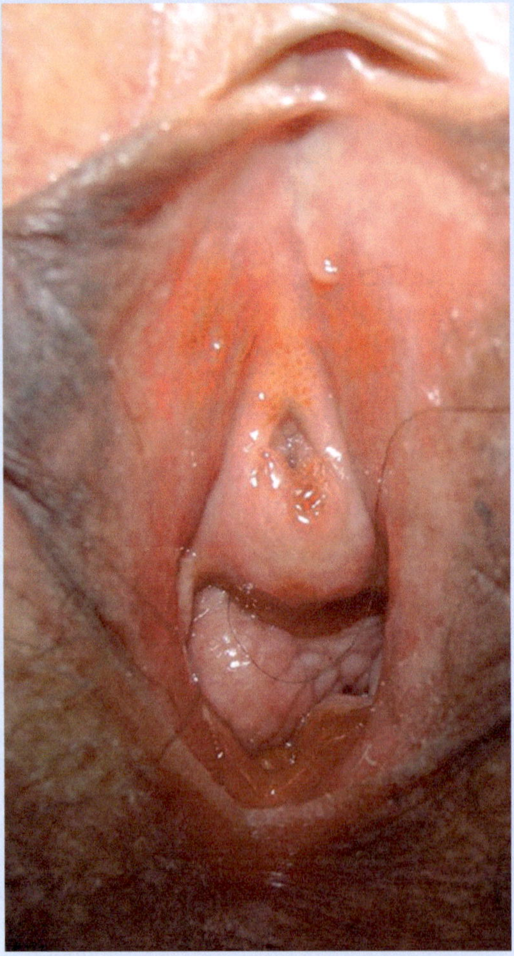

Fig. 8.1 Vestibule appears very thin with erosive appearance

Fig. 8.2 Atrophic changes of vulvar vestibule

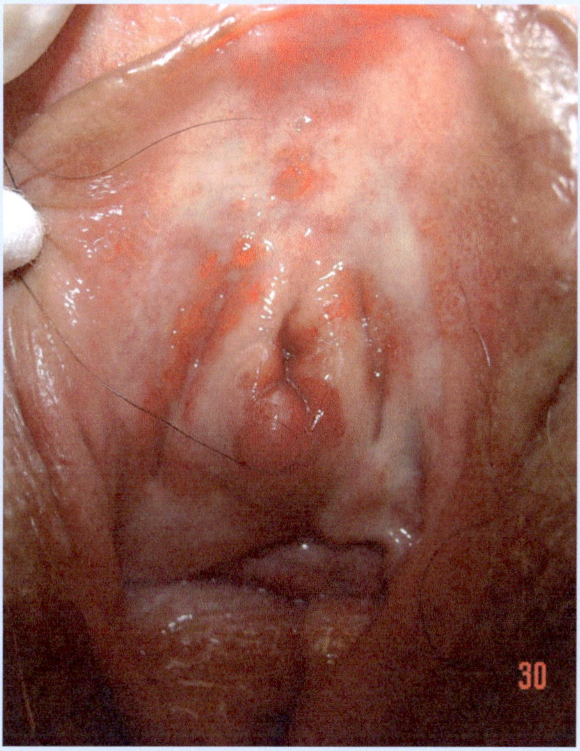

- Atrophy of vaginal epithelium
- Reduction of pubic hair
- Loss of fat and subcutaneous tissue from the mons pubis
- Atrophy of the labia majora
- Shortening and loss of elasticity of the vaginal barrel

8.7 The Vestibule: A Trigger of Vulvar Pain *also* After the Menopause

Very few studies on postmenopausal dyspareunia have been focused on location and quality of pain. It was reported that 95 % of menopausal women with dyspareunia also had localized provoked pain in the vestibule, despite the use of hormone supplements in 31 % of them (Kao et al. 2012a). The swab test remains a key for this specific diagnosis.

Vestibular pain is principally related to differences in nerve density between vagina and vulvar vestibule.

A rich nerve plexus within the vaginal submucosa was identified, but it is composed only of sympathetic and parasympathetic axons with smaller contributions by sensory fibers; in the vulvar vestibule, the sensory nerve endings are dense and shallow, making this region physiologically more sensitive.

The association of low estrogen levels and nerve proliferation in vaginas of rats has already been reported; at baseline estrogen levels in estrus cycles, nerves proliferate, and then these nerves retreat when estrogen is higher (Zoubina and Smith 2001). This is consistent with observations that postpartum women can exhibit entry dyspareunia in approximately 50 % of attempts at intercourse, and resolution is associated with the return of menstruation after lactation (Goetsch 1999).

Key Point

Many menopausal women with complaints of dyspareunia have vestibular tenderness with more pronounced atrophic changes in this region rather than in the vagina (Fig. 8.3).

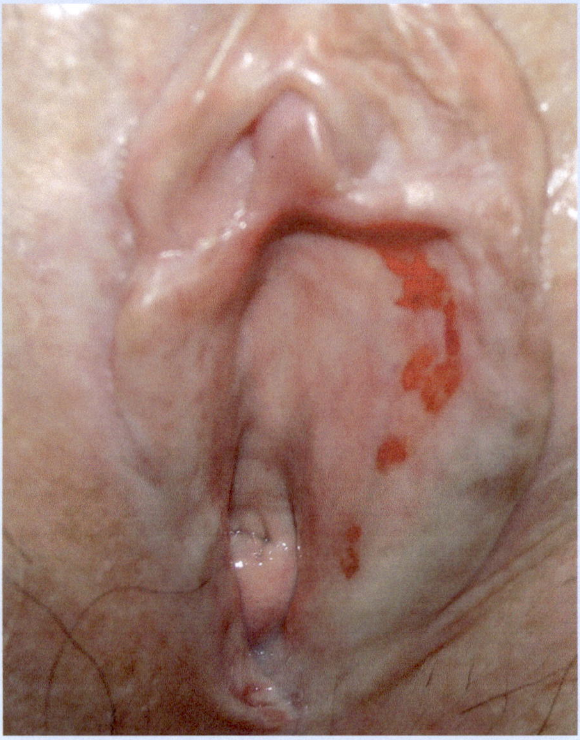

Fig. 8.3 Vestibule very thin with hemorrhagic area at Hart's line

Furthermore, it is likely, as Kao et al. suggests, that vulvovaginal atrophy alone does not adequately explain the findings of vestibular pain (Kao et al. 2012b). In 95 % of her postmenopausal cohort with vestibular pain and dyspareunia, women used a variety of estrogen supplements, and atrophy varied but vestibular pain persisted.

It was demonstrated that vaginal innervation in rats is also responsive to endogenous and exogenous estrogen, resulting in reductions in neurovegetative axons and in peptidergic sensory fibers.

Topical estrogen therapy is effective in reducing the density of vaginal autonomic and sensory nerves. Estrogen is known to affect inflammatory neuropeptides involved in chronic pain, in which the lack of estrogens is associated with an increased density of sympathetic, parasympathetic, and sensory nerve fibers in the vulva; acute or chronic estrogen administration may decrease the total and sympathetic fiber numbers (Straub 2007). We can conclude that *between the level of estrogen and vaginal innervation, there is an inverse relationship*.

Exogenous estrogen therapy has *multiple effects on the vagina*, including increased blood flow, improved epithelial thickness, reduced pH, normalization of the microbiota with prominent lactobacilli, reduced concentration of inflammatory molecules (such as IL-1 and IL-6), and increased secretions (see below).

However, many data have suggested that although these factors are important, they are incomplete as explicative mechanisms:

- Autonomic and sensory neurons express estrogen receptors and are responsive to estradiol in culture, supporting the idea that estrogens can act directly on neurons (Ting et al. 2004).
- Vaginal innervation was reduced in women receiving estrogen replacement; moreover, topical therapy is more effective than systemic therapy (Griebling et al. 2012).

8.8 Treatment Perspectives for VVA, GSM, *and* Vulvar Pain

Treatment perspectives include:

1. Raising women's awareness on the relationship between menopause and VVA/GSM and vulvar pain
2. Selecting a well-tailored pharmacologic treatment for vestibular/vulvar pain associated with VVA/GSM
3. Selecting other possible non-pharmacological therapies.

8.8.1 Raising Women's Awareness

This strategy includes:

- *To promote an open dialogue on genital, sexual, and urinary symptoms, to avoid the "collusion of silence"* (Graziottin et al. 2016): women feel often ashamed and embarrassed particularly to speak about sexual issues with their physician. The majority of women think that vaginal atrophy and vulvar pain are a normal and ineluctable event. It is the physician's responsibility to raise the subject in a respectful and constructive approach, with the goal of reducing the percentage of "underreported and underdiagnosed" cases of VVA, GSM, *and* Vulvar pain.

- *To promote a comprehensive treatment and to avoid a minimalistic approach*: what happens when a sexual problem is raised? Are we able to treat it? The majority of women affected with VVA, GSM, and vulvar pain receive a lubricant as an answer when they ask for treatment. This is perceived as humiliating by the woman, as a deception by the man, and as a frustrating *fiction of arousal* by the couple (Graziottin et al. 2016).

8.8.2 Pharmacologic Treatments

8.8.2.1 Hormones (Box 8.4)

Topical estrogens (estradiol, estriol, promestriene, conjugated estrogens) should be prescribed *soon after the menopause when vaginal dryness is the tip of the iceberg of VVA (*The North American Menopause Society Menopause 2013; Rahn et al 2014*)*. *Estriol* has 1/80 of estradiol potency, and it is the safest estrogen (as it has a prominent action on estrogen receptor beta, which has antiproliferative and reparative actions). It can be used in form of vaginal gel or vaginal suppositories, every other day, to maintain vaginal and bladder trophism. *Estrogens* have an effect on vaginal epithelium, diminishing postmenopausal VVA, protecting the normal pH and vaginal microbiota ("healthy biofilm") (Graziottin and Zanello 2015), and thus decreasing the incidence of *E. Coli's* vaginitis and lower urinary tract infections (UTIs). They also have a protective effect on the urethra and on the bladder, thus reducing urge urinary incontinence, overactive bladder, and recurrent postcoital cystitis that is complained of 24–72 h after the intercourse (Graziottin 2015b). Topical estrogens are still contraindicated in case of adenocarcinomata of the uterus and of breast cancer.

Systemic estrogens Women with uterus should use estrogens combined with progesterone/progestins, indicated to protect the endometrium, either in cyclical or continuous combined regimen. Tibolone is another option. After hysterectomy, women can use only estrogens. The WHI study clearly indicates that the postmenopausal treatment with only estrogens in hysterectomized women significantly *reduces the risk of breast cancer*, while it maintains all the benefits on cardiovascular system, brain, bones, joints, gastrointestinal system, urogenital system, and on sensory organs, skin and mucosae first. It can therefore be used in the long term, if symptoms persist. However, as the systemic administration may not be sufficient to guarantee a normal vaginal lubrication, topical estrogens should be considered to optimize the functional outcome in individual cases. Hormones are indicated as well after squamous cell carcinoma of the cervix or if bilateral ovariectomy (for cancers different from adenocarcinomas) has been performed.

Topical testosterone On the vulva and vagina, as cream of testosterone propionate (2%) or testosterone of vegetal origin, in galenic preparation. Topical testosterone improves *the vulvar trophism in the clinical setting*. The pathophysiological plausibility is consistent with the rich density of testosterone receptors of the vulvar tissue (Graziottin and Gambini 2015), due to its embryologic origin from the cloacal sinus. The (relative) anti-inflammatory activity of testosterone, in downregulating the hyperactive mast cells in case of introital vulvar pain (provoked vestibulodynia, PVD), is another plus to be considered. However a Cochrane evaluation of testosterone use in lichen sclerosus, a leading cause of itching/vulvar pain and introital dyspareunia, failed to show beneficial effects. The same review confirmed the benefits of clobetasol propionate 0.05 % in relieving lichen symptoms (Chi et al. 2011). After the natural menopause, by the age of 50, women loose more than 50 % of the total testosterone. This contributes to sexual symptoms (loss of desire/interest and drive, of systemic and genital arousal, reduced lubrication, and cavernosal congestion and impaired orgasm) (Davis et al. 2016) and systemic symptoms (depression, low vital energy, fatigue), unless testosterone is replaced. Consistent data were found during the research clinical studies on testosterone patches, excellent but currently not available in the market (DeRogatis et al. 2009). After 3 months of topical treatment, women report a more rapid genital congestion, more intense feelings of pleasure, and a reassuring orgasm "comeback." Authors' clinical experience suggests that *vulvar pain from vestibular atrophy is reduced, more so if rehabilitation of the pelvic floor is recommended*, when hyperactivity of the levator ani is a cofactor in the entry dyspareunia and vestibular pain (see below). Partner reports that the physical response of the woman is more gratifying for both partners ("a velvet vagina is definitely a most welcomed result after month/years of dry sex") (Graziottin et al. 2016).

Topical DHEA (prasterone), in cream applied in the vagina, is another useful tool to be explored in treatment of VVA and GSM. Preliminary data are very positive in terms of vaginal lubrication, with no changes in the systemic levels of prasterone (Bouchard et al. 2016; Davis et al. 2016; Labrie et al. 2016; Martel et al. 2016). Daily dosing is necessary as reduced efficacy has been shown when the treatment is reduced to two doses/week (Bouchard et al. 2016). Specific research on vulvar/vestibular pain has not been carried out so far in the Authors' knowledge. However the pharmacology and mechanism of action suggest that the effect could be positive, on daily dosing, as shown (still preliminary results) by Authors' experience.

DHEA systemic (10 or 25 mg) Evidence-based data suggest modest systemic effects on sexuality, mood, and cognition (Pluchino et al. 2015). Preclinical data suggest that DHEA may have positive effects on the immune system in modulating the aging process (Corsini et al. 2016). However in the clinical setting, many women report more energy, more positive feelings, and increased muscle tone and strength (contrasting the sarcopenia typical of aging and menopause). The potential synergy with topical hormonal treatments in improving vulvovaginal trophism, reducing VVA and GSM, and relieving vulvar pain deserves further prospective studies.

Box 8.4. Key Point: Time Is Key

- *Window of opportunity*: "The sooner, the better" is the motto for hopefully preventing and treating VVA, GSM, and vulvar pain, when they are complained of. The delay in the hormonal treatment, at least vaginal, leads to progressive (and non-completely reversible) atrophic changes, tissue retraction, and sexual dysfunctions.
- *Lifelong treatment is key,* as women need estrogens, at least topical, in the vagina, *until the end of their life* and not only for a short period of time. Would we use insulin "for the shortest period of time"? This is a biological nonsense for estrogens too, when they are not specifically contraindicated (in case of adenocarcinoma of the cervix or of the uterus, or in case of breast cancer). At least topical hormonal treatments (such as estriol in gel) should be considered lifelong, to prevent and cure the vaginal/bladder consequences of VVA and GSM (Graziottin et al. 2016).
- *Testosterone and prasterone* deserve long-term studies on efficacy, focusing also on treatment of vulvar pain, and safety.

8.8.3 Selective Estrogen Receptor Modulators (SERMS)

Ospemifene is an estrogen agonist and antagonist approved by the US Federal Drug Administration (FDA) for the treatment of "moderate to severe dyspareunia, a symptom of vulvar and vaginal atrophy, due to menopause" (Cui et al. 2014; Pinkerton and Kagan 2015). Its mechanism of action, typical of the SERM family, is protective for the breast. The drug is approved also for women treated for breast cancer who completed all the treatments, including the adjuvant ones. Ospemifene can be *the drug of choice for women who suffer from VVA, who do not want vaginal treatments (hormonal or nonhormonal) and would love to have a good vaginal health and responsiveness while being perfectly reassured about breast safety*. Ospemifene does significantly improve vaginal symptoms and underlying atrophy and symptoms of vulvar irritation/itching (Bruyniks et al. 2016), but not necessarily/specifically the vulvar atrophy, according to some very recent case reports (Goldstein and King 2016). *Published, peer-reviewed, placebo-controlled studies have shown objective improvement in dyspareunia, vaginal atrophy, and vulvar irritation/itching*. However, Goldstein and King state that there are no published data that have specifically assessed changes in vulvar atrophy after the use of ospemifene. Specific prospective, controlled studies are needed to better qualify its role in relieving vulvar atrophy and pain related/caused by the atrophic changes, by PVD and by intercourse experienced in such negative tissue conditions. Testosterone cream could be a better choice for nonresponsive cases given the rich testosterone receptor pool in the vulva, its androgen-sensitive embryology, and the underappreciated anti-inflammatory effect of testosterone on the inflammatory cascade. Prospective studies combining systemic ospemifene and topical testosterone should be carried out to evaluate the potential synergy, both in terms of improved tissue trophism and sexual function, while considering the long-term safety.

Bazedoxifene (BZA) and Conjugated Estrogens (CE) The combination between a SERM and CE has been shown effective in the control of menopausal symptoms, including VVA, while preventing osteopenia/osteoporosis (Bachmann et al. 2010; Kagan et al. 2010; Abraham et al. 2014). This combination does not cause an increase of breast cancer risk, thanks to the protective effect of bazedoxifene on the breast. This is very reassuring, after the worldwide concerns raised by the Women's Health Initiative study (WHI) when CE were used with medroxyprogesterone acetate (MAP). The BZA/CE combination can be considered when VVA is the tip of the iceberg of a more complex menopausal symptomatology in women who would like to address their systemic and genital symptoms in safety from the breast risk point of view. However, specific data focusing on the vulvar trophism and relief of vulvar pain require further controlled studies.

8.8.3.1 Nonhormonal Treatments

Hyaluronic acid in gel or ovules, colostrum gel, phytotherapic creams, and lubricants can be considered in women who do not want or cannot use hormonal treatments, systemic or local vaginal and vulvar.

8.8.4 Non-pharmacological Treatments

8.8.4.1 Physiotherapic Rehabilitation

Physiotherapists, but also specifically trained nurses and midwives, can have a still underappreciated role in the pelvic floor rehabilitation when a hyperactive pelvic floor contributes to introital dyspareunia and vestibular pain after the menopause (Graziottin and Gambini 2016; Mercier et al. 2016). Specific treatment care includes a preliminary and/or parallel pharmacologic treatment (either hormonal or nonhormonal) of vaginal dryness.

Physiotherapy includes:

- *Vaginal dilators, when the stenosis of the vagina is severe*. This complication is most frequently seen in VVA and vulvar pain after years of neglect. It worsens when lichen sclerosus further reduces the entrance of the vagina. Radiation therapy for gynecologic, anal, or bladder cancers is another worsening factor, to be carefully looked after particularly in young women who long for resuming a normal vaginal receptiveness and vulvar responsiveness after the threatening experience of a pelvic cancer. Dilators and topical estrogen and/or testosterone or prasterone therapy can synergize in reducing vaginal dryness and dyspareunia and improving vulvar trophism while reducing vulvar pain. In the Authors' practice, molds or dilators with progressive increase of dimensions can be used home daily for 5 min, twice a day. The combination with topical hormonal treatment, stretching of the levator ani "hands-on" (see below), and molds/dilators provides more rapid and better outcomes in terms of vaginal sexual elasticity, receptiveness, and vulvovaginal responsiveness. The option of combining physiotherapy with a systemic hormonal treatment, or with a SERM alone (ospemifene), or with a combination of BZA/CE, is to be decided with clinical wisdom to offer the best-tailored treatment to the individual woman.

- *Pelvic floor rehabilitation hands-on* may further contribute to maintain elasticity through appropriate stretching, massage, and physiotherapy (Graziottin and Gambini 2016).

8.8.4.2 Regular Sexual Activity

If desired, it has a great benefit in preventing vaginal atrophy, when at least a minimum physiologic response is in play. The trophic impact of the neurovascular response associated with genital arousal is likely to promote genital neuroplasticity, endothelial trophism, and vessel plasticity and improve the genital sexual self-schema as well. More so the genital and vulvar tissue anatomy and physiology are maintained with appropriate hormonal, SERM, or nonhormonal treatments.

8.8.4.3 Laser Treatments

Pulsed CO_2 lasers (Salvatore et al. 2015; Pieralli et al. 2016) (Monnalisa) and erbium laser treatment (Gambacciani et al. 2015) are increasingly used in the treatment of VVA after the menopause, particularly in women after breast cancer. These treatment options should be considered and proposed to the individual woman among the different treatment opportunities.

8.8.4.4 Psychosexual Therapy

Brief psychosexual interventions may be indicated when the persistence of sexual symptoms caused by a neglected VVA/GSM or vulvar pain has caused secondary loss of desire and/or relational problems. The focus is on physical, psychosexual, and relational aspects of sexuality and intimacy that goes far beyond a dry vagina and a painful vulva.

Conclusions

Postmenopausal vulvar pain may by the tip of the iceberg of different contributing conditions: VVA/GSM, postmenopausal provoked vestibulodynia, vulvar dystrophy, and associated comorbidities, such as lichen sclerosus, that can be isolated or present in comorbidity; vulvar cancer can cause pain in a subset of women; iatrogenic factors can contribute. The skilled physician should encourage the woman to disclose the bothersome symptoms of VVA/GMS and specifically of vulvar pain, make a comprehensive differential diagnosis of different etiological factors, and design a well-tailored treatment, offering an accurate follow-up.

The goal of increasing and improving women's health expectancy is of the highest importance, also from the genital, vulvar, and sexual point of view.

References

Abraham L, Pinkerton JV, Messig M, Ryan KA, Komm BS, Mirkin S. Menopause-specific quality of life across varying menopausal populations with conjugated estrogens/bazedoxifene. Maturitas. 2014;78(3):212–8. doi:10.1016/j.maturitas.2014.04.008. Epub 2014 Apr 26.

Alkatout I, Schubert M, Garbrecht N, Weigel MT, Jonat W, Mundhenke C, Gunther V. Vulvar cancer: epidemiology, clinical presentation, and management options. Int J Womens Health. 2015;7:305–13. doi:10.2147/IJWH.S68979. eCollection 2015.

Bachmann G, Bobula J, Mirkin S. Effects of bazedoxifene/conjugated estrogens on quality of life in postmenopausal women with symptoms of vulvar/vaginal atrophy. Climacteric. 2010;13(2):132–40.

Bouchard C, Labrie F, Derogatis L, Girard G, Ayotte N, Gallagher J, Cusan L, Archer DF, Portman D, Lavoie L, Beauregard A, Côté I, Martel C, Vaillancourt M, Balser J, Moyneur E, other participating Members of the VVA Prasterone Group. Effect of intravaginal dehydroepiandrosterone (DHEA) on the female sexual function in postmenopausal women: ERC-230 open-label study. Horm Mol Biol Clin Investig. 2016;25(3):181–90.

Bruyniks N, Nappi RE, Castelo-Branco C, de Villiers TJ, Simon J. Effect of ospemifene on moderate or severe symptoms of vulvar and vaginal atrophy. Climacteric. 2016;19(1):60–5.

Chi CC, Kirtschig G, Baldo M, Brackenbury F, Lewis F, Wojnarowska F. Topical interventions for genital lichen sclerosus. Cochrane Database Syst Rev. 2011;(12):CD008240.

Corsini E, Galbiati V, Papale A, Kummer E, Pinto A, Serafini MM, Guaita A, Spezzano R, Caruso D, Marinovich M, Racchi M. Role of androgens in dhea-induced rack1 expression and cytokine modulation in monocytes. Immun Ageing. 2016;13:20. doi:10.1186/s12979-016-0075-y. eCollection 2016.

Cui Y, Zong H, Yan H, Li N, Zhang Y. The efficacy and safety of ospemifene in treating dyspareunia associated with postmenopausal vulvar and vaginal atrophy: a systematic review and meta-analysis. J Sex Med. 2014;11(2):487–97.

Davis SR, Worsley R, Miller KK, Parish SJ, Santoro N. Androgens and female sexual function and dysfunction – findings from the fourth international consultation of sexual medicine. J Sex Med. 2016;13(2):168–78.

Del Pup L, Postruznik D, Corona G. Effect of one-month treatment with vaginal promestriene on serum estrone sulfate levels in cancer patients: a pilot study. Maturitas. 2012;72:93–4.

DeRogatis LR, Graziottin A, Bitzer J, Schmitt S, Koochaki PE, Rodenberg C. Clinically relevant changes in sexual desire, satisfying sexual activity and personal distress as measured by the profile of female sexual function, sexual activity log, and personal distress scale in postmenopausal women with hypoactive sexual desire disorder. J Sex Med. 2009;6(1):175–8.

Diagnostic and statistical manual of mental disorders fifth edition (DSM V). American Psychiatric Association Ed. 2015.

Freedman MA. Vaginal pH, estrogen and genital atrophy. Menopause Manag. 2009;17(4):9–13.

Gambacciani M, Torelli MG, Martella L, Bracco GL, Casagrande AG, Albertin E, Tabanelli S, Viglietta M, D'Ambrogio G, Garone G, Cervigni M. Rationale and design for the Vaginal Erbium Laser Academy Study (VELAS): an international multicenter observational study on genitourinary syndrome of menopause and stress urinary incontinence. Climacteric. 2015;18 Suppl 1:43–8.

Gass MLS, Cochrane BB, Larson JC, et al. Patterns and predictors of sexual activity among women in the Hormone Therapy trials of the Women's Health Initiative. Menopause. 2011; 18(11):1160–71.

Goetsch M. Postpartum dyspareunia – an unexplored problem. J Reprod Med. 1999;44:963–8.

Goldstein AT, King MA. Ospemifene may not treat vulvar atrophy: a report of two cases. Sex Med. 2016;4(3):e217–20.

Graziottin A. Recurrent cystitis after intercourse: why the gynaecologist has a say. In: Studd J, Seang LT, Chervenak FA, editors. Current progress in obstetrics and gynaecology, vol. 2. Mumbai: Suketu P. Kothari – TreeLife Media; 2014. p. 319–36.

Graziottin A. Unmet needs in vulvovaginal atrophy (VVA). Abstract book, 10th Congress of the European Menopause Society on "Promoting translation of science into clinical practice in midlife health and beyond", Madrid, Spain, May 20–22, 2015b, Maturitas 82(3):320–1, Nov 2015.

Graziottin A. Vaginal biological and sexual health – the unmet needs. Climacteric. 2015a;18 Suppl 1:9–12.

Graziottin A, Gambini D. Anatomy and physiology of genital organs – women. In: Vodusek D, Boller F, editors. Neurology of sexual and bladder disorders (Handbook of clinical neurology, vol. 130, 3rd Series). Edinburgh: Elsevier; 2015. p. 39–60.

Graziottin A, Gambini D. Female sexual dysfunction: treatment. In: Bø K, Berghmans B, Mørkved S, Van Kampen M, editors. Evidence-based physical therapy for the pelvic floor – bridging science and clinical practice. 2nd ed. Oxford: Elsevier; 2016 (in press).

Graziottin A, Lukasiewicz M. Female sexual dysfunction and premature menopause. In: Lipshultz L, Pastuszek A, Perelman M, Giraldi AM, Buster J, editors. Sexual health in the couple: management of sexual dysfunction in men and women. New York: Springer; 2015 (in press).

Graziottin A, Zanello PP. Pathogenic biofilms: their role in recurrent cystitis and vaginitis (with focus on D-mannose as a new prophylactic strategy). In: Studd J, Seang LT, Chervenak FA, editors. Current progress in obstetrics and gynaecology, vol. 2. 2nd ed. Mumbai: Kothari Medical; 2015 (accepted, in press).

Graziottin A, Gambini D, Bertolasi L. Genital and sexual pain in women. In: Vodusek D, Boller F, editors. Neurology of sexual and bladder disorders (Handbook of clinical neurology, vol. 130, 3rd Series). Edinburgh: Elsevier; 2015. p. 395–412.

Graziottin A, Lukasiewicz M. Psychosexual issues and quality of life after oncologic pelvic surgery, with focus on cervical cancer. In: Carbone A, Palleschi G, Pastore AL, Messas A, editors. Functional urologic surgery in neurogenic and oncologic diseases. Springer; 2016. p. 113–32.

Graziottin A, Lukasiewicz M, Serafini A. Sexual rehabilitation after gynecologic cancers. In: Gianotten W, Reisman Y, editors. Sexual rehabilitation. Springer; 2016 (in press).

Griebling TL, Liao Z, Smith PG. Systemic and topical hormone therapies reduce vaginal innervation density in postmenopausal women. Menopause. 2012;19(6):630–5.

Kagan R, Williams RS, Pan K, Mirkin S, Pickar JH. A randomized, placebo- and active-controlled trial of bazedoxifene/conjugated estrogens for treatment of moderate to severe vulvar/vaginal atrophy in postmenopausal women. Menopause. 2010;17(2):281–9.

Kao A, Binik YM, Amsel R, Funaro D, Leroux N, Khalife S. Biopsychosocial predictors of postmenopausal dyspareunia: the role of steroid hormones, vulvovaginal atrophy, cognitive-emotional factors, and dyadic adjustment. J Sex Med. 2012a;9:2066–76.

Kao A, Binik YM, Amsel R, Funaro D, Leroux N, Khalife S. Challenging atrophied perspectives on postmenopausal dyspareunia: a systematic description and synthesis of pain characteristics. J Sex Marital Ther. 2012b;38:128–50.

Kingsberg SA, Wysocki S, Magnus L, Krychman ML. Vulvar and vaginal atrophy in postmenopausal women: findings from the REVIVE (REal Women's VIews of Treatment Options for Menopausal Vaginal ChangEs) survey. J Sex Med. 2013;10:1790–9.

Labrie F, Cusan L, Gomez JL, et al. Effect of one-week treatment with vaginal estrogen preparations on serum estrogen levels in postmenopausal women. Menopause. 2009;16(1):30–6.

Labrie F, Archer DF, Koltun W, Vachon A, Young D, Frenette L, Portman D, Montesino M, Côté I, Parent J, Lavoie L, Beauregard A, Martel C, Vaillancourt M, Balser J, Moyneur É, VVA Prasterone Research Group. Efficacy of intravaginal dehydroepiandrosterone (DHEA) on moderate to severe dyspareunia and vaginal dryness, symptoms of vulvovaginal atrophy, and of the genitourinary syndrome of menopause. Menopause. 2016;23(3):243–56.

Lahaie MA, Amsel R, Khalifé S, Boyer S, Faaborg-Andersen M, Binik YM. Can fear, pain, and muscle tension discriminate vaginismus from dyspareunia/provoked vestibulodynia? Implications for the new DSM-5 diagnosis of genito-pelvic pain/penetration disorder. Arch Sex Behav. 2015;44(6):1537–50.

Lukasiewicz ME, Graziottin A. Women' sexuality after gynecologic cancers. In: Studd J, Seang LT, Chervenak FA, editors. Current progress in obstetrics and gynaecology, vol. 2. 2nd ed. Mumbai: Kothari Medical; 2015 (in press).

MacBride MB, Rhodes DJ, Shuster LT. Vulvovaginal atrophy. Mayo Clin Proc. 2010;85(1):87–94.

Management of symptomatic vulvovaginal atrophy: 2013 position statement of The North American Menopause Society. Menopause. 2013;20(9):888–902.

Martel C, Labrie F, Archer DF, Ke Y, Gonthier R, Simard JN, Lavoie L, Vaillancourt M, Montesino M, Balser J, Moyneur É, Prasterone Clinical Research Group. Serum steroid concentrations remain within normal postmenopausal values in women receiving daily 6.5mg intravaginal prasterone for 12 weeks. J Steroid Biochem Mol Biol. 2016;159:142–53.

Mercier J, Morin M, Lemieux MC, Reichetzer B, Khalifé S, Dumoulin C. Pelvic floor muscles training to reduce symptoms and signs of vulvovaginal atrophy: a case study. Menopause. 2016;23(7):816–20.

Nappi RE, Kokot-Kierepa M. Vaginal health: insights, views & attitudes (VIVA) – results from an international survey. Climacteric. 2012;15:36–44.

Nappi RE, Palacios S. Impact of vulvovaginal atrophy on sexual health and quality of life at postmenopause. Climacteric. 2014;17:3–9.

Nappi RE, Mattsson LÅ, Lachowsky M, Maamari R, Giraldi A. The CLOSER survey: impact of postmenopausal vaginal discomfort on relationships between women and their partners in Northern and Southern Europe. Maturitas. 2013;75:373–9.

Nappi RE, Biglia N, Cagnacci A, Di Carlo C, Luisi S, Paoletti AM. Diagnosis and management of symptoms associated with vulvovaginal atrophy: expert opinion on behalf of the Italian VVA study group. Gynecol Endocrinol. 2016;17:1–5.

Parish SJ, Nappi RE, Krychman ML, et al. Impact of vulvovaginal health on postmenopausal women: a review of surveys on symptoms of vulvovaginal atrophy. Int J Womens Health. 2013;5:437–47.

Phillips NA, Brown C, Foster D, Bachour C, Rawlinson L, Wan J, Bachmann G. Presenting symptoms among premenopausal and postmenopausal women with vulvodynia: a case series. Menopause. 2015;22(12):1296–300.

Pieralli A, Fallani MG, Becorpi A, Bianchi C, Corioni S, Longinotti M, Tredici Z, Guaschino S. Fractional CO2 laser for vulvovaginal atrophy (VVA) dyspareunia relief in breast cancer survivors. Arch Gynecol Obstet. 2016;294(4):841–6.

Pinkerton JV, Kagan R. Ospemifene for the treatment of postmenopausal vulvar and vaginal atrophy: recommendations for clinical use. Expert Opin Pharmacother. 2015;16(17):2703–14.

Pluchino N, Drakopoulos P, Bianchi-Demicheli F, Wenger JM, Petignat P, Genazzani AR. Neurobiology of DHEA and effects on sexuality, mood and cognition. J Steroid Biochem Mol Biol. 2015;145:273–80.

Portman DJ, Gass ML. Genitourinary syndrome of menopause: new terminology for vulvovaginal atrophy from the International Society for the Study of Women's Sexual Health and the North American Menopause Society. Maturitas. 2014;79(3):349–54.

Rahn DD, Carberry C, Sanses TV, Mamik MM, Ward RM, Meriwether KV, Olivera CK, Abed H, Balk EM, Murphy M, Society of Gynecologic Surgeons Systematic Review Group. Vaginal estrogen for genitourinary syndrome of menopause: a systematic review. Obstet Gynecol. 2014;124(6):1147–56.

Reissing ED, Borg C, Spoelstra SK, Ter Kuile MM, Both S, de Jong PJ, van Lankveld JJ, Melles RJ, Weijenborg PT, Weijmar Schultz WC. "Throwing the baby out with the bathwater": the demise of vaginismus in favor of genito-pelvic pain/penetration disorder. Arch Sex Behav. 2014;43(7):1209–13.

REVIVE EU, Abstract presented at EMAS 2015

Salvatore S, Stavros A, Candiani M. The use of pulsed CO2 lasers for the treatment of vulvovaginal atrophy. Curr Opin Obstet Gynecol. 2015;27(6):504–8.

Schneidewind-Skibbe A, Hayes RD, Koochaki PE, Meyer J, Dennerstein L. The frequency of sexual intercourse reported by women: a review of community-based studies and factors limiting their conclusions. J Sex Med. 2008;5(2):301–35.

Straub R. The complex role of estrogens in inflammation. Endocr Rev. 2007;28(5):521e74.
Sturdee DW, Panay N. Recommendations for the management of postmenopausal vaginal atrophy. Climacteric. 2010;13:509–22.
Ting AY, Blacklock AD, Smith PG. Estrogen regulates vaginal sensory and autonomic nerve density in the rat. Biol Reprod. 2004;71(4):1397–404.
Zoubina E, Smith P. Sympathetic hyperinnervation of the uterus in the estrogen receptor alpha knock-out mouse. Neuroscience. 2001;103:237–44.

9 Iatrogenic Vulvar Pain

Physicians and healthcare providers (HCPs) can contribute to vulvar pain with different pathophysiologic pathways and responsibilities. They seem to be often unaware of a dramatic truth, valid in every field of medicine: doctors can be cofactors in the pathogenesis of a disease (Graziottin 2006; Norian and Stratton 2008; Esparaz et al. 2015). Specifically, *HCPs* may contribute to *cause vulvar pain*, acting as:

- *Predisposing factor*, with two leading mechanisms:
  - First, when they increase the vulnerability of the vulvar organ, or the afferent nerves and muscle, to precipitating factors and/or of the emotional attitude toward genital pain, during diagnostic or therapeutic maneuvers (Graziottin 2006)
  - Second, when they do not recognize and diagnose conditions that may prelude, precipitate, or perpetuate vulvar pain (Graziottin 2015)
- *Precipitating factors*, with two other mechanisms:
  - First, through the inappropriate prescription of medications, the negative outcome of surgery, obstetrics, and/or chemotherapy, hormonotherapy, or radiotherapy (Graziottin 2011, 2014 Graziottin and Serafini 2012; Graziottin and Lukasiewicz 2016a, b; Lukasiewicz and Graziottin 2015; McDonald et al. 2015).
  - Second, when HCPs do not respect the professional boundaries in the clinician-patient relationship, with sexually abusive behaviors. This is another neglected precipitating cofactor of vulvar pain and sexual dysfunctions, especially for women who sought professional help in a vulnerable moment of their life (Gabbard et Anderson 1995; Plait 2003; Stewart et al. 2009). It is a problem still dramatically underdiagnosed and underreported, persisting in the shadow of medical misconducts (Stewart et al. 2009).
- *Perpetuating factors*, through the most frequent mistake in the field of vulvar pain: the lack of diagnostic recognition of its biological truth. Furthermore, the

A. Graziottin, F. Murina, *Vulvar Pain*, DOI 10.1007/978-3-319-42677-8_9

diagnostic omission encompasses occasional or systematic diagnostic neglects, particularly in the area of biological/medical etiology of vulvar pain. Typical omissions include:

- *Lack of diagnostic attention* to:
  - *Vulvar pain,* when even the name is missing, such as in vulvar pain in childhood or after female genital mutilation/cutting (FGM/C) (please see the dedicated chapters).
  - *Vestibulodynia/vulvodynia* complaint: the average diagnostic delay between the onset of symptoms and the correct diagnosis is of about 4 years in the author's personal series (Graziottin, unpublished data).
  - *Sexual pain,* and specifically *introital dyspareunia,* a persistently neglected complaint from adolescence onward and particularly after delivery (Glazener 1997; McDonald et al. 2015).
  - *Hyperactive pelvic floor*, as a predisposing, precipitating, and perpetuating factor of vestibular pain and introital dyspareunia (Graziottin 2015).
  - *Comorbidities* between vulvar pain and other medical conditions.
- *Lack of appropriate treatment* of all the abovementioned conditions. Conditions specifically critical for perpetuating vulvar pain include:
  - *Pelvic floor hyperactivity* that can be associated to vaginismus and introital dyspareunia and may turn into a serious perpetuating factor (Graziottin and Gambini 2015).
  - *Sexual pain disorders.*
  - *Comorbidities* between medical conditions, sexual problems, and vulvar pain. For example, the abuse of antibiotics in recurrent cystitis alters the intestinal and vaginal microbiota vaginal, predisposing and precipitating recurrent *Candida* infections, with consequent increased vulnerability to vulvar vestibulitis and provoked vestibulodynia (Graziottin 2014; Graziottin and Zanello 2015) (please see Chap. 6 for more details).

Key Point

"Iatrogenic" is not only what an HCP actively does, which causes vulvar damage (and sometimes sexual damage), but also what the *HCP omits to diagnose and treat.* In consequence of that, it causes one or more damages, as vulvar pain becomes chronic and/or because the natural course of the disease will not be changed due to the omitted diagnosis and treatment.

This chapter will discuss a few critical aspects in these three major areas of iatrogenic disorders, as a paradigm, to open a mental window that physicians all too often omit to consider.

9.1 Iatrogenic Factors *Predisposing* to Vulvar Pain in the Lifespan

It is difficult to provide an effective intervention, if there is no mention of a problem (Graziottin 2006). The omission of a frank and respectful discussion about sexual pain issues may contribute to vulvar pain with different dynamics, which will be briefly reviewed with a lifespan perspective.

9.1.1 Vulvar Pain in Childhood

The diagnostic omission is amazing as even the name of vulvar pain is omitted (please see the Chap. 4).

9.1.2 Vulvar Pain in Adolescents

In a retrospective case series of vulvodynia in preadolescent girls, Reed and Cantor found similar pain characteristics as in adulthood (Reed et Cantor 2008). The girls had many years of pain without a correct diagnosis and without an adequate physical examination.

In adolescence, causes of recurrent vulvovaginal pain have been associated with intercourse. The association with sexual activity and vulvodynia compromises future sexual functioning, psychological well-being, and quality of life. It was suggested that 30–50 % of adult women with provoked vestibulodynia experienced primary, i.e., lifelong, introital dyspareunia. It is often associated with undiagnosed lifelong vaginismus, not severe enough to prevent penetration, but sufficient to determine both fear of intercourse, poor/inadequate/absent arousal due to the phobic attitude, and a tightening/squeezing of the vaginal entrance, due to the associated hyperactive pelvic floor that predisposes to introital microtraumas with recurrent pain and vestibular inflammation at every sexual attempt, contributing to intermittent/chronic vulvar vestibulitis (Graziottin 2006). This neglected inflammation, gradually shifting from physiologic to pathologic, finally may contribute to the shift to pathologic/neuropathic inflammation, genital and in the brain, the hallmark of provoked vestibulodynia.

Vulvovaginal pain in adolescents was associated not only with intercourse but also with the nonsexual contextual factor such as the impossibility to tampon insertion in virginal adolescents. Vulvovaginal insertional pain is a red alert on a hyperactive pelvic floor (Graziottin 2006, 2015). It has been linked to chronic dyspareunia, as a powerful predisposing factor. Severe pain at first tampon insertion use was associated with a fourfold risk of reporting dyspareunia (Landry and Bergeron 2009).

The practical tip is just one: when a girl tells the HCPs (usually a "she") that she cannot use tampons, the correct answer must not be: "Well, use the external protection instead" but "Why she cannot?", to make the appropriate diagnosis. It is essential to examine gently the perineum and evaluate the contraction of the levator ani around the vaginal entrance and the condition of the hymen while thinking: "Is there an hyperactive pelvic floor? Is there a fibrous, cribrous, thick, tightened hymen? Are there signs of recurrent Candida vaginitis and inflammation?" (please see Chap. 6 for more details).

Key Point
In adolescents, the difficulty in using tampons for the menstrual protection is one of the first (neglected) signs of hyperactivity of the pelvic floor, predicting dyspareunia and vulvodynia.

9.1.3 After Female Genital Mutilation/Cutting (FMG/C)

Vulvar pain is not even mentioned in the majority of papers on FGM/C, in spite of the fact that the vulva itself is cut and sutured, often with primitive means. So an excruciating pain, due the extremely rich nervous vulvar network, goes totally unrecognized and undiagnosed. This neglect persists in spite of more than 20 % of women with FGM reporting severe introital dyspareunia with a subset that cannot accept/have penetration at all ("apareunia") because of pain (Berg et al. 2014) (see the chapter on vulvar pain in women with FGM/C for the analysis of the many implications of this diagnostic omission).

A serious issue is when *HCPs perform FGM/C themselves*. Medicalization of FGM/C refers to situations in which FGM/C is practiced by any category of healthcare provider, in a public or a private clinic, at home, or elsewhere (Abdulcadir et al. 2015). It also includes reinfibulation at any point of time in a woman's life. Medicalization of FGM/C has been condemned by WHO and medical associations, including the International Federation of Gynecology and Obstetrics (FIGO), United Nations agencies, international agencies, non-governmental organizations (NGOs), and governments (Abdulcadir et al. 2015).

The practice of FGM/C by HCPs should be considered as a serious misconduct, violating the basic, essential medical principle of *not harming* first, more so when the intervention implies involving partial or total removal of the external female genitalia or other injury to the female genital organs *for nonmedical reasons*. The serious responsibility of HCPs in causing permanent *iatrogenic health and sexual damages* when performing FGM/C should be more rigorously stigmatized and condemned by health organizations.

Ambiguities and controversies assimilating FGM/C to female genital cosmetic surgery (FGCS) deserve careful consideration and a more definite clear-cut position by scientific societies and health agencies.

9.1.4 In Pregnancy and After Delivery

Lack of professional recognition of the many biological etiologies of vulvar pain is still a serious issue all over the world. It persists with unmodified figures as well in the so-called high-income world (Glazener 1997; McDonald et al. 2015).

9.1.5 After the Menopause

After the menopause, a general lack of communication about female sexual health issues and specifically about vulvovaginal atrophy (VVA) in the clinical setting has been reported in many researches (please see Chap. 8 for a detailed discussion). In the recent Real Women's Views of Treatment Options for Menopausal Vaginal Changes (REVIVE) survey, postmenopausal women reported that *only 19% of healthcare professionals* addressed their sexual lives and only 13% specifically raised the issue of genitourinary symptoms, despite the fact that 40% of women expected their HCPs to initiate discussions related to menopausal symptoms (Kingsberg et al. 2013).

9.2 Iatrogenic Factors *Precipitating* Vulvar Pain in the Lifespan

Physicians may not only predispose women to vulvar pain, but they may actively precipitate or worsen a preexisting unrecognized vulvar disease, in their daily practice.

This negative effect may be due to the known, but not completely avoidable, side effects of a necessary treatment, medical and surgical, or to mistakes, negligence, and overall malpractice.

9.2.1 Pharmacologic Effects

- *Chemotherapy* has a complex effect: in prepubertal and fertile women, it may cause a permanent ovarian damage with, respectively, primary hypergonadotropic amenorrhea or premature menopause. This prolonged deprivation of sexual hormones, especially in women with hormone-dependent cancers, where hormone therapy is currently contraindicated, may negatively affect the whole sexual response, the younger the woman, the worse the effect, for the negative impact of the menopause on general and sexual health. When not adequately treated, particularly in women after breast cancer, when vaginal estrogens are still contraindicated, vulvovaginal atrophy (VVA) may become a critical predisposing and precipitating effect of vestibular pain, vaginal dryness, and introital dyspareunia (Graziottin 2001, 2006; Graziottin et Lukasiewicz 2016a;

Lukasiewicz et Graziottin 2015). Peripheral neuropathies consequent to chemotherapy may affect the pudendal nerve (Graziottin et al. 2015).

- *Hormonotherapy:* estrogenic receptor-positive breast cancer has been treated with tamoxifen for almost three decades. Although reasonably well tolerated, this worldwide used drug may specifically affect sexual function. Studies indicate that during tamoxifen therapy the most frequent complaints are hot flushes (85 %), disturbed sleep (55 %), vaginal dryness and/or dyspareunia (47 %), decreased sexual desire (44 %), and muscular-skeletal symptoms (43 %). Disturbed sleep correlates with hot flushes ($P<0.0005$) and concentration problems ($P<0.05$). Decreased sexual interest correlates with vaginal dryness ($P<0.0005$) and/or dyspareunia ($P<0.0005$). This is clinically obvious, as sexual pain is a major killer of sexual intimacy. After discontinuation of tamoxifen, symptoms decreased significantly (Merits et al. 2002; Graziottin e Lukasiewicz 2016a; Graziottin 2006, 2016).
- More recent treatments with *aromatize inhibitors* such as anastrozole, which inhibits the conversion of androgens to estrogens, may as well have a negative impact on the whole sexual response, specifically contributing to VVA and vestibular pain and, consequently, to introital dyspareunia (Derzko et al. 2007; Graziottin 2016)

9.2.2 Negative Outcomes of Surgery in Oncology

- *Cervical carcinoma* may require radical surgery, radiotherapy, and chemotherapy in the most aggressive and/or advanced stages. Radical surgery may shorten the vagina, thus reducing its "habitability," i.e., receptiveness, which may be further reduced by radiotherapy, unless early psychosexual rehabilitation and at least topical hormonal treatment are timely started. Cervical adenocarcinoma, being hormone dependent, is the only contraindication to hormonal treatment for 5 years after surgery.

  Assessment and treatment of a hyperactive, defensive pelvic floor, more frequent in nulliparous women or women who had cesarean section, is mandatory (Graziottin 2006, 2015; Graziottin and Gambini 2015, 2016). The sooner, the better.

  Dyspareunia is the most frequent complaint related to vaginal shortening, while loss of desire, arousal difficulties, and vaginal dryness may be related to the loss of estrogens and testosterone concomitant to oophorectomy and cancer-related problems (Graziottin 2001, 2006; Graziottin and Lukasiewicz, 2016a, b). This includes the severity and duration of neuroinflammation, which recognizes a multifactorial etiology. After cancer diagnosis and treatment, neuroinflammation is the leading contributor to sickness behavior, fatigue, and depression and major neglected contributor to loss of desire and global female sexual dysfunction. Concomitant bladder symptoms, if the nerve sparing technique has not been made or has not been adequate, may further negatively impact on the sexual outcomes (Graziottin 2001, 2006; Graziottin and Lukasiewicz 2016a, b).

- *Vulvar cancer*. Treatment modalities for vulvar carcinoma have greatly improved over the last three decades by providing improved cure rates with *more conservative surgery*. This carries decreased risk of morbidity (e.g., lymphedema, disfigurement, and sexual dysfunction) (Aerts et al. 2012).

  Surgical requirements for removal of clitoral areas and stenosis of the vaginal opening along with local pain from scarring create different patterns of sexual dysfunction post therapy (Graziottin 2006; Lukasiewicz et Graziottin 2015; Graziottin e Lukasiewicz 2016b).

  Surgical management of vulvar carcinoma must be individualized and tailored to the extent of disease. By optimizing care to the individual patient, psychological, sexual, and physical morbidity will be minimized (Graziottin e Lukasiewicz 2016b).

  However, these surgeries remain a major psychological trauma for women. Clinical attention, openness to discussing sexual and psychological functioning, and timely rehabilitative intervention, hormonal and physical, before and after surgery, can definitely improve the outcomes of vulvar cancer.

9.2.3 Negative Outcomes of Radiotherapy

- *Total body radiotherapy* may specifically damage sexuality through two major mechanisms:
  - Associated with bone marrow transplant, it may be associated with sexual dysfunction because of associated premature menopause, with the cohort of climacteric symptoms (Graziottin and Basson 2004; Graziottin et Lukasiewicz 2016a).
  - The negative impact on sexuality may be worsened by asthenia, fatigue, and immunodepression due to the primary neoplastic disease and the need of immunodepressants, when inadequate host/donor compatibility leading to graft versus host reaction requires chronic immunomodulating treatment (Graziottin and Basson 2004).
- *Pelvic radiotherapy* – for anal, cervical, or bladder cancers – may specifically damage vaginal habitability, causing retraction, vascular damage, loss of lubrication, vaginal dryness, and dyspareunia (Graziottin 2001, 2006; Graziottin and Lukasiewicz 2016b).

9.2.4 In Gynecology: For Benign Conditions

- Women are seeking care for *pelvic organ prolapse* (POP) in increasing numbers. A significant proportion of them will undergo *a second repair for recurrence* (Ellington and Richter 2013). This has initiated interest by both surgeons and industry to utilize and design prosthetic mesh materials to help augment longevity of prolapse repairs. Unfortunately, the introduction of transvaginal synthetic mesh kits for use in women was done without the benefit of level 1 data to determine its utility compared to native tissue repair (Ellington et Richter 2013).

- Moreover, *surgical treatment of POP* may correct the anatomical and mechanical causes of dysfunction, but surgical intervention may also cause *changes to vaginal anatomy* and *sexual dysfunction*. A common mistake is that surgeons do not ask women, especially after 70 years of age, if they are still sexually active. The surgeon then tightens the vagina ("Your vagina is new, now, like a virgin"). Unfortunately, too narrow! This may cause severe introital dyspareunia up to a frank impossibility to have sexual intercourse, further worsened when even a topical estrogenic treatment is not provided.
- Currently, the surgical management of POP involves vaginal and abdominal procedures with or without use of meshes or grafts for tissue reinforcement. The use of meshes is more common in cases of severe fascial defects, where reconstruction with native tissue cannot be achieved.

  The use of grafts or scar-tissue formation may cause genital, vaginal, and vulvar pain. Synthetic meshes used during repair may cause bleeding, discharge, pain, partner discomfort, vaginal shrinking, and sexual dysfunction with *dyspareunia* being the most frequent complaint, ranging *from 9 to 20 % of women after surgery* (Weber et al. 2000; Milani et al. 2005; Murphy et al. 2012; Ellington et Richter 2013).

  Warnings on the safety of use of synthetic mesh in transvaginal repairs have recently been issued. The US Food and Drug Administration (FDA) stated that, on the basis of an updated analysis of adverse events reported to the FDA and complications reported in the scientific literature, *surgical mesh for transvaginal repair of POP is an "area of continuing serious concern"* (Murphy et al. 2012).

  They identified adverse effects ranging from transient vulvar pain and dyspareunia, constipation, and small mesh erosions to larger vaginal mesh exposures or extrusions or perforations into the bladder or bowel. Shrinkage or contraction of mesh around pelvic organs, or excess tension on the mesh arms, can cause *vaginal pain* in some women. Furthermore, the insertion of mesh can make the vagina less pliable and perhaps more prone to pain or dyspareunia.

  The American Congress of Obstetricians and Gynecologists and the American Urogynecologic Society recommend that mesh augmentation be reserved for women at high risk in whom *the benefit of mesh placement outweighs the potential risks* (Johnsson Funk et al. 2013).

9.2.5 Electrosurgery: Laser or Cold Knife Surgery of Vulvar-Vestibular Lesions

They are dangerous for the development of vulvar pain. The two main conditions that require these treatments are genital warts and the high-grade squamous intraepithelial lesion of the vulva (VIN).

- *Genital warts*. Symptomatic warts are prevalent in at least 1 % of the population between the ages of 15 and 49, with estimates of up to 50 % of the population being infected with human papillomavirus (HPV), particularly genotypes 6 and

11, at some point in their lifetime (Workowski and Berman 2010). Psychosexual consequences of different vulvar treatment for HPV lesions are often underestimated (Graziottin et Serafini 2012).

Treatment of benign, symptomatic genital warts is aimed at alleviation of physical symptoms and cosmetic improvement. 40 to 60% of untreated warts will spontaneously be resolved in 9–12 months, but many patients are psychologically distressed by the presence of warts and require intervention to eradicate them (Wiley et al. 2002) (Box 9.1).

- *VIN* is a high-grade intraepithelial squamous lesion and precursor of invasive squamous cell carcinoma (SCC). The 2004 International Society for the Study of Vulvovaginal Disease (ISSVD) classification distinguished two types of VIN: usual type (HPV related) and differentiated type (not HPV related). The incidence of usual-type VIN is higher in younger women, while differentiated-type VIN is more common in older patients with chronic dermatologic conditions. Differentiated-type VIN has a greater invasive potential and shorter time between diagnosis and SCC than usual-type VIN (Darragh et al. 2013).

  Local excision of genital warts and VIN, consisting of removal of all visible lesions, can be performed with different techniques: scalpel, electrosurgery, or laser.

Key Points

- All destructive therapies can cause vulvar inflammation and leave scars and chronic vulvar sensitivity, particularly in the vestibular and the clitoral area.
- The "ablative" trauma can trigger vulvar pathologic inflammation, where an increase in the number and degranulated mast cells and hyperinnervation are pivotal. Persistence of vulvar inflammation may progressively contribute to neuroinflammation, with sickness behavior, depression, and sexual dysfunction.
- The *number, volume*, and *site* of lesions and the response to initial treatment have to guide the clinician to the most effective treatment option or combination of options for each individual patient.

Box 9.1. Imiquimod in the Treatment of Vulvar Condylomata and VIN: Is It Safer Than Surgery or Physical Treatment?

Imiquimod is a medical treatment used in the attempt to avoid surgery in patients with genital warts and VIN (Pepas et al. 2011):

- Imiquimod is thought to directly enhance immune recognition of HPV by inducing monocytes and macrophages to secrete cytokines such as interleukin-2 (IL-2), interferon alpha, and tumor necrosis factor, which serve as chemical signals that trigger a cellular immune response. The result is decreased HPV viral load, decreased wart volume, and significantly increased clearance of the external genital warts (EGWs).

- Imiquimod should be applied directly to the affected area at bedtime three times a week, ideally on an every-other-day basis, for up to 16 weeks. The treated area should be washed with mild soap and water the following morning, and a response is usually seen within 8 weeks and often much sooner.
- In three randomized, placebo-controlled trials of 5 % imiquimod cream, about half of all participants demonstrated complete clearance within 16 weeks (Gotovtseva et al. 2008; Moore et al. 2001; Yan et al. 2006).
- The primary adverse side effects of imiquimod occur secondary to induction of cytokine expression and immune stimulation.
- Mild-to-severe erythema, erosion, itching, and burning are common, but usually resolve within a few days of discontinuing the medication.
- Although it can be used as a stand-alone treatment, it may be most effective in clearing genital warts when used in conjunction with conventional therapies.

Warning is raised to avoid the treatment in the vestibular area for the risk of development of vulvar vestibulitis and neuroinflammation (Lopaschuk 2013).

9.2.6 Cosmetic Vulvar Surgery

It is a broad descriptor of numerous procedures designed to improve the appearance, function, or both of the vulvar structures (Mowat et al. 2015). Controversy regarding this type of interventions was amplified following an ACOG Committee Opinion advising caution due to a lack of data on safety and efficacy.

Women's search for a "perfect" vagina and vulva is stimulated via the Internet promotional messages promising extraordinary cosmetic and functional improvements (female genital cosmetic surgery, FGCS). An interesting recent research on the web promotion of cosmetic vulvar surgery identifies 5 major themes aimed to promote and normalize the practice of FGCS (Mowat et al. 2015):

- Pathologization of genital diversity.
- Female genital appearance as important to well-being.
- Characteristics of women's genitals are important for sex life.
- Female body as degenerative and improvable through surgery.
- FGCS as safe, easy, and effective.

Critical questions are arising among doctors and scientist more ethically focused on what is really appropriate when we consider (real) women's health and well-being first. All this emphasis on FGCS that focuses only on over-appreciated (and often not scientifically proven) benefits, while omitting to inform about potentially serious side effects, is manipulative of women's ability to make balanced decisions.

Indeed: "Is this public communication of the phenomenon of aesthetic genital surgery *decent, honest, balanced and ethical*?" (Ashong and Batta 2012).

An important point is that many of these procedures, while elective, are not limited to aesthetic goals alone. For example, the majority of women seeking labiaplasty also have a concomitant functional issue, whether it be discomfort from clothing or dyspareunia. Many procedures exist in the medical and marketing literature for correcting the *normal* vulva.

These include functional and aesthetic labia minora reduction, vaginal rejuvenation, designer vaginoplasty, G-spot amplification, and revirgination. Here, for the sake of concision, we will analyze only the most common FGCS request: the partial excision of the labia minora. General considerations on risks and pitfalls of different surgical goals of FGCS are summarized.

Partial excision of the labia minora is the first request to change genital morphology. Procedures are offered mainly by gynecologists and plastic surgeons (Liao et al. 2010).

Potential complications of labiaplasty include infection, wound separation, sinus formation, loss of natural contour or labial pigmentation, frenulum distortion, scarring, *painful intercourse*, and altered sensation (with vulvar pain) – all of which could affect up to 4 % of women undergoing these procedures (Liao et al. 2010). In the two larger case series, the reoperation rates were 2.9 and 7 % (Rouzier et al. 2000; Lynch et al. 2008).

Unfortunately a large number of procedures are performed on *adolescents* and even on young children (Jothilakshmi et al. 2009). This can be a real "disaster," because:

- The labia minora continue to develop in childhood and, especially, in adolescence. Any asymmetry may correct itself during pubertal development; if the contralateral labium starts to grow at this stage, previous procedures may lead to further asymmetry prompting more operations.
- The human anatomy is not a stable entity and continues to change throughout the lifespan; postoperative cosmesis is likewise impermanent.
- The amount of genital tissue removed in cosmetic labial surgery is comparable with type I and II female genital mutilation, which are associated with perineal trauma, postpartum hemorrhage, and potential long-lasting vulvar pain and introital dyspareunia. Careful information of patients and, when younger than 18, of parents on potential long-lasting health and sexual risk is mandatory.

Key Points

- Physicians should undergo proper training and provide appropriate information on limited outcome data and not be driven by monetary incentives.
- Before surgery, it is important to obtain a complete sexual history, including any type of abuse or other female sexual dysfunction relating to desire, arousal, orgasm, or pain.
- Surgeons performing cosmetic gynecologic procedures should have a clear understanding of the patient's desires and expectations, including her goals for surgery.

- Psychological evaluation for potential body dysmorphic disorder may be indicated.

(Hailparn 2012)

9.2.7 In Obstetrics

Perineal trauma is associated with postpartum dyspareunia and sexual dysfunction (Glazener 1997; McDonald et al. 2015). It was identified that women who underwent episiotomy, with or without additional perineal trauma, had higher rates of postpartum dyspareunia and vulvar pain when compared with women who delivered with an intact perineum or spontaneous perineal trauma (Klein et al. 1994). Therefore, it is essential to follow evidence-based guidelines for the prevention, identification, and repair of obstetric lacerations and for episiotomy. Practical recommendations to reduce the impact of perineal traumas on vulvar and genital health are summarized in Box 9.2.

The management of perineal trauma is an essential component of training in midwifery and obstetrics. Nevertheless, studies have reported a lack of knowledge of pelvic floor anatomy, assessment, and repair techniques in both midwives and doctors.

Iatrogenic damages during pregnancy, childbirth, and after delivery may be rooted in inadequate training, poor medical skills and knowledge, and underappreciation of the importance of caring about the woman's general, genital, and vulvar health.

Key Points

- Eighty-five percent of women will sustain perineal trauma after childbirth, and at least 70 % of these will require suturing.
- Around 6 % of affected women will experience important short-term complications such as infection and wound dehiscence.
- Problems can extend into the long term, such as dyspareunia, urinary, and fecal incontinence, pelvic organ prolapse, psychosocial problems, and postnatal depression.
- Timely assessment and repair of perineal trauma are necessary to ensure accurate repair.
- Women should be given help and advice about perineal care after the birth.
- Midwives, doctors, and health visitors caring for women in the postnatal period should ask appropriate questions and review the wound to ensure adequate healing (Webb et al. 2014).
- Any diagnostic omission of postpartum complications may translate into long-lasting vestibular/vulvar pain and persistent introital dyspareunia impacting the whole sexual function, sense of self-worth, and self-esteem and contributing to major marital/relationship crisis.

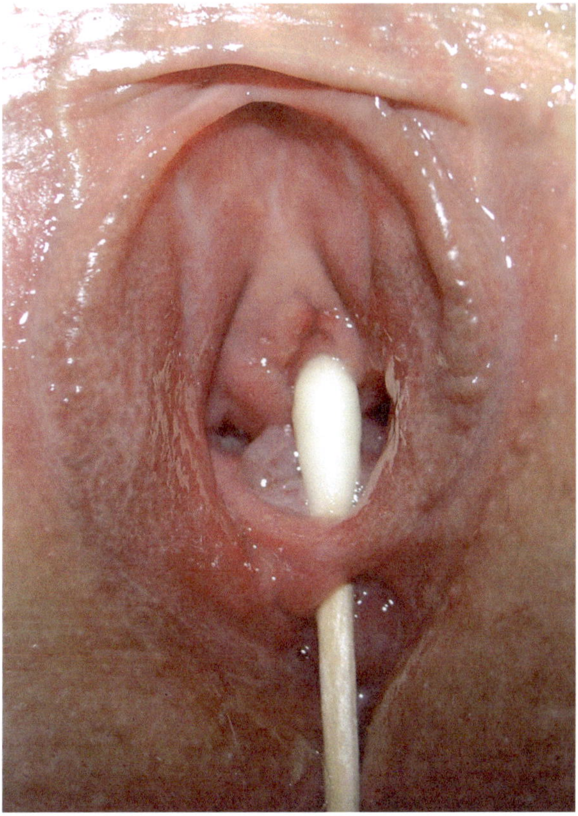

Fig. 9.1 Vestibular adhesions and areas of granulated tissue

Fear of perineal injury that requires suturing and worries about infection and wound breakdown are major concerns for women worldwide. In addition to infection, complications such as adhesions and areas of over-granulated tissue may arise and lead to longer-term morbidity, which can have detrimental effects on women's physical, psychosocial, and sexual well-being (Fig. 9.1).

The healing of perineal wounds by primary or secondary intention may result in the formation of excessive granulation tissue and persistent vulvar pain.

Continuous suturing of a second-degree laceration is preferred over interrupted suturing. A meta-analysis of 16 trials (8,184 women) that compared continuous versus interrupted absorbable sutures (for all layers or perineal skin only) for repair of episiotomy and second-degree perineal tears found that *continuous repairs are associated with less pain* for up to 10 days postpartum, less analgesia use, and a lower risk of having suture material removed postpartum (Kettle et al. 2012).

Box 9.2. Postnatal Advice for Women with Perineal Trauma

- Ensure good perineal hygiene, keeping the area clean and dry as much as possible and changing sanitary protection regularly.
- Wash hands regularly, especially before and after changing sanitary protection or during cleaning of the perineum.
- Take a daily bath or shower, making sure the perineum is washed with gentle soap and water only and rinsed with clear water. It is important that the wound is dried as much as possible by either patting gently with a soft and clean towel or using a hairdryer on a "cool" setting.
- Be vigilant for signs and symptoms of perineal infection, such as an increase in pain, excessive discharge that has changed in color or offensive smells, swelling, suture breakdown, and hematoma.
- Take any prescribed analgesia regularly and as directed.
- Maintain a well-balanced diet with adequate fluid intake to help promote healing and assist with breast milk production if required.

9.3 Iatrogenic Factors *Perpetuating* Vulvar Pain in the Lifespan

The neglect of asking about and listening to patient's report or complaint about his/her sexuality is a relevant maintenance factor of sexual pain. The belief that vulvar pain is substantially psychogenic or context dependent may induce the diagnostic omission of its potential biological etiology. This thinking dichotomy – maintaining that male sexual disorders are mainly biologically rooted while female sexual disorders are psychogenically driven – is partly responsible of the two-speed progress in sexual dysfunction research and approval of effective drugs.

The biological neglect is also responsible for the lack of recognition of the pathophysiology of vulvar pain. *This deprives the woman of the timely appropriate diagnosis and treatment of her complaint.*

Sometimes the medical or surgical intervention is credited to be fully responsible of the pain complaint, while it simply increased the woman's or couple's awareness of a preexisting problem.

Last but not least, vulvar pain can be caused or precipitated by medical malpractice, due to negligence, inexperience, and/or carelessness.

Key Point

Women's quality of sexual function and the potential presence of vestibular/vulvar pain and/or painful intercourse/introital dyspareunia should be reported in the medical record *before doing whatever type of genital/vulvar surgery.*

Conclusion

Iatrogenic factors are still systematically overlooked when vulvar pain is the woman's leading complaint. The purpose of this concise chapter is to draw clinician's attention to the underappreciated role of iatrogenic factors in predisposing, precipitating, and/or perpetuating vulvar pain.

The goal is to stimulate HCP attention to iatrogenic factors and to motivate them to improve their motivation to diagnose and treat vulvar and sexual pain with the most committed and unbiased clinical attention and to prevent and treat any damage HCPs may cause, for negligence, uncaring attitude, and/or primary economic personal interests.

References

Abdulcadir J, Irion O, Martinez de Tejada B. Female genital mutilation/cutting type IV in Cambodia: a case report. Clin Case Rep. 2015;3(12):979–82.

Aerts L, Enzlin P, Vergote I, et al. Sexual, psychological, and relational functioning in women after surgical treatment for vulvar malignancy: a literature review. J Sex Med. 2012;9:361e71.

Ashong AC, Batta HE. Sensationalising the female pudenda: an examination of public communication of aesthetic genital surgery. Glob J Health Sci. 2012;5(2):153–65. doi:10.5539/gjhs.v5n2p153.

Berg RC, Underland V, Odgaard-Jensen J, Fretheim A, Vist GE. Effects of female genital cutting on physical health outcomes: a systematic review and meta-analysis. BMJ Open. 2014;4(11):e006316.

Darragh TM, Colgan TJ, Cox JT, et al. LAST Project Work Groups. The lower anogenital squamous terminology standardization project for HPV-associated lesions: background and consensus recommendations from the College of American Pathologists and the American Society for Colposcopy and Cervical Pathology. Arch Pathol Lab Med. 2013;137:738.

Derzko C, Elliott S, Lam W. Management of sexual dysfunction in postmenopausal breast cancer patients taking adjuvant aromatase inhibitor therapy. Curr Oncol. 2007;14 Suppl 1:S20–40.

Ellington DR, Richter HE. The role of vaginal mesh procedures in pelvic organ prolapse surgery in view of complication risk. Obstet Gynecol Int. 2013;2013:356960. doi:10.1155/2013/356960. Epub 2013 Aug 28. Review.

Esparaz AM, Herts BA, Pearl JA, LeBlanc J, Kapoor B. Iatrogenic urinary tract injuries: etiology, diagnosis, and management. Semin Interv Radiol. 2015;32(2):195–208.

Gabbard GO, Anderson C. Professional boundaries in the physician-patient relationship. JAMA. 1995;273:1445–9.

Glazener CM. Sexual function after childbirth: women's experiences, persistent morbidity and lack of professional recognition. Br J Obstet Gynaecol. 1997;104(3):330–5.

Gotovtseva EP, Kapadia AS, Smolensky MH, Lairson DR. Optimal frequency of imiquimod 5% cream for the treatment of external genital warts in immunocompetent adults: a meta-analysis. Sex Transm Dis. 2008;35(4):346–51.

Graziottin A. Sexual function in women with gynecologic cancer: a review. Ital J Gynaecol Obstet. 2001;2:61–8.

Graziottin A. Iatrogenic and post-traumatic female sexual disorders. In: Porst H, Buvat J, editors. ISSM (International Society of Sexual Medicine) Standard Committee Book, Standard practice in Sexual Medicine. Oxford: Blackwell; 2006. p. 351–61.

Graziottin A. Psychogenic causes of Chronic Pelvic Pain and impact of CPP on psychological status. In: Vercellini P, editor. Chronic pelvic pain. Oxford: Blackwell Publishing; 2011. p. 29–39.

Graziottin A. Recurrent cystitis after intercourse: why the gynaecologist has a say. In: Studd J, Seang LT, Chervenak FA, editors. Current progress in obstetrics and gynaecology, vol. 2. Mumbai: Suketu P. Kothari – TreeLife Media; 2014. p. 319–36.

Graziottin A. Female sexual dysfunction: assessment. In: Bø K, Berghmans B, Mørkved S, Van Kampen M, editors. Evidence-based physical therapy for the pelvic floor – bridging science and clinical practice, 2nd ed. Oxford: Elsevier; 2015. p. 243–57. Available at www.alessandragraziottin.it.

Graziottin A. Sexual functions and breast cancer. In: Veronesi U, Goldhirsch A (Main editors), Veronesi P, Gentilini O, Leonardi MC (Associate editors). Breast cancer. Innovation in research and management. Springer; 2016.

Graziottin A, Basson R. Sexual dysfunction in women with premature menopause. Menopause. 2004;11:766–77.

Graziottin A, Gambini D. Female sexual dysfunction: treatment. In: Bø K, Berghmans B, Mørkved S, Van Kampen M, editos. Evidence-based physical therapy for the pelvic floor – bridging science and clinical practice, 2nd ed. Oxford: Elsevier; 2015. p. 258–70. Available at www.alessandragraziottin.it.

Graziottin A, Gambini D. Evaluation of genito-pelvic pain penetration disorder. In: Waguih WI, ed. The textbook of sexual medicine. Springer; 2016. Accepted.

Graziottin A, Gambini D, Bertolasi L. Genital and sexual pain in women. In: Vodusek D. Boller F, editors. Neurology of sexual and bladder disorders. Handbook of clinical neurology, vol. 130, 3rd Series. Elsevier; 2015. p. 395–412. Available at www.alessandragraziottin.it.

Graziottin A, Lukasiewicz M. Female sexual dysfunction and premature menopause. In: Lipshultz L, Pastuszak A, Perelman M, Giraldi AM, Buster J, editors. Sexual health in the couple: management of sexual dysfunction in men and women. New York: Springer; 2016a.

Graziottin A, Lukasiewicz M. Psychosexual issues and quality of life after oncologic pelvic surgery, with focus on cervical cancer. In: Carbone A, Palleschi G, Pastore AL, Messas A, editors. Functional urologic surgery in neurogenic and oncologic diseases. Verlag: Springer; 2016b. p. 113–32.

Graziottin A, Serafini A. HPV infection in women: psychosexual impact of genital warts and intraepithelial lesions. In: Takac I, editor. Recent advances in cervical cancer. Kerala: Transworld Research Network; 2012. p. 69–85.

Graziottin A, Zanello PP. Pathogenic biofilms: their role in recurrent cystitis and vaginitis (with focus on D-mannose as a new prophylactic strategy). In: Studd J, Seang LT, Chervenak FA, editors. Current progress in obstetrics and gynaecology, vol. 3, 2nd ed. Mumbai: Kothari Medical; 2015. p. 218–38. Available at: www.alessandragraziottin.it.

Hailparn TR. Cosmetic gynecology and the elusive quest for the "perfect" vagina. Obstet Gynecol. 2012;120(5):1207–8.

Jonsson Funk M, Edenfield AL, Pate V, et al. Trends in use of surgical mesh for pelvic organ prolapse. Am J Obstet Gynecol. 2013;208:79.e1–7.

Jothilakshmi PK, Salvi NR, Hayden BE, Bose-Haider B. Labial reduction in adolescent population – a case series study. J Pediatr Adolesc Gynecol. 2009;22:53–5.

Kettle C, Dowswell T, Ismail KM. Continuous and interrupted suturing techniques for repair of episiotomy or second-degree tears. Cochrane Database Syst Rev. 2012;(11):CD000947.

Kingsberg SA, Wysocki S, Magnus L, Krychman ML. Vulvar and vaginal atrophy in postmenopausal women: findings from the REVIVE (REal Women's VIews of Treatment Options for Menopausal Vaginal ChangEs) survey. J Sex Med. 2013;10(7):1790–9.

Klein MC, Gauthier RJ, Robbins JM, Kaczorowski J, Jorgensen SH, Franco ED, et al. Relationship of episiotomy to perineal trauma and morbidity, sexual dysfunction, and pelvic floor relaxation. Am J Obstet Gynecol. 1994;171:591–8.

Landry T, Bergeron S. How young does vulvo-vaginal pain begin? Prevalence and characteristics of dyspareunia in adolescents. J Sex Med. 2009;6:927.

Liao L-M, Michala L, Creighton S. Labial surgery for well women: a review of the literature. BJOG. 2010;117:20–5.

Lynch A, Marulaiah M, Samarakkody U. Reduction labiaplasty in adolescents. J Pediatr Adolesc Gynecol. 2008;21:147–9.

Lopaschuk CC. New approach to managing genital warts. Can Fam Physician. 2013;59(7):731–6.

Lukasiewicz ME, Graziottin A. Women' sexuality after gynecologic cancers. in: Studd J, Seang LT, Chervenak FA, editors. Current progress in obstetrics and gynaecology, vol. 3, 2nd ed. Mumbai: Kothari Medical; 2015. p. 95–116. Available at www.alessandragraziottin.it.

McDonald EA, Gartland D, Small R, Brown SJ. Dyspareunia and childbirth: a prospective cohort study. BJOG. 2015;122(5):672–9. doi:10.1111/1471-0528.13263. Epub 2015 Jan 21.

Merits MJ, Beckerman I, de Varies EG, van deer Zee AG, et al. Tamoxifen effects on subjective and psychosexual well being, in a randomized breast cancer study comparing high-dose and standard dose chemotherapy. Br J Cancer. 2002;86(10):1546–50.

Milani R, Salvatore S, Soligo M. Functional and anatomical outcome of anterior and posterior vaginal prolapse repair with prolene mesh. BJOG. 2005;112:107.

Moore RA, Edwards JE, Hopwood J, Hicks D. Imiquimod for the treatment of genital warts: a quantitative systematic review. BMC Infect Dis. 2001;1:3. Epub 2001 Jun 5.

Mowat H, McDonald K, Dobson AS, Fisher J, Kirkman M. The contribution of online content to the promotion and normalisation of female genital cosmetic surgery: a systematic review of the literature. BMC Womens Health. 2015;15:110–5.

Murphy M, Holzberg A, van Raalte H, et al. Time to rethink: an evidence-based response from pelvic surgeons to the FDA Safety Communication: 'UPDATE on Serious Complications Associated with Transvaginal Placement of Surgical Mesh for Pelvic Organ Prolapse'. Int Urogynecol J. 2012;23:5–9.

Norian JM, Stratton P. Labial fusion: a rare complication of chronic graft-versus-host disease. Obstet Gynecol. 2008;112(2 Pt 2):437–9.

Pepas L, Kaushik S, Bryant A, Nordin A, Dickinson HO. Medical interventions for high grade vulval intraepithelial neoplasia. Cochrane Database Syst Rev. 2011;(4):CD007924.

Plait S. Understanding and managing professional-client boundaries. In: Levine SB, Alto SE, Risen CB, editors. Handbook of clinical sexuality for mental health professional. New York: Brunner Rutledge; 2003. p. 407–24.

Reed BD, Cantor LE. Vulvodynia in preadolescent girls. J Low Genit Tract Dis. 2008;12:257.

Rouzier R, Louis-Sylvestre C, Paniel BJ, Haddad B. Hypertrophy of labia minora: experience with 163 reductions. Am J Obstet Gynecol. 2000;182:35–40.

Stewart DE, Venos E, Asraf IJ. Mental health policies on reporting child sexual abuse and physician-patient sexual relationships. World Psychiatry. 2009;8(1):45–8.

Webb S, Sherburn M, Ismail KM. Managing perineal trauma after childbirth. BMJ. 2014;349:g6829.

Weber AM, Walter MD, Piedmonte MR. Sexual function and vaginal anatomy in women before and after surgery for pelvic organ prolapse and urinary incontinence. Am J Obstet Gynecol. 2000;182:1610–5.

Wiley DJ, Douglas J, Beutner K, Cox T, Fife K, Moscicki AB, et al. External genital warts: diagnosis, treatment, and prevention. Clin Infect Dis. 2002;35 Suppl 2:S210–24.

Workowski KA, Berman S. Centers for Disease Control and Prevention Sexually transmitted diseases treatment guidelines, 2010. MMWR Recomm Rep. 2010;59(RR-12):1–110.

Yan J, Chen SL, Wang HN, Wu TX. Meta-analysis of 5% imiquimod and 0.5% podophyllotoxin in the treatment of condylomata acuminata. Dermatology. 2006;213(3):218–23.

How to Make a Comprehensive Diagnosis of Vulvar Pain

10

Vulvar pain is challenging for patients and healthcare providers. It can be acute, recurrent, chronic, and neuropathic with or without premenstrual flares. Patients may present with a variety of symptoms such as pain, burning, itching, irritation, soreness, and patterns continuous or intermittent, localized or generalized. Some critically differential aspects are summarized in Box 10.1.

Box 10.1. Differential Diagnostic Criteria in Different Types of Vulvar Pain

- *Duration* of vulvar pain: shorter than 3 months when acute, between 3 and 6 or more for chronic, more than 6 months neuropathic.
- *Etiology: usually objective, clear, and precise in the acute and chronic types,* it becomes progressively difficult to be objectified when the neuropathic pain is in play.
- *Type of inflammation associated:*
  - *In acute vulvar pain*, it is:
    - *Finalized* to restore the normal tissue cytoarchitecture and function ("resolving")
    - *Of short duration* (less than three months)
    - *Of severity proportional to the intensity of the tissue damage*
    - *Limited in intensity*
  - *In neuropathic vulvar pain,* it is:
    - *Non finalized, "non-resolving"*
    - Of duration lasting *more than 6 months*
    - *Of growing intensity*, disproportionate to the type/extension of the visible lesion

A. Graziottin, F. Murina, *Vulvar Pain*, DOI 10.1007/978-3-319-42677-8_10

- *Degree of neuroinflammation:*
  - *Limited*
  - *Progressively prominent with increasing neurogenic pain within the brain and in the peripheral tissues* (Xanthos et al. 2011; Xanthos and Sandkühler 2014)

Graziottin A., Presented at the 18th World Congress of Childhood and Adolescents Gynecology, Florence June 25–28, 2016

Vulvar pain often has a burning quality, while other patients describe their problem as "irritation," "stinging," "raw feelings," "crawling," or just "vulvar awareness." Sometimes discomfort has also been referred to as "the pain down there" or as "feminine pain."

Furthermore, vulvar pain can be *provoked*, when it occurs in response to stimulation, or *unprovoked*, if it occurs independently of stimulation. Some experience *allodynia*, which is defined as pain resulting from stimuli which would not normally cause pain, such as touch or pressure. Some suffer from *hyperalgesia*, or severe pain experienced from mild pain stimuli.

Virtually every condition of the vulva can be sore, raw, irritating, or burning at times. Even common problems such as vulvar dermatitis, which is usually only itchy, can become painful if scratching or splitting leads to open areas and ulcerations.

A simple general concept about the relationship between intensity of pain and meaning of it (useful to be explained to women and partners) is represented in Fig. 10.1.

The golden rules for an accurate diagnosis of vulvar pain include:

- *Report carefully in the clinical record the woman's wording about her symptoms*; do it "verbatim" that means reporting exactly the woman's words. Virtually every condition of the vulva can be sore, raw, irritating, or burning at times. Even common problems such as vulvar dermatitis, which is usually only itchy, can become painful if scratching or splitting leads to open areas, ulcerations, and infections.

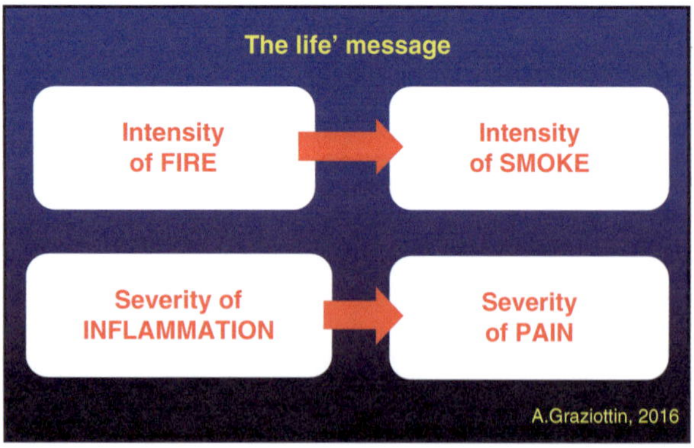

Fig. 10.1 Relationship between pain and inflammation

- *Record the precise narrative timing of the pain picture*. The symptom of vulvar pain must be fully evaluated. As pain is subjective, the *patient's history* provides the main evaluation. Useful questions include the following: When did pain start? Was there a specific damaging agent: a trauma, intentional (abuse) or unintentional, an infection, surgery (episiotomy, colporrhaphy), or the onset of pain that was not triggered by any specific event? Examination and investigations provide further understanding of the pain syndrome and exclude other conditions.
- *Quantify the intensity of vulvar pain*. Vulvar pain can only be measured subjectively. The most reliable and well-understood method is a numerical rating scale, from 0 (no pain) to 10 (extreme pain), with half-points marked. This is superior to the widely used visual analogue scale (VAS), which is a 10 cm line with "no pain" marked at one end and "extreme pain" at the other. Alternatively, a simple verbal rating scale can be used, e.g., "none," "mild," "moderate," and "severe." Both numerical and verbal scales can be used by patients without the need for paper and pen, unlike the VAS.
- Record *pain distress, and interference of pain with activities of daily life, besides pain intensity*. Because pain is multidimensional, a single rating scale combines these dimensions in unknown quantities. Depending on the clinical question, treatment, patient, and setting, it can be helpful to assess separately pain intensity, pain distress, and interference of pain with activities of daily life. It can also be helpful to ask about average pain, worst pain (as even if this only occurs rarely, it can still reveal what patients should avoid), and pain on, for example, bladder voiding. Pain reduction or relief is measured directly using a percentage, from 0 % = no relief up to 100 % = total relief.

Classically, pain can be considered to have *three dimensions*: sensory discriminative, motivational affective, and cognitive evaluative. The most used and validated multidimensional tools for the measuring pain are the long and short forms of the McGill Pain Questionnaire (Melzack 1987) (Fig. 10.2).

The questionnaire consists primarily of *three major classes of word descriptors* – sensory, affective, and evaluative – that are used by patients to specify subjective pain experience. It also contains an intensity scale and other items to determine the properties of the pain experience. The questionnaire was designed to provide quantitative measures of clinical pain that can be treated statistically. Vulvar pain analysis and quantification are optimal for a comprehensive understanding of the patient's experience and for effective treatment planning, and pre- and posttreatment quantification of vulvar sensitivity can lead to advances in the optimization of treatment success.

The audiovisual recording of the vulvar lesions either intentional or unintentional with the immediate description of the causative events in the child/adolescent/women should be accurately recorded at the first examination in the emergency department (Box 10.2).

Short-Form McGill Pain Questionnaire - Ronald Melzack

Patient's name: Date:

Pain definition	None	Mild	Moderate	Severe
Throbbing	0)	1)	2)	3) ....
Shooting	0)	1)	2)	3) ....
Stabbing	0)	1)	2)	3) ....
Sharp	0)	1)	2)	3) ....
Cramping	0)	1)	2)	3) ....
Gnawing	0)	1)	2)	3) ....
Not-Burning	0)	1)	2)	3) ....
Aching	0)	1)	2)	3) ....
Heavy	0)	1)	2)	3) ....
Tender	0)	1)	2)	3) ....
Splitting	0)	1)	2)	3) ....
Tiring-Exhausting	0)	1)	2)	3) ....
Sickening	0)	1)	2)	3) ....
Fearful	0)	1)	2)	3) ....
Punishing-Cruel	0)	1)	2)	3) ....

Fig. 10.2 The short-form McGill pain questionnaire (Adapted from Melzack 1987)

Box 10.2. Vulvar Pain from Intentional Trauma/Sexual Abuse: Recording Is Mandatory

At the very first visit in emergency units, every physician, especially those working in emergency departments, *should immediately do an audiovisual recording of any vulvar/genital lesion and of the child/adolescent/woman wording*. A mobile phone that everybody possesses today is sufficient if more sophisticated instruments are not available. This is mandatory when the type of lesions and/or the child/adolescent/woman's wording suggests sexual abuse.

The goal of the immediate accurate audiovisual recording at first visit is twofold:

- Avoid repeated questioning and examining, especially for legal purposes, as repeated investigations and examinations may trigger negative memories and exacerbate the emotional and physical suffering.
- Record an impeccable "fresh" documentation for legal reasons, if the author of the intentional lesions is to be suited.

10.1 The Sexual Correlate of Vulvar Pain: Introital Dyspareunia

Dyspareunia is a component of vulvar pain related to the "provocation" of sexual intercourse, and it may be the only symptom, especially in provoked vestibulodynia (Box 10.3). Dyspareunia is a genital pain experienced just before, during, or after sexual intercourse; patients with dyspareunia may complain of a well-defined and localized pain or express a general disinterest in and dissatisfaction with intercourse that stems from the associated discomfort.

Patients with dyspareunia are more likely than the general population to report pain with insertion of a tampon or finger, or during a gynecologic examination. Dyspareunia is an important component of vulvodynia, and it can occur as an isolated symptom.

If a woman reports difficulties with intercourse, it is important to determine whether pain on intercourse is *superficial*, at the point of penetration, which is likely to be related to a vulvar problem, or *deep inside* (deep dyspareunia), which is not caused by vulvar disease, but may be a component of a comorbid condition.

Box 10.3. Marinoff Dyspareunia Scale

0	No dyspareunia
1	Causes discomfort but does not interfere with frequency of intercourse
2	Sometimes prevents intercourse
3	Completely prevents intercourse (Marinoff and Turner 1992)

The *Female Sexual Function Index* (FSFI) is a 19-item multidimensional, self-report measure of sexual function. The measure has received empirical support for its reliability in several patient samples and for its ability to discriminate between samples of women with sexual dysfunction and healthy samples (Rosen et al. 2000).

The FSFI includes both *frequency items* ("Over the past 4 weeks, how often did you experience discomfort or pain during vaginal penetration?") and *intensity items*

("Over the past 4 weeks, how would you rate your level [degree] of discomfort or pain during or following vaginal penetration?"). Higher scores reflect better functioning.

10.2 How Should Patients with Vulvar Pain Be Evaluated?

10.2.1 Medical History

Obtaining *a history* is of paramount importance for a diagnosis, but the process may be hampered by the woman's embarrassment when discussing the topic. The manner of questioning requires *a nonjudgmental approach*, with a mixture of directed and open-ended questions (Box 10.4).

Personal habit is a fundamental aspect to consider: eliminating all possible irritants is an important step. If patients are using topical creams with an irritating base, as is often the case, they have to inform the clinician. The daily use of a potentially

Box 10.4. History of Vulvar Pain

Demographics	Age, occupation (sitting, standing), and leisure activities (bicycle riding, running)
Duration	Weeks, months, years
Timeline of pain	Start, factors at onset, what happened then and now, course
Site	Localized to one area or all over the vulva
Description	Burning, rawness, and irritation Spontaneous or provoked Intermittent or constant
Severity	0–10 scale (0 no pain, 10 most severe pain)
Factors that worsen or relieve pain	Cycling, sitting, pain with tampon insertion
All treatments	Over the counter and prescribed
Current sexual activity	Frequency, use of lubricants and devices
Contraception	Method, age of onset, duration
Pain with sexual intercourse	Pain on arousal, foreplay, touch, penetration, afterward, when the last time normal painless intercourse, if any, took place
OB/GYN history	Abortions, pregnancy termination, pregnancy, mode of delivery, complications, lactation, postpartum depression
Menstrual history	Last menstrual period, onset, duration, regularity, menstrual symptoms, menstrual worsening of vulvar pain, pads/tampons, douching
Trauma history	Vulvar, pelvic (including obstetric) or back trauma, sexual and/or physical abuse, motor vehicle, bicycle or equestrian accident
Family history	Vulvovaginal disease, skin diseases, atopy, autoimmune diseases, gastrointestinal diseases
Comorbid conditions	Migraines, endometriosis, irritable bowel syndrome, chronic constipation, interstitial cystitis, temporomandibular joint disease, fibromyalgia, chronic low back pain, anxiety, depression, stress

irritating mini-pad or panty liner is not healthy for any woman, and many lubricants also contain irritants as preservatives. It is also important to recognize *certain aspects of a patient's medical history* such as bladder and bowel function. It has been estimated that more than half of vulvodynia patients have symptoms of excessive urgency and frequency of urination and suprapubic pain. This condition is defined *painful bladder syndrome/interstitial cystitis* (PBS/IC). PBS/IC is a chronic, severely debilitating disease of the urinary bladder with a course that is usually marked by flare-ups and remissions. Dyspareunia is not uncommon in women with PBS/IC and may be related to the mechanical effects of intercourse on the inflamed bladder.

10.2.2 Physical Examination

The first important aspect of physical examination is the visual inspection of vulvar region. A systemic approach should be utilized, to make sure that all vulvar parts are included in the examination: this requires *a meticulous and methodical examination* of the vulva, including the perineum and perianal region. You should pay attention to skin texture, color, and the presence of lesions, ulcers, cysts, excoriations, *and anything else that attracts your attention as* "different."

It is extremely important to allow the patient to control over the situation, which means that *the patient must feel free to stop the examination at any time.*

There are some common normal variants which may be mistaken for pathology:

- Enlarged sebaceous glands, called *Fordyce spots*, present as multiple small yellow sebaceous glands along the inner aspects of the labia minora (Fig. 10.3). They can coalesce into cobblestone appearance, but have no clinical significance.
- A common normal variant is *vulvar papillomatosis*, which is found in 8–48 % of women in the reproductive age group. These are filiform soft projections often found in the vestibule. They can be mistaken for condylomas (Table 10.1). Vulvar micropapillomatosis should be left untreated: laser removal, for example, frequently results in an "iatrogenic" trigger for the development of a vestibulodynia (Fig. 10.4) (Cohen Sacher 2015).

Vulvoscopy, the colposcopic examination of the vulva, gives the examiner the ability to characterize any lesions with much greater detail (Box 10.5).

Box 10.5. Vulvoscopy: A Diagnostic Opportunity to "See" Better

- Vulvoscopy gives the examiner the ability to characterize any lesions with much greater detail. It helps to determine if:
  - A lesion is a raised plaque or just a flat macule.
  - The margins of the lesion can be characterized (e.g., are the lesions distinct or are the observed changes more diffuse/confluent?).
  - There is an area deserving a target biopsy for histologic examination.

- Vulvoscopy enhances the ability to detect:
  - Color changes associated with inflammatory or neoplastic diseases of the vulva:
    - Red areas can be visualized when there are stromal changes due to inflammation, vulvar dermatoses, or neovascularization in association with neoplasia.
    - White areas can be found when there are decreased vascularization, fibrotic changes in the stroma, and increased keratinization (lichenification)
  - Scarring and architectural changes: chronic inflammatory disorders of the vulva, such as lichen sclerosus and lichen planus, frequently cause structural changes such as the resorption of the labia minora and phimosis of the clitoris.
  - Subtle lesions such as tiny fissures, which may be very painful.

(Sideri et al. 2009)

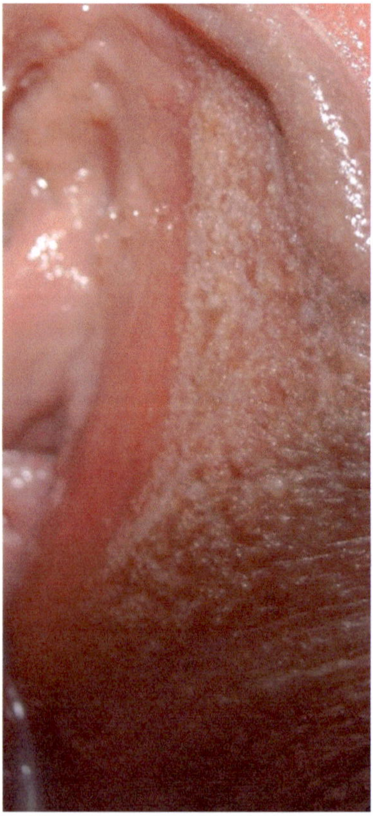

Fig. 10.3 Fordyce spots on labia minora

Table 10.1 Differentiating vulvar micropapillomatosis from vulvar condylomas

Vulvar micropapillomatosis	Vulvar condylomas
Regular shape and distribution	Small bumps
Uniform color	Flat or verrucous
Soft consistency	Reddish or brown, smooth
Lack of tendency to fuse	Dome-shaped lesion on keratinized skin

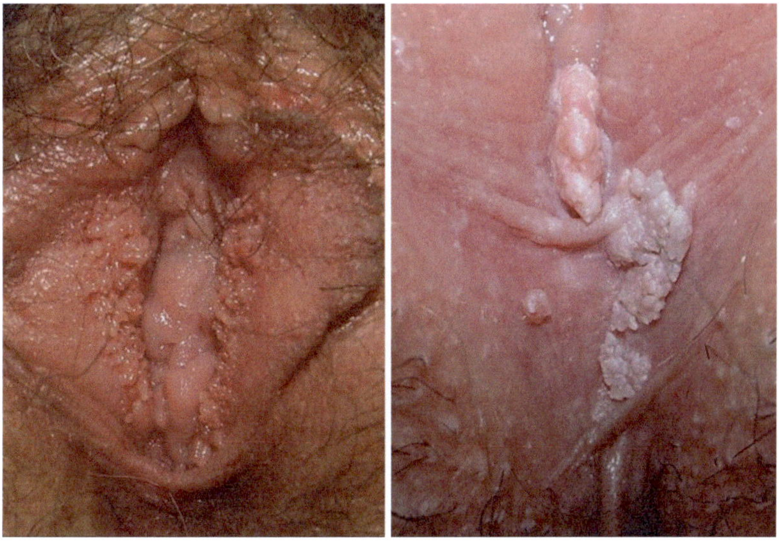

Fig. 10.4 Vulvar micropapillomatosis on the left and condylomas on the right

In premenopausal women a history of pain with entry is most commonly associated vulvar vestibulitis/provoked vestibulodynia, recurrent candida infections, and painful outcome of episiotomy to mention the most frequent.

In postmenopausal women entry dyspareunia is more frequently associated with the genitourinary syndrome of menopause (Portman and Glass 2014).

Atrophic changes from inadequate estrogen levels may also cause entry dyspareunia, although the pain typically extends into the vaginal area as well.

The patients complain with dyspareunia and signs of vestibular and vaginal atrophy including a thinned, dry, fragile, or pale mucosa (Fig. 10.5).

Vestibular tenderness is assessed by applying a cotton tipped swab (Q-tip test: Fig. 10.6) to the vulvar vestibule in a clock-like pattern. Gentle touch provokes either *hyperesthesia*, a heightened intensity relative the degree of applied pressure, or *allodynia*, the perception of a different sensation to that applied (e.g., pain rather touch). The Q-tip test is performed by touching gently with a cotton swab at the different vulva parts, from the labia majora gradually toward the introitus, where the pain is expected to be worse. *The Q-tip touch test has been validated* as useful in identifying the exact location of the pain and enabling the patient to classify the areas where it is mild, moderate, or severe. A diagram of pain locations is helpful in assisting the assessment of pain over time (Stockdale and Lawson 2014).

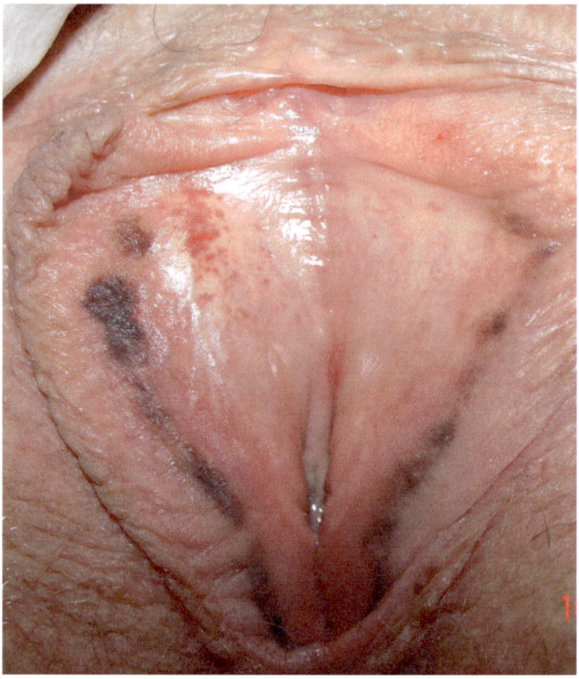

Fig. 10.5 Atrophic changes in menopausal women

10.3 Dermatological Disorders of the Vulva or Vagina Can Also Cause Pain

Lichen sclerosus, lichen planus, and lichen simplex chronicus are three of the most common *nonneoplastic epithelial disorders* of the vulva that can be painful (Box 10.6).

Box 10.6. The Most Important Questions to Have in Mind During the Examination

1. Is there a rash or lesion, taking into account subtle lesions such as tiny fissures which may be very painful? If there is an abnormality, one must query whether it could account for the patient's symptoms.
2. Is this a normal vulva, taking into account the patient's age? Take note of where the pain is and whether it radiates and whether the patient is able to localize the pain or indicates a general area of pain. Establish whether there is tenderness on palpation of the vestibule or on insertion of a finger or Q-tip.

10.3.1 Lichen Sclerosus (LS)

LS is an *inflammatory dermatosis of unknown etiology*. There is evidence to suggest that autoimmune factors may be involved in its pathogenesis, and recent evidence has shown autoantibodies to extracellular matrix protein 1; besides, there is an increased frequency of other autoimmune disorders in females with LS (Simonetta et al. 2015).

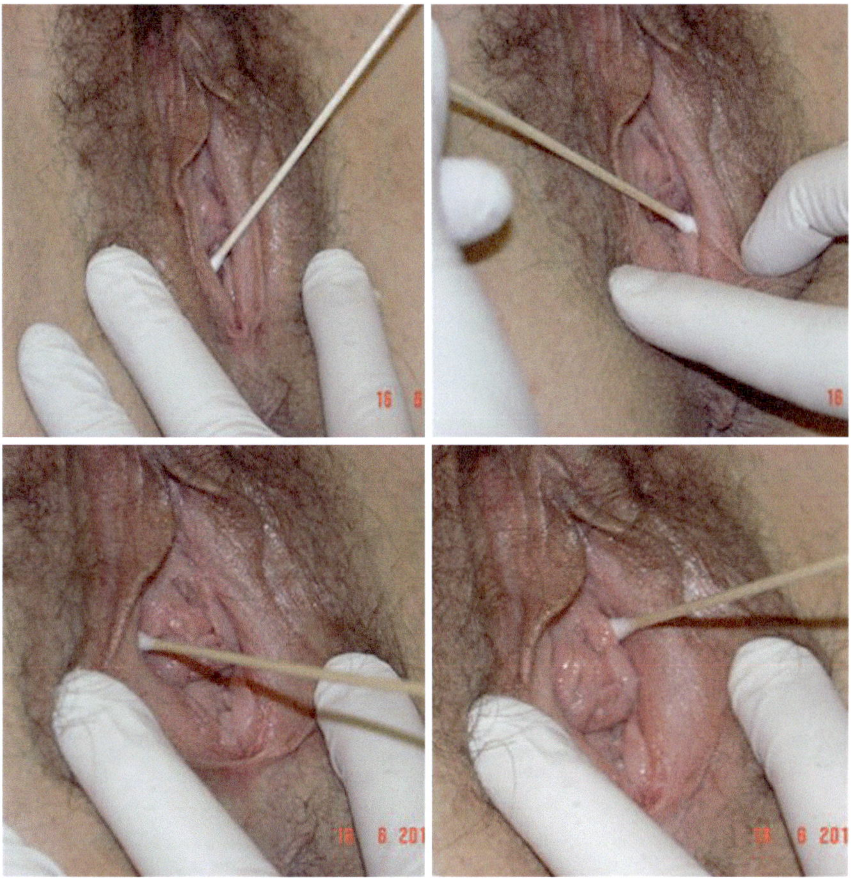

Fig. 10.6 Q-tip test

Itch is the main symptom, but pain occurs if there are erosions or fissures. There is typically no genital mucosal involvement, but the stenosis that may develop at the edge of mucocutaneous junctions can cause severe dyspareunia. The *clinical features* of lesions are variable, depending on the stage and severity of the disease. Patchy involvement is seen in some, while others have extensive, confluent disease (Fig. 10.7). Areas of pale, thinned, wrinkled, atrophic skin, possible telangiectasia, and hemorrhagic blisters may be evident at sites of lesions (Fig. 10.8).

Lichenification or hyperkeratosis may also be the prevalent pattern. Progressive sclerosis can lead to loss of normal genital structures. Labia minora may become fused or resorbed, the clitoris may be buried, and the introitus significantly narrowed.

LS in females has *two peak ages of presentation*. The first of these occurs in prepubertal girls, while the other one in postmenopausal women.

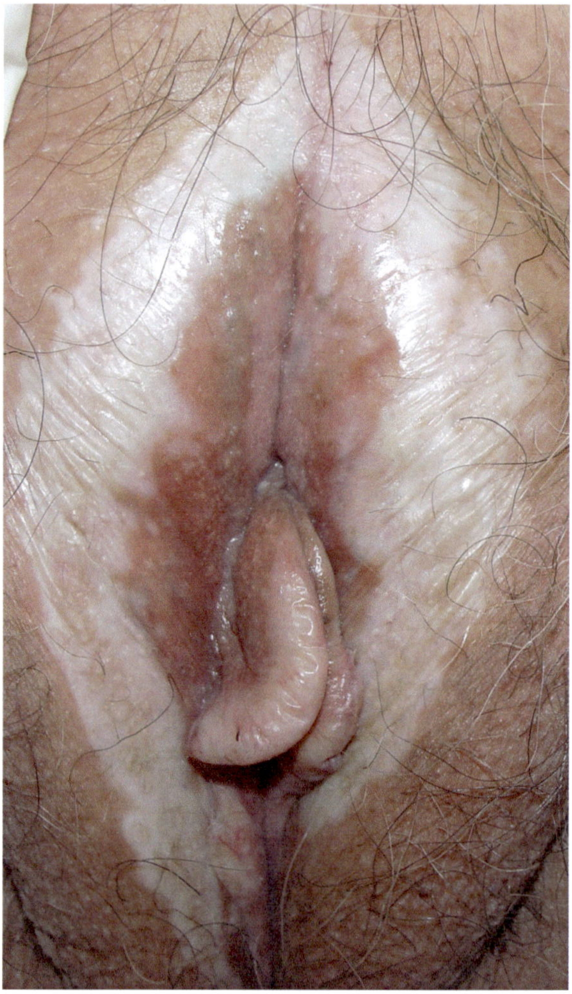

Fig. 10.7 Vulvar lichen sclerosus: confluent white areas

10.3.2 Lichen Planus (LP)

It is *an inflammatory condition* of unknown pathogenesis, but it is probably an immunological response by T cells activated by, as yet, unidentified antigens.

There are *three clinical variants* that affect the vulva: erosive lichen planus, papulosquamous lichen planus, and hypertrophic lichen planus. Vulvovaginal involvement can be associated with itching, burning, pain, dyspareunia, and destruction of the vulvar and vaginal architecture. The variant that typically affects the vulva and vagina is called *erosive LP*, and this is the most painful form of the disease (Fig. 10.9).

In LP the mucosa of the introitus is often denuded with a red, glazed appearance; there may be an erythema of the vestibular mucosa with varying degrees of

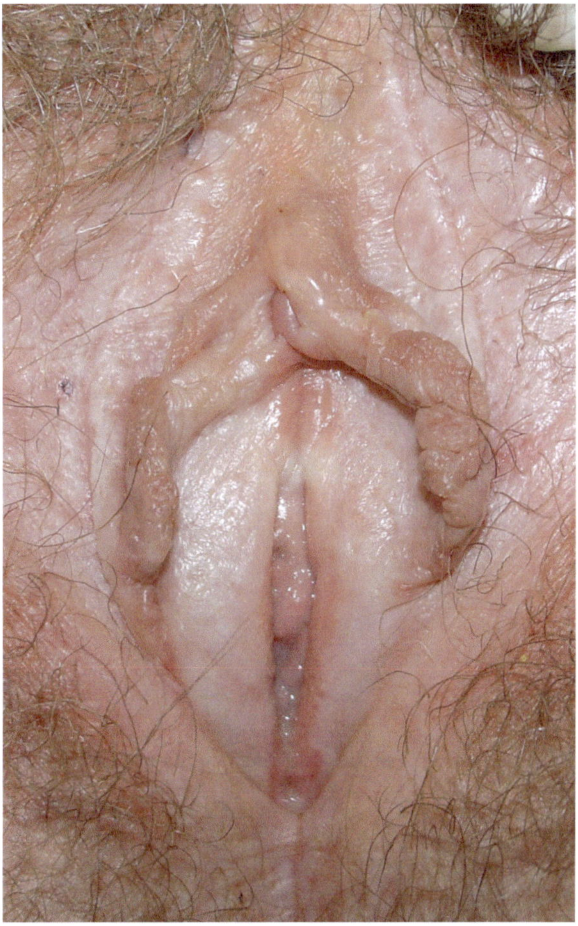

Fig. 10.8 Vulvar lichen sclerosus: atrophic skins with erosions

epithelial desquamation or frank erosions. In erosive lichen planus, it is important to recognize vaginal lesions early and start treatment immediately, as they can lead to scarring and complete stenosis. The lesions consist of friable telangiectasia with patchy erythema, which are responsible for the common symptoms of postcoital bleeding, dyspareunia, and a variable discharge which is often serosanguinous (Zendell 2015).

10.3.3 Lichen Simplex Chronicus

It is not a specific entity, but rather describes *lichenification of the vulva caused by persistent itching and scratching*. The skin can become leathery and thickened or, in severe cases, may be excoriated (Fig. 10.10). Vulvar pain, if present, is usually a result of irritation from open lesions.

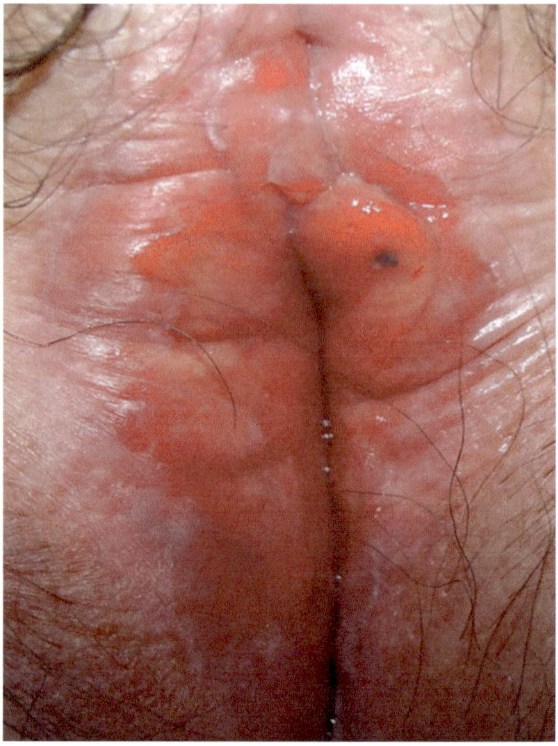

Fig. 10.9 Erosive lichen planus

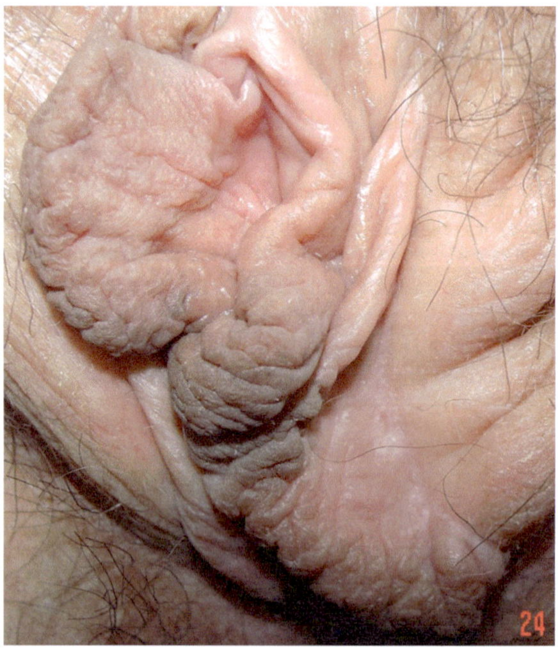

Fig. 10.10 Vulvar lichen simplex

Key Points

Many different diseases may produce *erosive, ulcerative, or desquamative lesions* of the vulva. These conditions tend to present with a relevant pain for the patients.

Vulvar aphthae are small, shallow ulcers with a yellow base and erythematous rim. They occur acutely and resolve over a few days and are quite painful. Although attacks tend to be intermittent, they can be very frequent or almost continuous in some patients. Women with vulvar aphthosis frequently have oral aphthae (Fig. 10.11). Initially, the ulcers are covered by either a pseudomembrane or necrotic eschar, then slough to exhibit a yellow/white fibrinous base.

Vulvar aphthae are commonly confused with *genital herpes*, and this is hardly surprising, given that they are painful, acute, recurrent ulcers. The difference is that genital herpes, once past the very brief blister stage, has the appearance of an erosion rather than the typical deeper, ulcerative lesions that

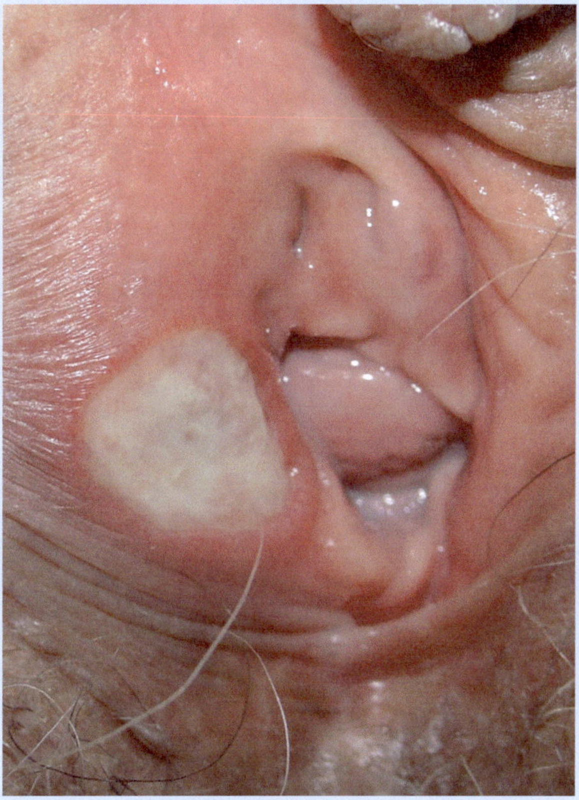

Fig. 10.11 Vulvar aphthae

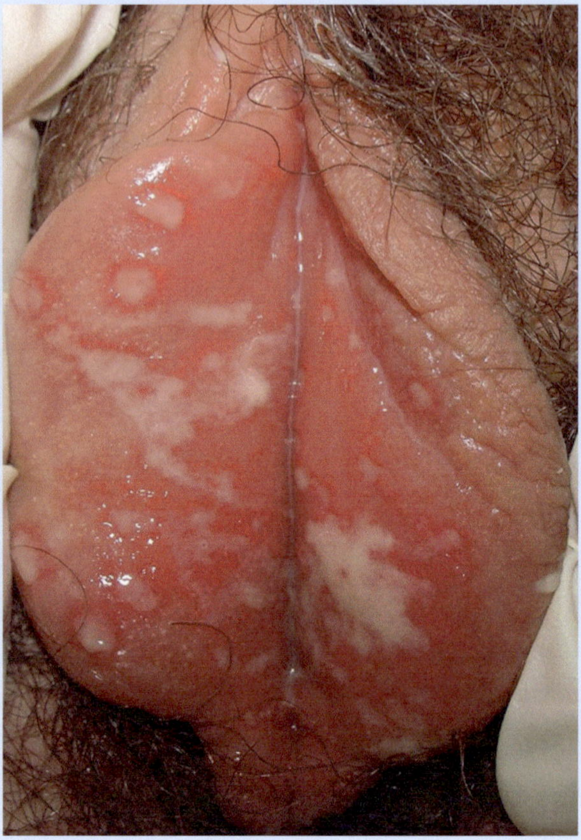

Fig. 10.12 Genital herpes

are seen in the mouth (Fig. 10.12). These painful ulcers can appear as a single ulcer or in a grouping of multiple ulcers. They are shallow with sharply demarcated borders and erythematous edges. Isolated episodes of childhood aphthae are mostly linked to viruses and are unlikely to recur or represent underlying conditions. Adult aphthae behave differently: in 5 recently published case series, 32 % of women had recurrences and 47 % had oral ulcers at some point and, therefore, met criteria for complex aphthosis (Huppert et al. 2006; Farhi et al. 2009).

Vulvar intraepithelial neoplasia (VIN) does not have a characteristic presentation. Some patients may have pruritus or burning, while others will notice an asymptomatic abnormality on the vulvar skin. The lesions may be raised or flat with a rough surface. The lesions may appear white or red or of mixed color (Fig. 10.13).

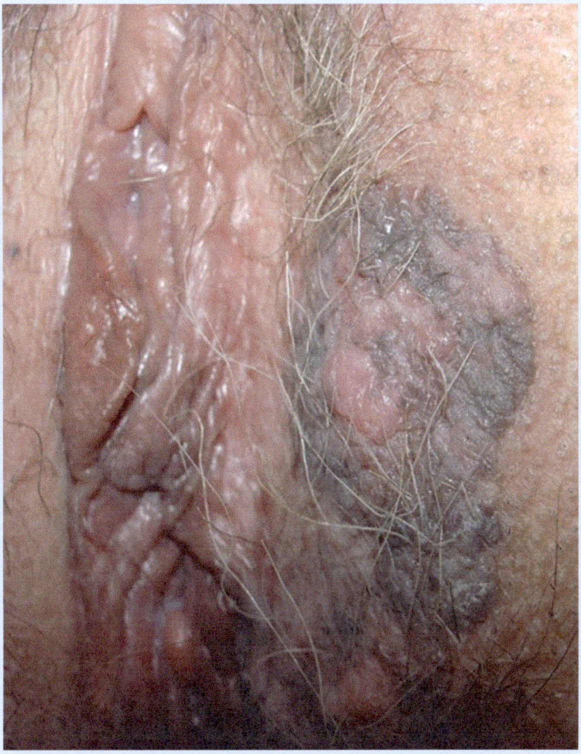

Fig. 10.13 Vulvar intraepithelial neoplasia

10.4 Pelvic Floor Evaluation

10.4.1 Observation of the Pelvic Floor

Clinical evaluation of the pelvic floor begins with *simple observation of pelvic floor muscle activity* during the process of squeezing and relaxation. The simple observation of the perineum and introital area in the dorsal lithotomy position during the performance of a Kegel squeeze is often quite revealing:

- When the *centrum tendineum of the perineum is retracted* (sometimes up to 6–7 cm inner to the line passing above/tangent to the glutei), the immediate diagnosis of an hyperactive pelvic floor can be made.
- The presence of a *hemorrhoid at 12 o'clock* suggests an inadequate command: this means that the woman usually pushes without relaxing the pelvic floor. In other words, when she tries to evacuate, she pushes the stool without relaxing the levator ani. Over time this causes the protrusion of an increasing part of the

hemorrhoids, a specialized type of engorged vessels located just inside the anal sphincter, finalized to increase the anal continence to liquid feces and gas. The hyperactivity of the pelvic floor contributes to the so-called obstructive constipation, exacerbated when a hyperactivity/hypertonicity of the anal sphincter is in play. The latter may contribute to *Escherichia coli* inflammation of the vestibular/vaginal tissues and/or of the bladder, contributing to recurrent vaginitis and cystitis. Comorbidity between hyperactivity of the pelvic floor, lifelong obstructive constipation, recurrent cystitis, and introital lifelong dyspareunia with vestibular pain is frequently diagnosed when the examining physician can blend together a careful clinical history, a skilled physical examination, and a multisystemic pathophysiologic reading of the symptoms the woman is complaining about.

- An "inverted command" of the pelvic floor is appreciated when the woman is requested to push. Instead, she pulls, increasing the retraction and the contraction, thus tightening/narrowing the entrance of the vagina even more. This is a mandatory indication to perform pelvic floor rehabilitation with electromyographic biofeedback to educate to woman to master a perfect control and command of the contraction and relaxation process.

10.4.2 Palpation of the Pelvic Floor

Muscular pain can be assessed with insertion of one finger at the introitus as the patient slowly performs a series of contraction and relaxation exercises while breathing deeply with the "abdominal breathing," i.e., using the diaphragm, a movement that helps to relax the posterior part of the pelvic floor (Fig. 10.14).

The woman squeezes the muscles used to stop the flow of urine for about 10 s and then relaxes them for about 10 s. Patients with pelvic floor hypertonic dysfunction often have so much muscle tension at "rest" that they are unable to produce

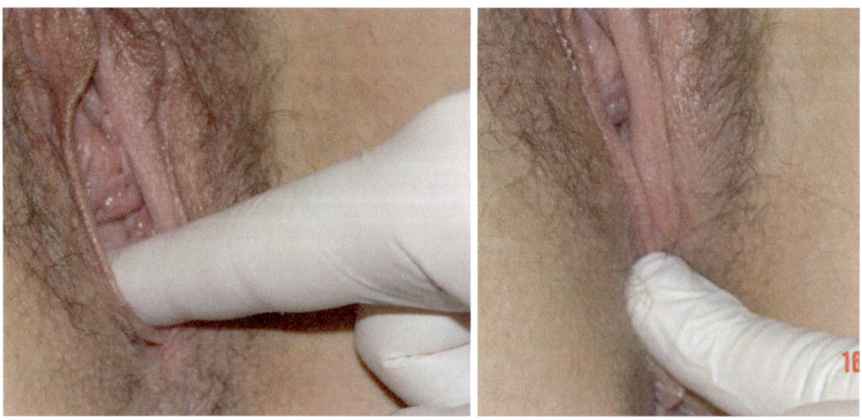

Fig. 10.14 Pelvic floor muscle examination

Box 10.7. Pelvic Floor Hypertonicity Score

0	No hypertonicity
1	Mild hypertonicity
2	Moderate hypertonicity
3	Severe hypertonicity

more contractile strength and therefore cannot produce an effective squeeze. It can be revealed by a "short perineum," conventionally with a length inferior to 2 cm.

At this point the examiner, if accepted by the patient, should place a generously lubricated single finger in the vagina to assess pelvic floor awareness and the ability to squeeze and relax the levator ani. Many scales are available to document strength, tone, and tenderness; yet all these scales are subjective and nonvalidated. Authors usually used a simple empiric score that allows to reproduce pelvic floor hypertonus with an acceptable reliability (Box 10.7).

The *lateral walls* of the vagina should be palpated accurately:

- Laterally, focusing at the insertion of the pubococcygeus to the spine. A light pressure can elicit no pain (normal finding) or a localized mild/moderate pain ("tender point," indicating a levator ani myalgia) or a more intense pain that can be referred also to the vulva or to the pelvis, in a nonmetameric fashion ("trigger point" of the elevator ani, often associated with fibromyalgia findings in other body muscles).
- Along the bladder and urethra anteriorly: pain can be elicited when symptoms suggestive of urethralgia and/or trigonitis are complained of.
- Along the posterior wall and fornices. Any tenderness or nodules, more often endometriotic, and the position of the uterus should be noted.

Many patients will be found to be most tender along the lateral border of the levator ani, which is where the levator muscles insert onto the arcus tendineus levator ani. Spontaneous or elicited pain in the lower third of the anterior vaginal wall should be carefully explored, as it may be associated with bladder-related comorbidities (cystalgia, urethralgia, postcoital cystitis, interstitial cystitis) that are reported in one third of vulvodynia patients.

10.5 Vaginal Inspection

The vagina should be evaluated using a narrow and well-lubricated *speculum*. During assessment of mucosal integrity, the presence or absence of vaginal rugae, fissures, or friable tissue should be noted. The fornices should be palpated around the cervix for *nodules suggestive of endometriosis* and may also be the etiology for fixed adnexa or may result from pelvic inflammatory disease. The vagina should also be examined for possible evidence of abnormal discharge.

The *discharge* is collected with a cotton swab from the posterior fornix or vaginal lateral walls for the purpose of *checking the pH and performing microscopy examination* (Box 10.8).

Box 10.8. pH Evaluation

A normal vaginal pH for women in the reproductive age is below 4.5.

It is higher for premenarchal girls and postmenopausal women with vaginal atrophy.

Measuring vaginal pH is a good way to rule out several conditions, such as bacterial vaginosis and trichomoniasis that elevate the pH.

10.5.1 Wet Mount Microscopy

An important diagnostic tool is *wet mount microscopy*. This is performed by smearing vaginal fluid collected by a cotton swab onto one slide. A drop of normal saline is mixed with the discharge on the slide. The fluid wet mount or saline preparation should be done routinely to identify the presence of yeast cells and mycelia, but also to exclude the presence of so-called clue cells indicative of bacterial vaginosis and motile trichomonads (Fig. 10.15).

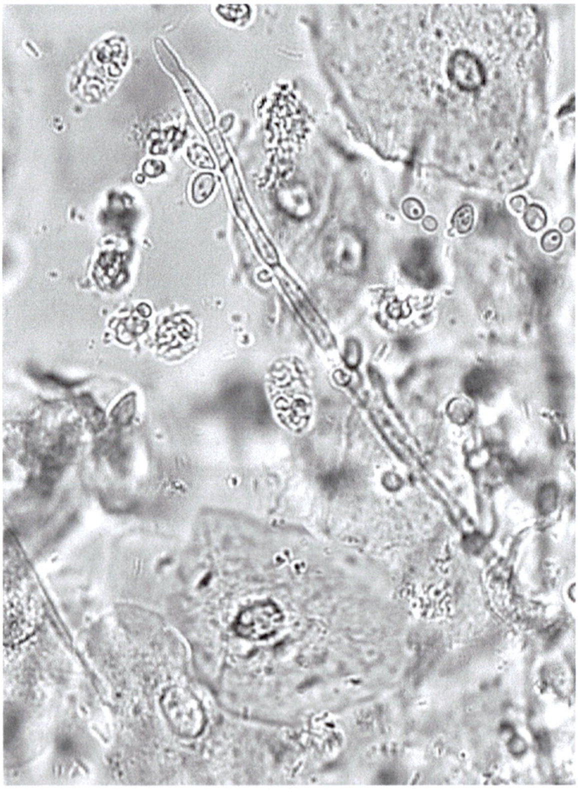

Fig. 10.15 Wet mount microscopy: presence of yeast cells and mycelia

Table 10.2 Testing for causes of vaginitis

Condition	Vaginal pH	Saline microscopy
Normal	<4.7	Unremarkable, white blood cells, bacillary flora
Vulvovaginal candidiasis	<4.7	Hyphae, blastospores
Bacterial vaginosis	>4.7	Clue cells, coccobacillary flora
Trichomoniasis	Varies	Trichomonads
Atrophic vaginitis	>5.5	Parabasal cells, decreased mixed flora

Modified from Nyirjesy (2014)

Microscopy was found to have a wide range of reported sensitivity for diagnosing candidiasis (between 38 % and 83 %) and high positive predictive value for diagnosing *Trichomonas*.

Diagnosis of *bacterial vaginosis* requires microscope examination as part of the Amsel diagnostic criteria. However, other signs in the wet mount may point to the diagnosis, as lack of lactobacilli-like rods, presence of numerous small rod-shaped bacteria, and paucity of white blood cells.

In other forms of vaginitis, abnormal wet mount may suggest an infection (Nyirjesy 2014) (Table 10.2).

10.6 Tests

- *Target biopsy of the vulva*: the main reason for taking a biopsy is to rule out premalignancy or malignancy and to establish a histopathologically based diagnosis. Biopsies are not generally performed when the physical examination and history have ruled everything else out. Local anesthesia should be performed, and a designated skin punch instrument preferred. The biopsy should be taken from a representative part of the lesion, preferably from its edge. Vulvoscopy may be useful in targeting the biopsy to select the most informative tissue sample.
- *Pelvic floor surface electromyography (EMG)* is a test that should not be performed routinely. Objective identification of pelvic floor hypertonic dysfunction can be obtained using various techniques. The most common is surface EMG, which is often performed as a part of a pelvic floor evaluation by physical therapists and nurse clinicians trained in the evaluation and management of patients with pelvic floor dysfunction.

In patients with *hypertonic dysfunction*, we find the following (listed in order of prevalence):

- Elevated and unstable resting baseline activity
- Poor recovery, poor postcontraction, and relaxation
- Spasms with sustained contractions and poor strength

10.7 Pudendal Neuralgia

Pudendal neuralgia is a painful, neuropathic condition involving the dermatome of the pudendal nerve. The distribution of the pudendal nerve, in the perineum, is mediated by 3 branches derived from the sacral roots S2–S4. These branches are the dorsal nerve of the penis or clitoris, the perineal nerve, and the inferior anal nerve. On the basis of this pattern of distribution, damage to the pudendal nerve can result in either unilateral or bilateral pain in the female vulva, vagina, or clitoris.

Electromyography is part of instrumental exams.

The "Nantes criteria" are now widely accepted for the diagnosis of pudendal neuralgia. They are grouped into four categories:

- Inclusion criteria
- Complementary diagnostic criteria
- Exclusion criteria
- Associated signs

To be diagnosed with pudendal neuralgia, a patient must exhibit all five inclusion criteria, without any symptoms of the exclusion criteria (Labat et al. 2008) (Box 10.9).

Box 10.9. Physical Examination in Pudendal Neuralgia

- Bimanual pelvic examination then follows, with attention to the pelvic floor muscles, in particular the levator and obturator muscles, as well as tenderness of the bladder and sacrospinous ligaments.
- In patients with pudendal neuralgia, maximum tenderness, or a trigger point, can be produced by applying pressure to the ischial spine, which serves anatomically as the insertion site for the sacrospinous ligament. Palpation of this area can reproduce pain and symptoms as a positive Tinel's sign.

10.7.1 Inclusion Criteria

- Pain in the area innervated by the pudendal nerve extends from anus to clitoris, is more severe when sitting, and does not awaken patients from sleep, with no objective sensory impairment; it is relieved by diagnostic pudendal block.

10.7.2 Complementary Diagnostic Criteria

- Pain characteristics: burning, shooting, stabbing, numbing, allodynia, or hyperesthesia
- Sensation of foreign body in the rectum or vagina (sympathalgia)
- Pain progressively worse throughout the day, predominantly unilateral, and triggered by defecation

- Significant tenderness around ischial spine on vaginal or rectal examination
- Abnormal neurophysiology testing (pudendal nerve motor latency testing) in men and nulliparous women

10.7.3 Exclusion Criteria

- Pain located exclusively in the coccygeal, gluteal, pubic, or hypogastric area (without pain in the area of distribution of pudendal nerve)
- Pruritus and pain exclusively paroxysmal
- Abnormality on the imaging test (magnetic resonance imaging, CT, and others), which can account for the pain

10.7.4 Associated Signs

- Buttock pain (area around ischial tuberosity) with sitting
- Referred sciatic pain and pain referred to the medial side of the thigh or suprapubic pain
- Urinary frequency or pain with full bladder
- Pain after orgasm and dyspareunia or pain after intercourse
- Normal pudendal nerve motor latency

Conclusions

The careful examination of the vulva and of the pelvic floor, in static and dynamic conditions, is essential to qualify the diagnosis and evaluate potential comorbidities, with the goal of tailoring the best treatment for that woman complaining of vulvar pain in that phase of her life.

References

Cohen Sacher B. The normal vulva, vulvar examination, and evaluation tools. Clin Obstet Gynecol. 2015;58(3):442–52.

Farhi D, Wendling J, Molinari E, et al. Non-sexually related acute genital ulcers in 13 pubertal girls: a clinical and microbiological study. Arch Dermatol. 2009;145(1):38–45.

Huppert JS, Gerber MA, Deitch HR, Mortensen JE, Staat MA, Adams Hillard PJ. Vulvar ulcers in young females: a manifestation of aphthosis. J Pediatr Adolesc Gynecol. 2006;19(3):195–204.

Labat JJ, Riant T, Robert R, Amarenco G, Lefaucheur JP, Rigaud J. Diagnostic criteria for pudendal neuralgia by pudendal nerve entrapment (Nantes criteria). Neurourol Urodyn. 2008;27:306–10.

Marinoff SC, Turner MLC. Vulvar vestibulitis syndrome. Dermatol Clin. 1992;10:435–44.

Melzack R. The short-form McGill pain questionnaire. Pain. 1987;30:191–7.

Nyirjesy P. Management of persistent vaginitis. Obstet Gynecol. 2014;124(6):1135–46.

Portman DJ, Gass MLS. Genitourinary syndrome of menopause: New terminology for vulvovaginal atrophy from the International Society for the Study of Women's Sexual Health and The North American Menopause Society. Maturitas. 2014;79(3):349–54.

Rosen R, Brown C, Heiman J, Leiblum S, Meston C, Shabsigh R. The Female Sexual Function Index (FSFI): a multidimensional self-report instrument for the assessment of female sexual function. J Sex Marital Ther. 2000;26:191–208.

Sideri M, Murina F, Bianco V, Radici GL. The role of vulvoscopy in the evaluation of dyspareunia. In: Goldstein AC, Pukall CI, Goldstein I, editors. Female sexual pain disorders. 1st ed. Oxford: Blackwell Publishing; 2009. p. 32–42.

Simonetta C, Burns EK, Guo MA. Vulvar dermatoses: a review and update. Mo Med. 2015;112(4):301–7.

Stockdale CK, Lawson HW. 2013 vulvodynia guideline update. J Low Genit Tract Dis. 2014;18:93–100.

Xanthos DN, Gaderer S, Drdla R, Nuro E, Abramova A, Ellmeier W, Sandkühler J. Central nervous system mast cells in peripheral inflammatory nociception. Mol Pain. 2011;7:42. doi:10.1186/1744-8069-7-42.

Xanthos DN, Sandkühler J. Neurogenic neuroinflammation: inflammatory CNS reactions in response to neuronal activity. Nat Rev Neurosci. 2014;15(1):43–53. doi:10.1038/nrn3617. Epub 2013 Nov 27.

Zendell K. Genital lichen planus: update on diagnosis and treatment. Semin Cutan Med Surg. 2015;34(4):182–6.

Vulvar Pain: From the Diagnosis to Treatment Strategies

11

Vulvar pain is often multifactorial in origin. Therefore, a multimodal approach to treatment should be considered. Multimodal interventions include the use of more than one type of therapy for the care of patients with acute, chronic, or pathologic/neuropathic pain (Graziottin 2006; Graziottin and Murina 2011; Graziottin and Gambini 2015a; Graziottin et al. 2016).

A committed trustworthy relationship with the patient is essential: the woman affected with the challenging vulvar pain needs to know, see, and feel, at any age, that the healthcare provider (HCP) *trusts the biological truth of her pain* and will do his/her best to diagnose the cause(s) of it and treat them in the most effective ways. Avoiding a minimalist approach is the first challenge (Box 11.1) (Graziottin et al. 2016).

Box 11.1: The Vulvar Scenario First: The Challenge of Avoiding a Minimalistic Approach

- *The missing listening or the collusion of silence*:
  - Women feel often ashamed and embarrassed to speak about vulvar pain and sexual issues with the physician. The majority of women think that vulvar pain is "too intimate to be spoken of" until it becomes invalidating. This is why HCPs should *routinely ask about vulvar and sexual pain as a normal part of the clinical history*. Otherwise it is difficult to provide an effective intervention if there is no mention of a problem
  - One third of women would not even speak about their vulvar pain, and/or vulvovaginal atrophy (VVA), with their partner. It is even more the physician's responsibility to raise the problem and, if present, ask the proper questions (Box 11.2) and analyze vulvar complaints with an *investigative mindset* and a *pathophysiologic reading* of the woman's narrative of symptoms.

A. Graziottin, F. Murina, *Vulvar Pain*, DOI 10.1007/978-3-319-42677-8_11

- *The missing diagnosis*:
  - The physician superficially examines the woman and concludes: "You have nothing, pain is all in your head," or "It is psychogenic." To improve the examining skills is mandatory! (Box 11.3)
- *Minimalistic treatments*:
  - What happens when vulvar and/or sexual pain are overtly reported? The majority of women facing vulvar and sexual pain, and associated comorbidities, receive a lubricant as an answer for their sexual concerns. This is frequently perceived as humiliating by the woman, as a deception by the man, as a *fiction of arousal* by the couple.
  - To address vulvar symptoms in a *comprehensive multimodal approach* is essential if vulvar pain is to be effectively and definitely cured.

Modified from Graziottin et al. (2016)

The second challenge is to distil an essential history taking, useful for every physician in his/her practice (please see the Chap. 10 on diagnosis of vulvar pain). Here the key questions and examining issues are summarized to ease the younger readers to systematize their vision of vulvar pain diagnostic basis, essential to design an effective treatment, and/or readers interested just on this chapter.

Box 11.2: Vulvar Pain: The Basic Mindset in the History Taking

- *Careful listening of spontaneous woman's wording*, rich of critical informations to design a personalized protocol and to prevent recurrences
- *Mandatory questions*:
  1. When did your vulvar pain initiate? Is it recent (lasting 3 months or less) or not?
  2. Do you recall any specific event triggering it (vulvar trauma, vaginitis, cystitis, antibiotics, intercourse, childbirth, sexual abuse, surgical operations, etc.)?
  3. How would you describe your vulvar pain: pain, burning, itching, irritation, dryness, or soreness? Is it continuous or intermittent, localized, or extended to the whole vulva ("generalized")? Is it worse at night or not? Please indicate as many key words as you feel appropriate.
  4. Do you specifically suffer from burning vulvar pain?
  5. Is it spontaneous or provoked (by the use on tampons, or the intercourse, or the clinical examination, or stress, or what else)?
  6. Does intercourse hurt at the entrance of the vagina ("introital dyspareunia")?
  7. Is there any pattern of recurrence: after intercourse or not?
  8. Does it worsen during the menstrual period?
  9. Do you suffer from recurrent vaginitis (particularly from *Candida*), recurrent or postcoital cystitis, irritable bowel syndrome (i.e.,

diarrhea/constipation), obstructive constipation, endometriosis, fibromyalgia, or headache?
10. Are you taking hormonal contraceptives (pill, patch, vaginal ring)?
11. Are your periods regular or are you without periods (amenorrhea: hypothalamic, postpartum, menopausal)?
12. Are you diabetic? How is your glycemic control? Do you have relatives with diabetes?
13. Since your vulvar pain has become chronic, did you have other symptoms such as fatigue, mood swings/depression, sleep difficulties, concentration, and memory problems?

Modified from Graziottin (2014)

Box 11.3: Vulvar Pain: The Mandatory Gynecological Examination

1. *Examine the vulva and the perineum*: is there any vestibular/vulvar erythema? Scratching signs? Scars? Dermatosis? Any discharge? Is there any sign of retracted/hyperactive pelvic floor (usually so in nulliparous women reporting positive answer to questions 1–6 (Box 11.2)) Hemorrhoids (suggestive of an hyperactive pelvic floor and/or chronic constipation)?
2. *Perform the swab test*, at five and seven, looking at the entrance of the vagina like a clockface and then *random* all over the vulva. The test is usually positive when the woman answers yes to two out of three questions 4–6 (Box 11.2). Is the clitoris painful?
3. *Examine the pelvic floor*: is it tense? Are there tender and/or trigger points at the insertion of the levator ani on the ischiatic spine bilaterally? How's the perineal command (absent, correct, inverted, i.e., when the woman is requested to push and relax the levator ani/perineal floor, she automatically pulls and retract it even further)? A hyperactive pelvic floor is usually present in case of at least four positive answers to questions 1–6 (Box 11.2). Examine the obturator muscle and the Alcock canal, bilaterally.
4. *Perform an accurate gynecological examination*: are there other areas of pain (along the anterior vaginal wall, in case of comorbid urethritis; deep in the posterior fornix and along the uterosacral ligaments in case of comorbid endometriosis; laterally, in the adnexal area in case of pelvic inflammatory disease [PID], etc.)?
5. *Evaluate the vaginal pH*: a pH of 4 is physiologic, but associated with recurrent *Candida*; pH of 4.6–5 or more is associated with bacterial vaginosis and increased vulnerability to invasion/infection from colonic germs, uropathogenic *Escherichia Coli* (UPEC) most. Usually the vaginal pH is elevated in case of positive responses to question 11 (Box 11.2) (i.e., in case of prolonged amenorrhea).

Modified from Graziottin (2014)

When women affected with chronic or pathologic/neuropathic vulvar pain finally meet a dedicated and committed HCP, they (and their families!) are usually devastated by *years of unaddressed inflammation and vulvar pain*, of diagnostic neglect, and the frequent appearance of other painful comorbidities (Graziottin and Murina 2011).

Moreover, the inflammation peripherally modulated by mast cells (Graziottin 2009) has reached the brain (please see the Chap. 3 on pathophysiology of vulvar pain). Chronic neuroinflammation induces:

- *Neurogenic neuroinflammation*, with massive upregulation of the microglia, whose role shifts from neuroplastic to neurotoxic (Graziottin et al. 2013, 2014a, b, 2015; Xanthos et al. 2011; Walker et al. 2013; Skaper et al. 2015). *Behavioral correlates* include maladaptive sickness behavior, depression (which is first of all the epiphenomenon of a massive neuroinflammation (Derry et al. 2015), not just a "black cloud over the head"), fatigue, sleep disorders, memory difficulties, and concentration problems. These symptoms are frequently reported to the listening physician. The treatment should address them and their pathophysiologic basis as well.
- *Neurogenic peripheral inflammation*, with persisting vulvar pain (and increasing comorbidities, worsening over time).

Key Point

When vulvar pain becomes neuropathic, it is just the tip of the iceberg of a massive systemic and brain inflammation. Treatment cannot be minimalistic, focused only on the vulva, but must address the neuropathic complexity with a strategic, pathophysiologically based vision.

A careful evaluation of *lifestyles and behaviors* potentially contributing to vulvar pain is a vital part of the diagnosis and treatment. Unfortunately it is often omitted, thus impairing the potential for a full recovery. A well-designed treatment should therefore address first of all the modification(s) of inadequate lifestyles to maximize the benefits in a well-designed therapeutic plan (Box 11.4).

The simple example that works to motivate many patients in improving their lifestyles is that *the river of pain originates from the river of inflammation* (that means *to set a biochemical fire*), like the intensity of smoke depends on the intensity of fire in the real world.

The river of inflammation has many tributaries, including but not limited to:

- *Overweight/obesity*, as the adipose tissue produces massive amounts of cytokines and other inflammatory molecules that flood the body and the brain (Pedersen 2009).
- *Physical inactivity* that is a major contributor of systemic diseases. The majority of them have inflammation and pain as leading characteristics (Booth et al. 2012).

- *Unhealthy diet*: women with unhealthy diet have more than twice the risk of widespread chronic pain (Vandenkerkhof et al. 2011), through different pathophysiologic pathways.
- *Reduced quality of sleep*, a major biological stress and cause of neuro and systemic inflammation when chronic, through the hyperactivation of the corticotrophin releasing pathway (CRP) (Finan et al. 2013).
- *Chronic stress:* biological, psychological, and/or context dependent (Derry et al. 2015).

Key Point
Neuroinflammation should first be addressed through the improvement of lifestyles, when inadequate, or altered by pain itself and associated behavioral changes.

Box 11.4: Vulvar Pain: Improve Lifestyles to Reduce Systemic and Brain Inflammation

- *Weight reduction* may improve the treatment outcome of vulvar (and any other) pain. Reducing adipose tissue:
  – Reduces in parallel the associated systemic and neuroinflammation, decreasing the risk of maladaptive sickness behavior, typical of neuropathic pain, of fatigue and depression (Pedersen 2009; Derry et al. 2015)
  – Improves body image, self-perception, vital energy, mood, and sex drive, especially if combined with daily physical activity. All these positive changes may contribute to the "healing project" in a comprehensive and rewarding way. As a patient said: "I'm so glad, doctor, that you are looking at me and curing me *as a woman*, not just as a *painful walking vulva*"
- *Physical exercise*: the anti-inflammatory effect of regular exercise can be mediated via:
  – An induction of an anti-inflammatory environment with each bout of exercise.
  – A reduction in visceral fat mass. The finding that muscles produce and release myokines provides a conceptual basis to understand the mechanisms whereby exercise influences metabolism and exerts anti-inflammatory effects (Pedersen 2009).
  – A reduction of the consequences of psychosocial and physical stress, a major contributor of depression (Slavich and Irwin 2014) and worsening of pain perception.

- A reduction of systemic inflammation, neuroinflammation, and depression, and a better immune functioning and a better sleep, the great and underappreciated guardian of health and sexuality, reduced fatigue and distress.
- A mental and psychological *redesign of the woman's body map*, giving the correct importance to all the body parts and not focusing only on the sick vulva.
- A modulation of the *dopaminergic system*, increasing dopamine secretion. It is likely that all these factors positively impact the recovery of sexuality as well.

- *Healthy diet:* increasing evidence supports the role of a healthy diet as a substantial health promoter and specifically as a pain reducer/controller, through the reduction of the inflammation induced by inadequate quality of food intake (Vandenkerkhof et al. 2011). Recommendations include limit alcohol to no more than one drink/day and avoid smoking. Alcohol and smoke may exacerbate inflammatory condition and have a detrimental mental effect.
- *Sleep quality and duration*: to maintain low levels of systemic inflammation, human being (with few exceptions) should sleep 1 h every 2 h wake. To improve quality and duration of sleep reduces inflammation, pain, and pain perception. Even napping may significantly reduce pain (Faraut et al. 2015). Protecting/improving the quality of sleep may significantly reduce pain (Finan et al. 2013). This can be achieved also with the help of melatonin, a natural circadian sleep hormone which has an anti-inflammatory effect.

11.1 The Start-Up: Explain the Diagnosis of Vulvar Pain and Realistic Treatment Goals

Any treatment approach should begin with a discussion including an explanation of the diagnosis and realistic treatment goals. A general guiding principle is *to begin with those treatment options with the fewest side effects or potential complications*.

Discussion of *lifestyles* must be included.

The patient should be counselled that *follow-up is needed* to evaluate treatment responses and adjust the therapeutic plan as needed to maximize pain reduction. A *multidisciplinary intervention* should be part of a treatment strategy for patients with vulvar pain. Multidisciplinary interventions are multimodality approaches in the context of a treatment program that includes more than one discipline.

The team of HCPs may involve gynecologist, dermatologist, psychosexual counselors, urologist, and physical therapists, plus other specialists when indicated. It is crucial to maintain communication among all the involved treating providers to avoid duplication of therapy and optimize a cohesive treatment plan.

Key Point

The three golden steps for a well-designed and effective treatment of vulvar pain are:

- To listen openly to health and sexual concerns focused on the vulva
- To encourage the dialogue on vulvar pain and associated sexual issues and comorbidities
- To address them with structured, comprehensive, and effective pharmacologic/rehabilitative therapeutic strategies, including improvement of inadequate lifestyles, directed at curing the underlying vulvar and systemic pathophysiology.

11.1.1 Vulvar Care Guidelines

Multiple studies have been conducted to show that there are important differences between vulvar tissue and other skin surfaces. Such characteristics as tissue structure itself, hydration status, occlusion, friction, and permeability make vulvar tissue more susceptible to inflammation as well as friction-related injuries (Podorozhansky et al. 2012).

We recommend that the patient should initially be encouraged to follow a few general advices for minimizing vulvar irritation. This is the first specific level of treatment that each physician must recommend to any patient with acute vulvar pain, chronic vulvar pain, and, even more so, provoked or spontaneous vestibulodynia/vulvodynia. By following vulvar care guidelines with regard to personal hygiene and product use, patients in whom contact dermatitis potentially contribute to vulvar pain should be able to see improvement in their symptoms.

Although vulvar care guidelines are not enough to constitute the entire scope of treatment of various vulvar disorders, they can serve as an important adjunct to conventional treatment (Box 11.5).

Box 11.5: Vulvar Care Measures to Minimize Vulvar Irritation

- Avoid vulvar irritants (perfumes, dyes, shampoos, detergents) and douching.
- Use adequate lubrication for intercourse.
- Wear all-white cotton or medicated silk fibroin underwear.
- Wear loose-fitting pants or skirts; do not wear pantyhose or jeans.
- Use dermatologically/gynecologically approved intimate detergents.
- Use soft, white, unscented toilet paper.
- Avoid getting shampoo on the vulvar area.
- Do not use bubble bath, feminine hygiene products, or perfumed creams or soaps.

- *Avoid penetration until vestibular inflammation and pain are resolved* (Box 11.6).
- *Do not use anesthetic cream to ease intercourse, as this will perpetuate the vestibular trauma and inflammation.*
- Apply ice, or a frozen blue gel pack (lunchbox size), wrapped in a single layer of towel to relieve burning after intercourse (if accepted in spite of pain).
- After sexual intercourses, urinate to prevent infection and rinse vulva with cool water.
- Avoid exercises that put direct pressure on the vulva, such as bicycle riding and horseback riding.
- Limit intense exercise that creates a lot of friction in the vulvar area (try lower-intensity exercises such as brisk daily walking).

Adapted from "Self-Help Tips for Vulvar Skin Care", National Vulvodynia Association, http://www.nva.org/

Box 11.6: The Amletic Dilemma: To Have Intercourse or Not to Have it?
A special note is to be made about having intercourse while vestibular pain is complained of:

- Many women accept intercourse, in spite of the burning pain persisting for days after penetration and worsening over time because of the repeated intercourse, for fear of losing the partner.
- Many partners insist that having intercourse is a normal part of the couple relationship.
- Many physicians recommend *the use of an anesthetic cream to reduce coital pain* and allow intercourse, "to help the couple to have a normal sexual life."
- This is *absolutely wrong from the pathophysiologic point of view.* Which physician would recommend/prescribe an anesthetic to a man or a woman with a broken leg (or whatever other fracture), "so that you can use it"?!
- With a broken leg, everybody would agree that the first goal is to heal the fracture, do the proper rehabilitative therapy, and *then* start walking and doing sport again.
- Why the vulva and the vagina should be treated differently? A woman is more than a vulva to be enjoyed and a vagina to be "used" while being penetrated.

Women and partner should be informed that pain (vestibular and sexual) is not just a disturbing symptom. It is the tip of the iceberg of a *real, severe inflammatory disease* of the *vulva*, with *increased proliferation of pain fibers* that multiply pain and *make it chronic and pathologic/neuropathic, if the microtraumas of the vestibular mucosa are further repeatedly caused by insisting on having intercourse.* Inflammation often extends to neighbor organs such as the bladder, causing cystitis 24–72 h after the intercourse in 60 % of cases (Salonia et al. 2013). A process called "comorbidity" that causes pain of progressive severity.

11.2 Therapy of Specific Disorders Causing Vulvar Pain in the Lifespan

11.2.1 Labial Adhesion

This term is used when the labia minora fuse together in prepubescent girls. Other nomenclature used to describe the condition includes *labial agglutination, labial fusion*, and *vulvar synechiae*. It is not a rare condition and has been reported to occur in up to 1.8 % of female prepubertal patients. It mainly affects girls 5 years of age, with a peak incidence around the age of 13–23 months (Simpson and Murphy 2014).

The etiology of the condition is unknown but it is believed to be associated with the low estrogenic state in prepubertal girls (Davis 2003). Less commonly, it occurs secondary to vulvar inflammation and irritation in which the skin becomes excoriated and denuded leading to fusion of the labial edges during the healing process. This condition can be distinguished from imperforate hymen or labioscrotal fusion (androgen associated, midline fusion of external genitals) by the inability to visualize the urethra (Davis 2003).

11.2.1.1 Management

- Explaining how the fusion has arisen, reassurance that it is a self-limiting condition and that the internal anatomy is normal is helpful for most parents.
- If more than 75 % of the labia are closed, and/or if the child complains of burning pain, and/or dysuria, urinary tract infection, and obstruction, it is appropriate to treat this with topical estrogen applied sparingly to the line of adhesion, twice daily, until separation occurs. Estrogen treatment should be continued until the urethra is visualized, as long as there is no evidence of systemic estrogenization (breast bud). Therapy may take up to 6 weeks (Davis 2003). Treatment can be repeated in case of recurrence.
- There is no consensus about the type of estrogen, the preferable frequency and duration of the application. In our experience, treatment may be required for several weeks to achieve separation of the labia minora, and the application of estriol gel 0.05 % once a day can prove to be very effective.
- Adhesions tend to recur if preventive measures are not taken (i.e., gentle labial separation to visualize the urethra with the application of petroleum jelly or barrier cream to reduce labial adherence). Additional management includes daily baths, avoidance of irritants such as soapy water or bubble baths, and vulvar "airing" (a daily period of time when the diaper is removed or not wearing underwear during the night). The surgical release of labial adhesions is rarely required.

- Underwear made of medicated silk fibroin, indicated for different atopic dermatoses in children, can complement the effectiveness of treatment, as it reduces dermatitis and associated bacteric infections.
- Surgical intervention should be reserved for severe cases resistant to conservative management in girls presenting with urinary retention and/or voiding difficulties and/or recurrent cystitis due to the stenosis induced by the tight central labial fusion.

11.2.2 Vulvovaginal Infections

1. *Childhood vulvovaginitis*

It is one of the most common gynecological conditions encountered in pediatric outpatient clinics, in both prepubertal and pubertal children.

Group A beta-hemolytic streptococcus (ABHS) is the most common cause of *prepubertal* vulvovaginitis. ABHS can cause a burning red rash in the vulva, and/or perineum, and/or perianal area, with or without fissures.

11.2.2.1 Management

- Treatment is with oral penicillin in adequate pro/kg doses (to be prescribed by the pediatrician) for 10–14 days, or clindamycin cream 2 % per vagina for 7–10 days. Nevertheless a recent randomized controlled trial compared oral penicillin against cefuroxime for Group A beta-hemolytic *Streptococcus pyogenes* perianal dermatitis in children under 16 years of age. Successful eradication of infection, as determined by a posttreatment swab, was greater in the cefuroxime group compared with the penicillin group (93 % vs. 47 %, $p<0.01$).
- The authors therefore concluded that 7 days of cefuroxime was more efficacious than 10 days of penicillin and should therefore be considered the treatment of choice for this condition (Meury et al. 2008).
- The opportunity to integrate the antibiotic treatment with probiotics should be discussed with the pediatrician who looks after the child. Probiotics are increasingly utilized in the lifespan to restore the normal intestinal microbiota, usually devastated by high-dose antibiotic treatments.

2. *Vulvovaginal candidiasis*

Candida albicans is rare in childhood and is usually diagnosed only in severely immunodepressed children. Candida vaginitis is increasingly frequent in *postpubertal girls*, when estrogens play a critical role as "permitting" factors in the transition of *Candida* from the "sleeping" phase of spore to the vegetative phase of hypha. Cardinal symptoms of vulvovaginal candidiasis include vulvovaginal pruritus, irritation, soreness, dyspareunia, and vaginal "cheese-like" white discharge.

Clinical signs are best exemplified by vulva erythema, edema, excoriation, and fissure formation together with introital and vaginal erythema.

It is essential to treat adequately the recurrent vulvovaginal candidiasis because infection or a hypersensitivity reaction to subclinical candidiasis is believed to play a prominent role in the development of vulvar pain and vestibulodynia (please see Chap. 6 on vulvar pain in adolescents).

11.2.2.2 Management

- It is not necessary to treat an asymptomatic colonization, because *Candida* is a commensal of human vagina.
- Topical treatment of acute vulvovaginal candidiasis can be performed for a period of 3 to 5 days using imidazoles with different preparations such as creams or vaginal tablets or suppositories, if the girl has already had intercourse; oral triazoles (3-day treatment) and antimycotic creams for the vulva may also be used. All of the different treatment regimens produced similarly good clinical and mycological results.
- Management of recurrent vulvovaginal candidiasis can be problematic, and current guidelines clearly indicate both the relative high incidence of relapse in the follow-up and poor compliance of the patients. Different regimens are summarized in Table 11.1.
- Attention to adequate lifestyle, including improving the diet by reducing yeast-containing foods (bread, pizza, biscuits, etc.), glucose, and excess calories, increasing fresh food, and having daily aerobic exercise (1 h brisk walking or any other sport of preference) to optimize the peripheral use of insulin, is part of a strategic management.

Table 11.1 Proposal of therapy for vulvovaginal candidiasis

Drug	Formulation	Dose
Acute		
Clotrimazole	1–2 % cream	3–5 g daily for 5–7 days
Miconazole	2–4 % cream	4 g daily for 5–7 days
Fenticonazole	600 mg vaginal suppository	q 72 h for 3 doses
Fluconazole	150–200 mg oral pills	q 72 h for 3 doses
Recurrent		
Fluconazole	150–200 mg	Induction, 150–200 mg q 72 h for 3 doses Maintenance regimen, 150 mg q weekly for 6 months or 200 mg weekly for 2 months, followed by 200 mg biweekly for 4 months, and 200 mg monthly for 6 months or 200 mg weekly for 4 weeks, then 1 after 10–15 to 20–30 days
Itraconazole	100–200 mg	Induction, 200 mg bid × 3 doses Maintenance, 100–200 mg/d for 6 months

Sobel (2016), Murina et al. (2011)

- The oral weekly administration of a single dose of 150 mg of fluconazole for a period of 6 months proved to be successful in 91 % of the cases, but decreased to 43 % during the observation period 6 months after the cessation of the therapy (Sobel et al. 2004).
- Other regimen with a personalized and decreasing administration of 200 mg fluconazole doses, often for rather long periods (4 months on average), has been proposed. This therapeutic scheme has shown no evidence of clinical recurrence in 75–90 % of women and reduced to 70–75 % after 1 year (Donders et al. 2008).
- Probiotic bacteria have been targeted as potential therapeutic agents of recurrent vulvovaginal candidiasis. Possible mechanisms of this protection include inactivation of pathogens by different *Lactobacillus* products (lactic acid, H_2O_2, and bacteriocins), competition for epithelial cell attachment sites, and creation and maintenance of a vaginal biofilm that hinders the persistence of an infection caused by *Candida*.
- It is crucial to interfere with biofilm formation early after the drastic reduction of the *Candida* concentration (e.g., induction phase with fluconazole) and then to maintain the "positive" biofilm with a greater interval of use of the lactobacilli. It was demonstrated that a product formulated in slow-release, slightly effervescent vaginal tablets containing live cells of *Lactobacillus fermentum* LF10 and *Lactobacillus acidophilus* LA02 is effective in the treatment of recurrent vulvovaginal candidiasis: 72 % of patients experienced no clinical recurrence throughout the 7-month follow-up period (Murina et al. 2014).

11.2.3 Herpes Simplex Virus Infection

It is a very common cause of vulvar pain, particularly recurrent pain. It may become a challenging infection when recurrences are frequent and/or trigger neuropathic pain (Graziottin et al. 2015).

Women usually present with recurrent disease, often with unilateral episodic burning and discomfort. Standard treatment regimens for initial either primary or non-primary genital HSV include acyclovir, valacyclovir 1 g bd, and famciclovir (Box 11.7).

Box 11.7: Treatment Regimens for Herpes Simplex Virus Genital Infections

First Clinical Episode of Genital Herpes

- Acyclovir 400 mg orally three times a day for 7–10 days
- Acyclovir 200 mg orally five times a day for 7–10 days
- Famciclovir 250 mg orally three times a day for 7–10 days
- Valacyclovir 1 g orally twice a day for 7–10 days

The treatment may be extended if healing is incomplete after 10 days of therapy.

Episodic Therapy for Recurrent Genital Herpes
- Acyclovir 400 mg orally three times a day for 5 days or 800 mg orally twice a day for 5 days
- Acyclovir 800 mg orally three times a day for 2 days
- Famciclovir 125 mg orally twice a day for 5 days or 1000 mg orally twice daily for 1 day
- Valacyclovir 500 mg orally twice a day for 3 days or 1.0 g orally once a day for 5 days

Recommended Regimens for Suppressive Therapy (Immune-Competent Patients)
- Acyclovir 400 mg orally twice a day
- Famciclovir 250 mg orally twice a day
- Valacyclovir 500 mg orally once a day or 1.0 g orally once a day

Romero and Nygaard (2015)

11.2.4 Vulvar Dermatosis

They are inflammatory conditions responsible for chronic or recurrent itching and pain. Pain and itch are thought to be closely related in that weak activation of nociceptors mediates itch, while strong activation of the same receptors results in weak pain. Moreover, there is a broad overlap in neuromediators of pain and itch signal processing. Interestingly, scratch-induced pain can abolish itching, suggesting reciprocal control of pain and itch (Lee et al. 2013). The lesions are either circumscribed to the vulva or associated with extragenital localizations which may help to assess the diagnosis. The most frequent vulvar dermatoses are lichen sclerosus, lichen simplex chronicus, and lichen planus.

1. *Vulvar lichen sclerosus (VLS)*

It is a chronic inflammatory disease with considerable impact on health-related quality of life (Simonetta et al. 2015). Patients with VLS complain mainly of itching, burning, pain, dyspareunia, and sexual dysfunction.

11.2.4.1 Management

- A definitive cure does not currently exist. The ideal treatment for VLS should aim at inducing relief of symptoms, reversing signs, and preventing further anatomical changes.
- Topical potent and ultrapotent corticosteroids represent the recommended first-line treatment for vulvar lichen sclerosus, both in the active phase and in maintenance treatment (Fistarol and Itin 2013).

- No trials comparing different treatment regimens are available. Clobetasol propionate 0.05 % ointment or cream for 12 weeks is the most used. Recent studies have shown that the less potent corticosteroid mometasone furoate 0.1 % (MMF) is effective in treating VLS as well. MMF is a potent glucocorticoid with greater anti-inflammatory activity and duration of action than other steroids of similar potency, characterized by a low potential to cause side effects and the convenience of once-daily administration (Virgili et al. 2014; Murina et al. 2015).
- Both tapering and continuous application of mometasone furoate 0.1 % ointment showed similar efficacy and tolerability in the treatment of active VLS, without any difference in patient adherence to therapy (Borghi et al. 2015) (Box 11.8).

Box 11.8: Lichen Sclerosus Practice Points

- Topical steroid regimens:
  - Clobetasol propionate 0.05 % ointment applied once daily, at night, for 4 weeks, then on alternate nights for 4 weeks, and then twice weekly for further 4 weeks.
  - MMF 0.1 % ointment initially once daily for 5 days a week for 4 weeks, then on alternate days for 4 weeks, and, for the final third month, twice weekly.
  - MMF 0.1 % ointment daily for 4 weeks and then twice weekly for another 4 weeks in combination with a moisturizing cream.
- The use of an emollient, in addition to the topical steroid during the initial treatment phase, and then as maintenance therapy, is very beneficial.
- For the very rare cases of resistance to topical steroids of VLS, therapeutical alternatives should be investigated (topical calcineurin inhibitors, topical and systemic retinoids, and photodynamic therapy).
- Prevention of squamous cell carcinoma associated with VLS relies on detection of precursors which should be suspected in the case of a circumscribed white raised lesions or pink patches.
- The 5 % risk of neoplastic progression makes mandatory a regular follow-up, yearly or more frequently when clinically indicated in individual cases.

Davis (2003), Kirtschig et al. (2015)

2. *Lichen simplex chronicus*

   It is usually treated with the therapeutic strategy used for lichen sclerosus.

3. *Lichen planus (LP)*

It is far less common than LS and commonly causes vulvar pain. Classically, painful LP is scarring and erosive with a glazed erythema, usually on the vulvar vestibule and posterior fourchette.

LP, unlike LS, can involve the vagina (with or without vulvar involvement) with erosions and/or desquamative vaginitis resulting in a vaginal discharge.

Evidence-based data on the treatment of LP are limited, and management choices mainly rely on clinical experience (Box 11.9).

Box 11.9: Treatment of Lichen Planus

- Clobetasol or mometasone ointment
- Triamcinolone acetonide intramuscular
- Prednisone 40–60 mg orally once a day, taper as clinically indicated
- Topical tacrolimus 0.03, 0.1 % ointment
- Other systemic treatment for very severe LP
  - Methotrexate 5–10 mg/week orally
  - Cyclosporine 4–5 mg/kg/day orally for 3–4 months
- Intravaginal hydrocortisone acetate suppository 25 mg (available) or 100 mg (compounded) 10 % compounded vaginal cream

Zendell (2015)

11.3 Management of Vulvovaginal Atrophy (VVA)/ Genitourinary Syndrome of Menopause (GSM)

GSM is a more descriptive term than VVA, which is part of it. It is defined as a collection of symptoms and signs associated with a decrease in estrogen and other sex steroids involving changes to the labia majora/minora, clitoris, vestibule, vagina, urethra, and bladder.

The syndrome may include, but is not limited to, genital symptoms of dryness, burning, and irritation and sexual symptoms of lack of lubrication, discomfort or pain, and impaired sexual function (please see the Chap. 8 on vulvar pain after the menopause for a detailed discussion of different treatment options).

The characteristic vulvovaginal changes that occur during and after the menopause are due to the combination of pathophysiologic aging, hypoestrogenism, and hypoandrogenism (Graziottin and Gambini 2016).

Estradiol, the primary form of estrogen produced by a woman's ovary during her reproductive years, plays an essential role in maintaining the elasticity and health of her genital tissues, including *an appropriate vaginal ad vulvar microbiota and adequate low vaginal pH* (Graziottin and Zanello 2015).

The genital involution is more rapid and anticipated in women affected by a premature ovarian insufficiency (Graziottin and Lukasiewicz 2016). A iatrogenic menopause after gynecologic cancers may have an even more dramatic impact on anatomy and function of genital organs, when the premature or anticipated menopause is complicated with the side effect of vaginal/pelvic radiotherapy (Lukasiewicz and Graziottin 2015; Graziottin et al. 2016; Graziottin and Gambini 2016).

Testosterone loss is responsible for the hormone-dependent involution of the cavernosal bodies (clitoral, bulbocavernous, and part of the equivalent of the male corpus spongiosum, around the urethra), of the androgen-dependent cells of the skin, of the connective tissue (fibroblasts and myocells), and of the androgen-dependent nitrergic nerve fibers, present at vaginal (1/3 is nitrergic, 2/3 are vipergic) and vulvar level (Graziottin et al. 2015b). This is the pathophysiologically based reason why topical estrogen and testosterone are the leading treatments for the VVA and GSM, with special focus on vulvar dystrophy and associated symptoms (Box 11.10).

GSM is a chronic condition and therefore requires long-term therapy as symptoms tend to return when treatment is stopped.

Box 11.10: Management of GSM/VVA

Topical Treatments

- *Topical estrogens* include estradiol-containing tablets and rings; estriol pessaries, creams, and ovules; and promestriene and conjugated estrogens. Compared with placebo, vaginal estrogens improved dryness, dyspareunia, urinary urgency, frequency, and stress urinary incontinence (SUI) and urgency urinary incontinence (UUI). Urinary tract infection rates decreased. The various estrogen preparations had similar efficacy and safety; serum estradiol levels remained within postmenopausal norms for all except high-dose conjugated equine estrogen cream (Rahn et al. 2014). The literature supports the efficacy of lower doses while minimizing adverse effects.
- The efficacy of vestibular use of 0.005 % estriol for the treatment of postmenopausal dyspareunia has recently been demonstrated. The tenfold reduction in dose of estrogen currently administered was effective in significantly normalizing vestibular innervation sensitivity. Its formulation as a highly mucoadhesive hydrating gel provides a reservoir effect for lengthy maintenance of active estriol on the vestibular surface (Murina et al. 2016a).
- *Topical testosterone* (testosterone propionate 2 % or, in alternative, testosterone of vegetal origin) is very effective for the treatment of VVA and GMS in the Author's experience in *otherwise healthy postmenopausal women*. Topical testosterone applied daily for 3 months improves vulvovaginal trophism and relieves symptoms of VVA and GSM. It definitely improves the genital sexual response, both in the arousal and orgasm dimension, with great satisfaction of the woman and of her partner.
- *Topical testosterone* has been used in *patients with breast cancer* under aromatase inhibitor treatment. Preliminary data are encouraging (Witherby et al. 2011). More recent data indicate that 300 microgram of testosterone applied in the vagina has a very significant impact on women's sexuality:

when compared with baseline FSFI scores, there was a statistically significant improvement for individual domain scores of desire ($P=0.000$), arousal ($P=0.002$), lubrication ($P=0.018$), orgasm ($P=0.005$), satisfaction ($P=0.001$), and pain ($P=0.000$). Total domain scores reflecting sexual health quality of life also improved when compared with baseline ($P=0.000$). Long-term controlled studies on the safety profile are needed (Dahir and Travers-Gustafson 2014).

- *Vaginal dehydroepiandrosterone* (DHEA). Daily intravaginal administration of 0.5 % (6.5 mg) DHEA for 52 weeks significantly improves dyspareunia, vaginal dryness, and irritation/itching. Cream applied in the vagina is another useful tool to be explored in treatment of VVA and GSM. Preliminary data are very positive in terms of vaginal lubrication, with no changes in the systemic levels of prasterone (Bouchard et al. 2016; Davis et al. 2016; Labrie et al. 2016). Daily dosing is necessary as reduced efficacy has been shown when the treatment is reduced to two doses/week (Bouchard et al. 2016). However, the pharmacology and mechanism of action suggest that the effect on vestibular pain could be positive, on daily dosing, as shown by Author's experience (still preliminary results).
- *Nonhormonal vaginal lubricants and moisturizers.* Lubricants, in general, give only temporary relief of symptoms. They must be applied frequently for more continuous relief and require reapplication before intercourse.
- *Fractional laser.* Laser therapy may result in remodeling and thickening of vaginal connective tissue. It improves glycogen storage of the vaginal epithelium in women with vaginal atrophy. Improvement in VVA symptoms (vaginal dryness, burning, itching, and dyspareunia) and vaginal health index scores have been reported. Pulsed CO_2 lasers (Monnalisa) (Pieralli et al. 2016) and erbium laser treatment (Gambacciani et al. 2015) are increasingly used in the treatment of VVA after the menopause, particularly in women after breast cancer.

Systemic Therapies

- *Systemic estrogens:* women *with* uterus should use estrogens combined with progesterone/progestins, indicated to protect the endometrium, either in cyclical or continuous combined regimen. Tibolone is another option. After hysterectomy, women can use only estrogens. The WHI study reanalysis clearly indicates that the postmenopausal treatment with only estrogens in hysterectomized women significantly *reduces the risk of breast cancer* while it maintains all the benefits on cardiovascular system, brain, bones, joints, gastrointestinal and urogenital system, and on sensory organs, skin, and mucosae first (Gurney et al. 2014). It can therefore be used in the long term, if symptoms persist. However, as the systemic administration may not be sufficient to guarantee a normal vaginal lubrication, topical estrogens should be considered to optimize the functional outcome in individual cases. Hormones are indicated as well after squamous cell carcinoma of the cervix or if bilateral ovariectomy (for cancers different from adenocarcinomas) has been performed (Graziottin and Lukasiewicz 2016; Lukasiewicz and Graziottin 2015).

- *Ospemifene*, a selective estrogen receptor modulator (SERM), has been approved for the treatment of VVA in postmenopausal women. The daily dose is 60 mg once a day, after the most important meal of the day, to optimize the drug absorption (please see the Chap. 12 on clinical cases) (Bruyniks et al. 2016). Subjects in these studies reported statistically significant improvement and relief for vaginal dryness ($p < 0.00001$), dyspareunia ($p < 0.001$), and statistically significant improvement and relief for vaginal and/or vulvar irritation/itching ($p < 0.01$) from baseline to week 12 with ospemifene compared with placebo. A similar trend was observed for women who reported substantial improvement of vaginal and/or vulvar irritation/itching (Bruyniks et al. 2016).
- *Bazedoxifene (BZA) and conjugated estrogens (CE)*: the combination between a SERM and CE has been shown effective in the control of menopausal symptoms, including VVA, while preventing osteopenia/osteoporosis (Bachmann et al. 2010; Kagan et al. 2010; Abraham et al. 2014). This combination does not cause the increase of breast cancer risk, associated with "classic" estrogen + progesterone/progestin menopausal therapies, thanks to the protective effect of bazedoxifene on the breast. This is very reassuring, after the worldwide concern raised by the Women's Health Initiative study (WHI), when CE were used with medroxyprogesterone acetate (MAP). The BZA/CE combination can be considered when VVA is the tip of the iceberg of a more complex menopausal symptomatology in women who would like to address their systemic and genital symptoms in safety from the breast risk point of view. However, specific data focusing on the vulvar trophism and relief of vulvar pain require further controlled studies.

Key Point

Currently, GSM/VVA can be perfectly addressed with a highly personalized treatment strategy. Topical estrogens have high efficacy and excellent safety profile. Topical testosterone seems to offer a specific advantage for the reduction of vestibular/vulvar pain symptoms after the menopause, with significant improvement of vestibular and vulvar trophism. SERMs offer increased safety profile, with significant improvement of VVA.

11.4 Vulvar Pain Without Clear Identifiable Cause: The Vulvodynia Therapy

Vulvodynia may be a final result of or common pathway for several pathological processes, such that any one-management strategy may not be adequate for all women complaining of pathologic/neuropathic vulvar pain. There is no consensus regarding the best treatment available, except that treatment should be tailored to fit the specific patient (Box 11.11).

Many women with vulvodynia experience loss of hope, which can further contribute to depression – specifically triggered by the neuroinflammation (please see the Chap. 3 on pathophysiology of vulvar pain) – and psychological and emotional issues.

Treatment should be multisystemic, i.e., focused not only on the primary site of pain but on neuroinflammation and on the subsequent impact of vulvar pain on the patient's quality of life and sexual functioning. It should include a detailed discussion focused on explanation of the diagnosis and determination of realistic treatment goals.

Box 11.11: The Aims of Therapy for Vulvodynia

- Optimize pain control, recognizing that a complete and definitive pain-free state may not be (always) achievable.
- Enhance functional abilities, and physical and psychological well-being.
- Enhance the quality of life of patients.
- Minimize adverse outcomes.

Treatment guidelines recommend a standard treatment algorithm for all women with vulvodynia, but we believe that a more personalized guided approach is needed, constructed using "end points" that reflect differences within patients with vestibulodynia or generalized vulvodynia (Box 11.12).

The proposal is derived from a cluster analysis of patients that explored whether subgroups exist among women with vulvodynia with respect to pain-related and personality variables.

Box 11.12: End Points for Vulvodynia Therapy

- Reduction of triggers and irritating stimuli
- Peripheral nociceptive blockade
- Central inhibition and modulation/reduction of neuroinflammation
- Treatment of associated pelvic floor dysfunction
- Treatment of the psychosexual ramifications of the syndrome
- Treatment of partner's issues and couple dynamics, when indicated

Topical agents in general should be avoided in order to prevent the problem of irritation and exacerbation of symptoms. Vulvar reactions to topical medications are not uncommon. They are often due to an allergic response to the base of the cream or gel, rather than the active ingredient.

The most commonly prescribed topical medication for the *symptomatic* short-term treatment of dyspareunia and vestibulodynia is *lidocaine* (2 and 5 %) in the form of a gel, cream, or ointment. Some physicians prescribe it as a palliative measure for sexual intercourse. However *these Authors disagree*, because:

- This will perpetuate the vestibular mucosal microtrauma, thus maintaining the inflammation and making it chronic.
- It goes against the protective meaning of pain.

In the case of sexual intercourse, physicians who prescribe it recommend that the topical anesthetic should be applied 20 e 30 min prior to penetration or on an as-needed basis. Although application of 5 % lidocaine ointment nightly for a mean of 7 weeks reduced dyspareunia in 57 % of patients with vestibulodynia, in a randomized, placebo-controlled trial, lidocaine 5 % cream was found to be less effective than topical placebo (20 % vs. 33 % response rate, respectively) (Zolnoun et al. 2003; Foster et al. 2010). Scientists should ask themselves why the placebo is most effective than the topical anesthetic then!

Stinging, erythema, and edema are skin and mucosal reactions, *indicators of a worsening local inflammation*, associated with topical anesthetics. The side effects of lidocaine include burning sensation at the site of application and toxicity which can be minimized by the use of the smallest effective dose of lidocaine 5 % ointment (or 2 % jelly).

Benzocaine, an anesthetic frequently found in over-the-counter topical preparation, should be avoided due to its frequent association with allergic contact dermatitis. It is also important to warn patients of the potential effects on the partner, such as penile numbness (male partners may prefer to wear condoms). Partners, if loving and well informed on the negative, perpetuating consequences of insisting in having intercourse with an inflammated vestibulum, would prefer to have other forms of sexual intimacy until a complete healing is obtained.

Transcutaneous electrical nerve stimulation (TENS) is a simple, noninvasive analgesic technique that is used extensively in healthcare settings by physiotherapists, nurses, and midwifes. TENS was originally developed in the early 1970s as a screening technique for the selection of women with chronic pain most likely to achieve satisfactory pain relief by the implant of an electrical stimulator (Box 11.13).

A significant number of women with chronic pain achieved pain relief through the screening itself and less stimulators needing to be implanted. The management of chronic pain – such as in chronic neuropathies, postherpetic neuralgia, and trigeminal neuralgia – by TENS is supported by a large number of clinical trials (Carroll et al. 2012).

It has been demonstrated that TENS is of significant benefit in the management of vulvar and sexual pain and vulvodynia. It can also have a relevant role in the treatment of vaginismus, a sexual dysfunction predisposing to dyspareunia and vestibulodynia/vulvodynia, when pelvic floor dysfunctions with hyperactive/hypertonic muscles are leading the pathophysiologic picture, together with the phobic attitude.

Electro-analgesia with diphasic currents of frequencies between 2 and 100 Hz and 50–100 μs pulse duration has been used in the treatment of localized vulvodynia, with a high improvement (75 %), superior to placebo (Murina et al. 2008). The stimulation was delivered through plastic vaginal probe inserted into the vagina for 20 mm, in all trials using TENS in vulvodynia.

TENS treatment can also be self-administered in the privacy of a woman's home after a short period of supervision, using an inexpensive device. This would help to gradually reduce the hyperactivity, reaching a more physiologic set point of the muscle, allowing a gentle penetration without further microtraumas.

Box 11.13: The Use of TENS in the Treatment of Vestibulodynia

Potential mechanisms for its effectiveness include:

- "Pain gate control," that is, blocking the information travelling along the nociceptive fibers through stimulation of the large-diameter afferent cutaneous Aβ fibers, at the level of the posterior horn of the medulla
- "Extrasegmental action," based on the release of endogenous opioids by stimulation of small-diameter afferent and motor fibers

A standard TENS protocol was applied in a trial with patients complaining of postpartum perineal pain and entry dyspareunia. TENS consisted of a 30-min weekly session of biphasic pulses with modulation 0/10–50 Hz of frequency and 300/100/3000 μs of pulse duration, in addition to a physical therapy program "hands-on". After five sessions of TENS, 84.5 % of women improved. At the end of the treatment period (ten sessions in total), 95 % of women had achieved a complete resolution of symptoms (Dionisi and Senatori 2011).

Oral medication used for neuropathic and chronic pain has been found useful in patients with chronic vulvar pain. Most medications used are for other neuropathic conditions and pain syndromes such as diabetic neuropathy, postherpetic neuralgia, fibromyalgia, headache, and irritable bowel syndrome (Leo and Dewani 2013; Watson and Dyck 2015).

A large body of evidence suggests that women who have unprovoked pain can be managed in a similar way to those with other neuropathic pain conditions.

The National Institute for Health and Clinical Excellence (NICE 2010) recommends the use of a tricyclic antidepressant or pregabalin (or both) for neuropathic pain. Although it does not list unprovoked vulvodynia in the list of neuropathic conditions, tricyclic antidepressants, gabapentin, and pregabalin have shown benefit in the treatment of unprovoked vulvodynia.

Oral *tricyclic antidepressants* (TCAs) are a common treatment for vulvar pain. Often, amitriptyline is used as a first-line agent. Amitriptyline should be started at a low dose (1 drop = 2 mg), with slow titration (1 drop increase per day, starting in the evening), until either the patient responds or has unacceptable side effects. Furthermore it cannot be abruptly stopped and needs to be tapered according to the side effects.

Side effects in some patients might influence compliance with treatment to a level that can cause withdrawal. Side effects of TCA treatment should be discussed with the patient. Common side effects are fatigue, dry mouth, weight gain, constipation, and somnolence; occasionally, cardiac and arrhythmic effects can occur, so TCAs should be used with caution in the elderly (Box 11.14).

Key Point

Antidepressants such as amitriptyline are effective in reducing both depression and neuropathic pain because they target and reduce the neuroinflammation that is the common denominator for both conditions.

Box 11.14 Trycyclic Antidepressant (TCAs)

- Amitriptyline is the most widely used TCA in vulvodynia patients.
- Start with a low dosage and slowly increase: ideally 1 drop = 2 mg with slow titration (1 drop increase per day, starting in the evening), particularly in patients with low BMI (20 or less). In patients with BMI above 25, Author's clinical experience suggests to start with a 10 mg tab, cut in ½.
- Increase in steps of 5 mg, as tolerated, every 3–7 days up to 125–150 mg.
- The average dosage ranges from 30 to 60 mg daily.
- Dose should be taken at approximately at 1–2 h before bedtime to help counteract morning sedation and fatigue.

It is important to communicate to the patient that although these medications are typically used for depression, they are also used to treat vulvar pain because they target the neuroinflammation responsible for both depression and neuropathic pain, as stated above.

Leo and Dewani (2013) conducted a systematic review of antidepressant therapy for vulvodynia. Although descriptive analyses showed some benefit from antidepressants, there were a number of methodological limitations.

No report directly compared pain-relieving effects of antidepressants or anticonvulsants of different classes, prohibiting detection of any appreciable benefit to any one agent group when compared with another.

Among *anticonvulsant*, gabapentin, the best-studied drug for vulvodynia, has the advantage of efficacy for chronic neuropathic pain (Watson and Dyck 2015), as well as for short-term effects upon non-neuropathic pain, such as postsurgical pain. Gabapentin has shown positive antalgic effects in patients affected by fibromyalgia (Moore et al. 2011).

Success ranges from 50 to 82 %, and the doses required range up to 1200 mg three times a day. While there are many dosing regimens, beginning at 100 mg a day and increasing as tolerated by 100 mg a day is a conservative schedule. Disadvantages include the thrice-daily dosing regimen and the large size of the tablets and capsules. The medication is increased until the patient is comfortable, reaches 3600 mg a day, or has objectionable side effects, whichever occurs first.

Side effects include dizziness, drowsiness, and, less often, dependent edema. Pregabalin, a related newer-generation medication, has the advantage of twice daily dosing, but also the disadvantage of unavailability as a generic.

There are no published data on its benefit for vulvodynia, except for an abstract that reported upon an open-label trial with 28 women: 12 of whom reported improvement (on a visual analogue scale) that averaged at 62 %, ten discontinued medication due to side effects, and four had no improvement.

Pregabalin can be started at 50 mg twice daily and titrated up to 150 mg twice daily over 2 weeks. Side effects of pregabalin, just like gabapentin, include dizziness, sleepiness, and fatigue (Spoelstra et al. 2013; Aranda et al. 2007).

Serotonin-norepinephrine reuptake inhibitors (SNRIs, such as venlafaxine and duloxetine) have proven to be effective in neuropathic pain (Watson and Dyck 2015), but have not been well studied in vulvar pain. The best results for pain are achieved with daily doses of venlafaxine 225 mg and duloxetine 60 mg.

The strength of the pain-relieving action of SNRIs is lower than that of tricyclic antidepressants, with a combined NNT (number needed to treat) value in painful neuropathies of about five for the two SNRIs and 2.3 for tricyclic antidepressants. Indeed, for this very reason, the European Federation of Neurological Societies guidelines recommend SNRIs as second-line treatment.

Key Points

- Amitriptyline drop formulation allows an easy, slow titration (1 drop = 2 mg).
- Combination therapy should preferably use drugs with complementary mechanisms.
- The synergistic interactions between antidepressants and gabapentin/pregabalin, for example, are not only logical but also encouraged by a reduction of side effects by the use of lower doses.

The use of *trigger point injections* in the management of vestibulodynia can be useful, in selected patients. The main objective is the inactivation of the trigger points, thereby reducing pain. The therapy should be used in combination with other approaches as a complementary treatment or like treatment of a residual disease.

Table 11.2 Trigger point injections

Corticosteroid plus anesthetics	*Botulinum toxin*
Methylprednisolone and lidocaine	*Botulinum toxin type A*
Rationale Corticosteroid acts via inflammatory/cytokine alterations (decreased numbers of mast cells degranulated) Anesthetic agents act by blocking sodium channels and can be effectively used for pain modulation at low doses that do not block complete nerve impulse propagation	*Rationale* Inhibition of pelvic floor hyperactivity/tonicity: injection into the pelvic floor muscles Direct antinociceptive effect: injection in painful area of vestibular epithelium
Characteristics of patients eligible for therapy Patients with dyspareunia (provoked pain) Pain *only* with sub-urethral localization and *very localized* (two or three sites)	*Characteristics of patients eligible for therapy* Patients with dyspareunia (coital pain and provoked vestibular pain), not (completely) responsive to the rehabilitation of the pelvic floor Patients with associated pelvic floor dysfunction

Modified from Stockdale and Lawson (2014)

Various combinations of drugs have been suggested, but we currently think that only two regimens should be used: corticosteroid plus anesthetics and botulinum toxin (please see Sect. 11.4.1 on pelvic floor dysfunction) (Table 11.2).

11.4.1 Pelvic Floor Dysfunction: Treatment Strategies

Currently, physical evaluation and therapy for pelvic floor muscle dysfunction should be *the* basic part of any treatment plan for vulvodynia (Graziottin and Murina 2011). Chronic pelvic floor dysfunctions are critical aspect of genital and vulvar pain (Hartmann and Sarton 2014).

According to the American Physical Therapy Association, the overall goal of physical therapy intervention is to restore normal function while working to reduce the negative psychological impact associated with the disease, pain, or dysfunction being addressed (Hartmann and Nelson 2001). Indeed, physical therapy markedly improves both physical and psychosexual aspects of vulvodynia. There are many beneficial measures to help relaxing the pelvic floor muscles (Graziottin and Gambini 2015a). The relaxation is the prerequisite for empowering the woman's motivation and interest in discovering a more gratifying sexual life (Box 11.15). Author's (AG) clinical experience suggests that women can be taught to listen to their mouth as well (Box 11.16).

Physical therapy is effective in lowering pelvic floor hyperactivity/hypertonus. A variety of techniques can be used, including:

- Pelvic floor exercises
- External and internal soft tissue self-massage
- Internal muscle stretching and massage "hands-on"
- Trigger point pressure

- Electromyographic biofeedback
- Use of vaginal trainers (molds)

Box 11.15: From Pain to Pleasure

Self-knowledge, muscle awareness, pain reduction, and sexual empowerment

- Often patients have no awareness of their pelvic floor muscles nor of the possibility of a voluntary control over these muscles and, even less, of the possibility of using the pelvic floor muscles as an *instrument to play the music of sex*. This is a very important positive message as (almost) all these patients are experiencing the dark, painful side of sex where they feel more victims of sexual pain than active players of pleasure.
- Instructing them to "check" their pelvic floor tension throughout the day is helpful in their understanding of the importance of keeping the pelvic floor relaxed under voluntary control.
- They can be taught to imagine the pelvic floor as a double door. The two half-doors can be kept tightened, a little opened or completely opened, just by breathing deeply with the abdominal breath (that should be taught).
- The instruction is that they can move from an involuntary constant tightened/retracted defensive contraction (often with an inverse command, where the woman further pulls when she is requested to push) to a voluntary relax, to an active participation to intercourse through sweet contractions and rhythmic relaxations, to move from pain to pleasure, as feminine protagonist of their pursuit of pleasure.
- Biofeedback techniques and accurate psychosexual wording are key to attaining a sensual motivation and pursue the target of a (re)discovered happier sexual life.

(a) Graziottin, content presented in a lecture on "Sexual Pain Disorders and Sexual Rehabilitation" at the Master Course in Andrology and Sexual Medicine, University of Florence (Italy), June 2016

Box 11.16: The Secret of the Marilyn Sensual Mouth

Why Marilyn Monroe Is an Icon of Sensual Seduction and Charming Invitation to Play Sex?

- Look at her face (besides the relaxed, sensual body language): her mouth is half-closed, the masseter muscle relaxed, the tongue is low and relaxed, the eyelids are half-closed, and the sight is looking lateral. The message of the mouth is very explicit, though sweet and not at all threatening: "I'm ready to surrender to pleasure. I'm ready to surrender to your desire and (hopefully) to your love!" The eyelids half-closed say: "I trust you, I do not need to control everything, I can surrender to your love."

- This is a useful example to discuss (with a mirror) the body language of patients with lifelong sexual pain disorders (vaginismus and dyspareunia) and associated lifelong provoked vestibulodynia.
- The nonverbal language of women with these disorders, namely, lifelong primary vaginismus and/or introital dyspareunia, is just the opposite: the mouth is kept very closed, the masseter muscle is tightened, the tongue is pushed against the palate, and the eyes are wide opened to check and control everything, in a body context of general muscle tension, superficial breathing, high adrenalin, and emotional tension and fear (please see the Chap. 6 on vulvar pain in adolescents).
- The nonverbal message clearly reveal their fear to abandon themselves to the emotions of love and sexual availability, not to mention their more or less unconscious fear of the "aggressiveness" implicit in penetration.
- "Your mouth reveals (and your brain commands) your body language of fear of sex and intimacy." With a tightened pelvic floor, pain at the entrance of the vagina is confirming that "sex is dangerous and painful," reinforcing the vicious circle of fear-pain-muscle contraction.
- "Fear can gradually be mastered and dissolve while you learn to master your own body (still hidden) sensuality through deeper breathing, increasing self-awareness and sexuality, mindfulness techniques, sexual fantasies, body and pelvic floor relaxation."

(a) Graziottin, content presented in a lecture on "Sexual Pain Disorders and Sexual Rehabilitation" at the Master Course in Andrology and Sexual Medicine, University of Florence (Italy), June 2016

Key Point

A parallel psychosexual work is therefore useful to give the *pelvic floor rehabilitation* its deeper sexual meaning in a context of a substantial change not only in the muscle tension but, even more important, in the *emotional opening to sex and love, helping the shift from pain to sexual pleasure.*

With a *vaginal probe*, levator ani activity can be monitored by the patient and her therapist. With careful coaching, the patient can be taught how to contract and then relax her pelvic floor using various protocols. Generally the goal is to teach muscle awareness and relaxation.

Typically sessions last 20–30 min and a success rate in the 60–80 % has been reported.

Manual therapy techniques are especially important for patients with myofascial pain disorders and include myofascial release, trigger point release, soft tissue mobilization, and massage. These internal techniques can be complemented by the patient being educated in the use of vaginal dilators for self-massage.

Sexual partners should also be educated in these techniques in order to encourage and provide further supportive therapy at home. The presence of the dilator provides proprioception to the musculature during exercise, augmenting improved pelvic floor contraction and relaxation. Vaginal dilatation can also diminish the anxiety associated with penetration, as the woman has/perceives/feels complete control of vaginal entry. With therapy, pelvic visceral tension can be eased and muscle hypertonicity reduced. At this stage, there is usually a reduction in the pain level at the introitus.

The advantages of regular pelvic floor muscle exercise are increased blood flow, improved pelvic floor support, decreased posterior fourchette fissuring, improved proprioception of the pelvic floor muscle position, and increased intensity of orgasm (Goldstein et al. 2009; Graziottin and Gambini 2016). Increased self-awareness, self-confidence, and self-esteem are translated in a more assertive and rewarding approach to different aspects of the general life.

The "social mirror", say, relatives, acquaintances, or colleagues, who do not know what is going on, nevertheless witness the change: "Oh, you look so much better, so feminine now," "What a change, you are so self-confident and charming now." A perfect endorsement of the substantial change that is going on when treatment of vulvar pain is combined with care of the sexual pain, of the emotional and physical fears, with a medical and psychosexual approach, and a gentle human touch.

Key Point

- Every center dedicated to the diagnosis and cure of vulvar pain and every physician individually committed to treat vulvar pain should have at least one experienced physiotherapist, midwife, or nurse as standard member of the therapeutic team.
- The clinical (and emotional) impact of these precious therapeutic figures is empowered if they have a quality training in sexual medicine.

11.4.2 Botulinum Neurotoxin (BoNT)

- The primary mode of action of BoNT is a reversible, time-limited chemodenervation of muscles via blockade of presynaptic acetylcholine release at the neuromuscular junction, with subsequent temporary paralysis or reduced contraction.
- In therapeutic use, BoNT has also demonstrated effectiveness in the treatment of pelvic pain disorders characterized by functional abnormalities of muscle tension and relaxation, such as vaginismus (Bertolasi et al. 2009).
- BoNT can be injected into the bulbospongiosus and pubococcygeus muscles. The majority of studies of BoNT in vulvar pain syndrome are targeted at pelvic floor spasm or inhibition of muscle spasticity.

- These trials represent some optimistic preliminary data that warrants further research in order to standardize dosing and optimize the number of injections (Pelletier et al. 2011).
- BoNT can be synergized with pelvic floor rehabilitation in patients with severe myogenic hyperactivity of the pelvic floor to optimize the outcome (Bertolasi et al. 2009; Graziottin and Gambini 2016).

Key Points

Synergy in Pelvic Floor Rehabilitation

- EMG biofeedback
- Myofascial release: manual therapy technique that uses light stretch to restore myofascial mobility and muscle length
- Myofascial trigger point release: manual therapies include skin rolling, strumming, and stripping of the affected muscle fibers

Surgical excision of the vestibule (vestibulectomy) may be considered in patients with local provoked vulvodynia (vestibulodynia) when all the other nonsurgical measures have been *competently but unsuccessfully* tried. The rational is to remove the vestibular mucosa layer of proliferated pain fibers, thus reducing/eliminating the amplified peripheral source of vestibular pain.

Surgical success rates range from 50 to 90 % (Bohm-Starke and Rylander 2008), with success defined as much improved (for how long?) or completely cured. Unfortunately, long-term follow-ups are not that positive. Eanes et al. in their retrospective long-term follow-up found that only eight patients out of 37 were completely free of pain, while those with unprovoked vestibular pain and other pain syndromes (typical of neuroinflammation) were the least likely to respond (Eanes et al. 2011), confirming Bohm-Starke and Rylander considerations.

Factors that limit direct comparison are differences in numbers of patients, the presence of associated comorbidities such as painful bladder syndrome, other medical treatments at the time of surgery, the technique used, the definition of success, and the length of follow-up (Eva et al. 2003; Eanes et al. 2011).

Nevertheless, the reported 70 % average success rate for surgery makes it a credited option for this debilitating condition. First and foremost, however, patient selection is crucial. In addition, adequate counselling and support should be given to the patient both pre- and postoperatively.

Surgical excision of the vestibule (vestibulectomy) may benefit a minority of patients with provoked pain and is performed more commonly in the United States. The procedure that yields the best result is *the modified vestibulectomy*, in which a horseshoe-shaped area of the vestibule and inner labial fold is excised, followed by advancement of the posterior vaginal wall.

Patients with provoked pain may have complex psychosexual and psychological problems, and outcomes after surgery can be poor if these problems are not dealt with.

Surgery should not be the first-line treatment for women with provoked vulvodynia, and those who do undergo surgery will need psychosexual support preoperatively and postoperatively to ensure the best outcome.

Surgery for women with unprovoked vulvodynia is not appropriate because it does not deal with the complex chronic pain issues that these women experience (Bohm-Starke and Rylander 2008; Tommola et al. 2011).

11.4.3 Critical Points to be Considered

- Removal of the vestibular area in case of provoked and, even worse, unprovoked vestibulodynia seems to be a minimalistic approach. It dismisses the complex pathophysiologic inflammatory process that is moving from the painful vulva to the brain.
- It negates/does not appreciate the progressive shift from acute inflammation and acute vulvar pain to chronic pathologic vulvar inflammation and brain neuroinflammation with neuropathic pain.
- *It is like removing the tip of the iceberg, hoping – and promising – that the iceberg would magically disappear.*
- In medical history former amputation of limbs with chronic neuropathic pain has ended into dramatic results: loss of the limb and persistence of pain, leading to the so-called phantom limb syndrome, exactly because the huge central component of neuropathic pain, caused by the progressive neuroinflammation, cannot be addressed with the minimalistic peripheral approach of cutting the limb.
- Does the average 30 % of patient with persisting pain after vestibulectomy present with and suffer from "phantom vestibular pain"? The question has not (yet) been arisen nor investigated in the Authors knowledge.
- On the opposite end, the question is: what are the characteristics of patients that do really well after vestibulectomy, with complete and persistent disappearance of vestibular pain? In other words, who are the patients where the removal of the peripheral input may downregulate neuroinflammation until the complete silencing of pain?
- How to select them?
- Why vestibulectomy is so popular in the United States, and much less in Europe, if it were so "resolving"?
- Is the combination of rehabilitation of the pelvic floor, systemic drugs for neuropathic pain, and vestibulectomy a better combination than surgery alone?

11.5 Management of Vestibulodynia/Vulvodynia by Anesthetic Blocks

The principles of treatment of chronic painful diseases have to be understood in the context of the sophisticated warning mechanisms that exist between the brain and peripheral tissue. Current pharmacological approach to pain control is essentially based on acute, nociceptive pain. Chronic *nonmalignant* neuropathic pain is different: it involves a *restructuring of both peripheral and central neural networks*, leading to wider cerebral integration and interpretation (Vincenti and Graziottin 2006; Vincenti 2014).

New plans of treatment must be developed according to recent pathophysiological data on neuropathic pain, neuroinflammation, and neuroplasticity. Repeated harmful afferent inputs may induce a chronic pathologic condition difficult to resolve by standard medical therapy: systemic opiates may only represent a way to relieve symptoms, but they are unable to offer a definitive resolution of the chronic painful state. Increased intraepithelial innervation by mast cell hyperactivation and microglia activation in nervous system lead to modifications of central circuits (Graziottin 2009; Graziottin et al. 2013, 2014a, b; Xanthos et al. 2011; Walker et al. 2013; Skaper et al. 2015); these structural and functional variations may explain allodynia and hyperalgesia and burning sensations as well (please see the Chap. 3 on pathophysiology of vulvar pain). In vivo studies demonstrate morphological changes in the brain, as a consequence of pain perception. These central changes, based on massive neuroinflammation, may be reversible in nature if a correct treatment is provided.

One of the best methods to reach a persistent amelioration of painful sensations until complete healing is based on periodic *anesthetic blocks* of the main nervous structures involved in innervation of the vulvar and perineal area (Vincenti and Graziottin 2006; Vincenti 2014). The clinical experience has shown that anesthetic blocks with bupivacaine (0.25 %) on sacral nerves (from S2 to S5), pudendal nerves, and particularly ganglion impar offer optimal results within a standard period between 6 and 9 months, when the frequency of treatment is maintained every 3–4 weeks (Vincenti 2014). The periodic reversible induced absence of nociceptive/painful sensations from hypersensitive areas may firstly modify the function and successively the anatomical central and peripheral neural organization.

Brain reorganization associated with chronic pain has also been investigated by comparing morphology between chronic pain and healthy controls. Altered brain morphology was shown in many pain conditions, including fibromyalgia, complex regional pain syndrome (CRPS), osteoarthritis, irritable bowel syndrome, headaches, chronic vulvar pain, and in women suffering from menstrual pain. However, many of the gray matter changes observed in chronic pain patients subside with cessation of pain. In addition, it has been shown that the observed morphological differences in chronic pain conditions often correlate to the duration of pain-related suffering as well as its intensity, thus suggesting that the brain morphological changes may be reversible in nature and are a consequence of pain perception (Vincenti 2014).

Chronic pain impacts morphology of whole brain structures. Treatment, in order to be effective, must recognize the importance of cerebral reorganization; but above all, it must induce the return to the status quo ante, i.e., to the preexisting peripheral and central anatomical and functional neural state.

In conclusion, it seems that repeated peripheral anesthetic blocks may favorably affect healing processes provided that causative factors are eliminated and without disabling amputation of the vestibular tissue, i.e., without vestibulectomy (Vincenti and Graziottin 2006; Vincenti 2014).

11.6 Supplements in the Treatment of Vestibulodynia/Vulvodynia

Fundamentally, inflammation is a protective cellular response aimed at removing injurious stimuli and initiating the healing process. However, when prolonged, it can override the bounds of physiological control. It becomes progressively pathologic, finalized ("non-resolving"), and destructive (Xanthos et al. 2011; Graziottin et al. 2013, 2014a, b; Skaper et al. 2015).

Inflammation is a key element in the pathobiology of chronic pain (please see the Chap. 3 on pathophysiology of vulvar pain). Inflammation is the common denominator ("the secret killer") of other neurological pathologies, including neurodegenerative diseases, stroke, spinal cord injury, and neuropsychiatric disorders.

Glial cells are key players in such nervous system disorder: they express a pro-inflammatory phenotype, but respond also to inflammatory signals released from cells of immune origin such as mast cells.

Neuropathic pain (NP), a condition due to diseases or lesions affecting the somatosensory nervous system pathways, either in the central or the peripheral nervous systems, remains a challenge from the therapeutic point of view (Nascimento et al. 2016).

Practical recommendations for the general treatment of neuropathic pain and peripheral neuropathies have been recently published (Watson and Dyck 2015) (Box 11.17).

Box 11.17: Neuropathic Pain: The Mayo Clinic Recommendations

First-Line Treatments

1. Anticonvulsants
   - Gabapentin (from 300 to 3600 mg/die)
   - Pregabalin (from 150 to 60 mg/die)
2. Antidepressants
   - Amitriptyline/nortriptyline (from 10 to 100 mg/die)
   - Duloxetine (from 20 to 60 mg/die)
3. Supplements
   - Alpha-lipoic acid (600 mg/die)
   - Acetylcarnitine (3000 mg/die)
4. Topical drugs
   - Lidocaine
   - Capsaicin

Second-Line Treatments

1. Antidepressants
   - Venlafaxine (75–375 mg/die)
2. Synthetic opioids
   - Tramadol (50–400 mg/die)

Third-Line Treatments

1. Opioids
   - Tapentadol (150–300 mg/die)
   - Other opioids

Modified from Watson and Dyck (2015)

11.7 Targeting Neuroinflammation in Neuropathic Pain

Currently the research is focusing (also) on molecules that can specifically target the inflammation that maintains the disorder of the somatosensory nervous system.

Chronic inflammatory processes causing pain may be counteracted by a program of resolution that includes the production of *lipid mediators* endowed with the capacity to *switch off inflammation* (Skaper et al. 2015).

These *naturally occurring lipid signaling molecules* include the N-acylethanolamines, N-arachidonoylethanolamine (an endocannabinoid), and its congener N-palmitoylethanolamine (palmitoylethanolamide or PEA) (Impellizzeri et al. 2014; Skaper et al. 2015).

Mast cells and glia play a key role in neuroinflammation associated with vulvodynia (Graziottin 2009; Graziottin et al. 2013, 2014a, b). Current research is focused on strategies to modulate their activation based on leveraging natural mechanisms with the capacity for self-defense against inflammation. Molecules particularly promising in animal and clinical studies include the palmitoylethanolamide (PEA) and the alpha-lipoic acid (ALA).

11.7.1 Palmitoylethanolamide (PEA)

- An increasing body of evidence suggests that the endogenous lipid amide belonging to the N-acylethanolamine family exerts neuroprotection in central nervous system (CNS) pathologies (Skaper et al. 2015).
- PEA plays a role in maintaining cellular homeostasis when faced with external stressors provoking, for example, inflammation.
- It is efficacious in mast cell-mediated models of neurogenic inflammation and neuropathic pain and is neuroprotective in models of stroke, spinal cord injury, traumatic brain injury, and Parkinson disease.

- In micronized/ultramicronized form, it shows superior oral efficacy in inflammatory pain models when compared to naïve PEA.
- PEA significantly reduces inflammatory pain in animal models (Impellizzeri et al. 2014).

11.7.1.1 PEA in the Treatment of Vestibulodynia and Vulvodynia

- In a multimodal treatment strategy, TENS was used in combination with palmitoylethanolamide (PEA) combination in patients with vestibulodynia (Murina et al. 2013).
- The premise was that PEA may contribute to a downregulation of hyperactivated mast cells responsible for the proliferation and sprouting of vestibular pain fibers.
- The study confirms that TENS is of significant benefit in the management of vestibulodynia, also in a home environment.
- PEA can be a value-added treatment adjunct when the onset of vestibulodynia is more recent or when the disease relapses.

11.7.2 Alpha-Lipoic Acid (ALA)

- Alpha-lipoic acid (ALA) – or 1,2-dithiolane-3-pentanoic acid – is a naturally occurring dithiol compound synthesized enzymatically in the mitochondrion from octanoic acid. ALA is a necessary cofactor for mitochondrial α-ketoacid dehydrogenases and thus serves a critical role in mitochondrial energy metabolism.
- ALA is also absorbed intact from dietary sources, and it transiently accumulates in many tissues. There is growing evidence that orally supplied ALA may not be used as a metabolic cofactor, but instead elicit a unique set of biochemical activities with potential pharmacotherapeutic value against a host of pathophysiologic insults.
- ALA has been implicated as a modulator of various inflammatory signaling pathways. It acts (also) as potent biological antioxidant, a detoxification agent, and a diabetes medicine.
- Elevated levels of oxidative stress play an important role in chronic inflammation. Oxidative stress-associated inflammation is thought to provoke early vascular events in atherogenesis, including the upregulation of vascular adhesion molecules and matrix metalloproteinase activity. These events require the activation of NF-kappaB, a transcription factor that induces expression of many genes involved in inflammation and endothelial cell migration. Given the oxidative nature of inflammation, therapeutic strategies aimed at mitigating oxidant production and oxidative damage have been investigated for decades in various models of inflammation (Shay et al. 2009).
- The anti-inflammatory properties of ALA have been documented on numerous animal studies, while studies in humans are ongoing.
- Its efficacy in pain reduction has been proven in diabetic neuropathy (Ziegler et al. 2011).

- ALA supplement has been included in the first-line treatment of neuropathic pain in the practical recommendations of Watson and Dyck (2015) of the Mayo Clinic

11.7.2.1 ALA in the Treatment of Vestibulodynia and Vulvodynia

- A study assessed the effectiveness of alpha-lipoic acid plus omega-3 polyunsaturated fatty acids (omega-3 PUFA) in combination with amitriptyline therapy in patients with vestibulodynia/painful bladder syndrome (VBD/PBS).
- Women with VBD+PBS were randomized to receive amitriptyline or amitriptyline plus a commercially available preparation containing, in two capsules, ALA 600 mg plus docosahexaenoic acid (DHA) 250 mg and eicosapentaenoic acid (EPA) 16.67 mg.
- Pain, as assessed by both the pain rating index of the VAS and of the short-form McGill Pain Questionnaire, decreased significantly in both trial groups, with a greater effect seen with the addition of ALA and n-3 PUFAs.
- The addition of ALA/omega-3 PUFAs to amitriptyline treatment in patients with VBD+PBD appears to improve outcomes and may allow for a lower dosage of amitriptyline, which may lead to fewer adverse effects (Murina et al. 2016b).

11.7.3 Psychosexual Approach to Vulvovaginal Pain

Women with vulvovaginal pain show important impairments in many life domains, primarily their sexuality, intimate relationships, and mental health. Specifically, controlled studies have shown that they report significantly less sexual desire, arousal difficulties, invalidating dyspareunia and reduced satisfaction, more difficulties in reaching orgasm, as well as lower frequencies of intercourse and more negative attitudes toward sexuality than pain-free controls.

The *goals* of most psychosexual interventions include:

- To help patients view their vulvovaginal pain as a multidimensional problem influenced by a variety of factors including thoughts, emotions, behaviors, and couple interactions
- To modify those factors associated with vulvovaginal pain with the goal of increasing adaptive coping and decreasing pain intensity
- To improve the quality of the sexual functioning, including sexual desire which is often significantly low in this population, steering the focus away from intercourse while developing a more positive attitude toward other pleasurable sexual activities
- To reduce avoidance of physical intimacy by working with the fear of pain (when pain has been adequately cured! If not [yet], fear of pain is a self-protective healthy mechanism to prevent further mucosal damage and inflammation that must be respected!)

Mental health professionals working with these women also aim to facilitate adherence to other treatment regimens or procedures, such as gynecological examinations or physical therapy. There is growing evidence that cognitive behavioral therapy, as treatment targeting these different psychological factors, can effectively reduce vulvovaginal pain and associated psychosexual difficulties.

Combining this type of care with concurrent medical management is thought to represent the most optimal model for treating vulvovaginal pain and the significant distress that it generates in patients and their partners, although this model has not (yet) been empirically validated (Bergeron et al. 2014).

11.8 Considerations on Sexual Partner Issues and Needs

When the woman has chronic and/or neuropathic vestibulodynia/vulvodynia, the partner (either a he or a she) may present with difficulties or problems that need to be addressed in a comprehensive treatment plan (Graziottin et al. 2016). The most important issues are summarized in Box 11.18. The psychosexual support offered to the couple during the treatment of vulvar pain (acute, chronic, or neuropathic) may translate in a powerful medical and psychosexual treatment enhancer.

In the Authors' experience, explaining to the partner the biological reasons why she has real pain, with simple words and examples, is a critical step for a successful management.

Partners may become very supportive *treatment assistants*, once they have received clear and simple explanations on the inflammatory and neuropathic causes of pain, a well-explained treatment plan, honest success rate, and average time to pursue the resolution of pain.

Key statement and explanations include:

- "She is not refusing you, she has a real pain that needs to be cured with appropriate drugs."
- Explaining why her pelvic floor muscles are tightened: excellent to show the tightened pelvic floor and the "biomechanics of the narrowing of the vaginal entrance."
- Men love biomechanical explanation and may turn into very supportive partner in treatment, once they have understood the "biomechanics" of the pelvic floor hyperactivity and why it is so important to relax the muscle with appropriate treatments.
- Why rehabilitation of those tightened muscles is needed and precious "to open the door" and to enter the vagina, without any more pain.

A motivated and supportive partner may greatly reduce the distress of vulvar pain while feeling important in contributing to a successful treatment. Temporary non-penetration will be more accepted when the example of the "broken leg" is made (see above). Gentle partners are also willing to be trained in the "hands-on" massage and may prove very helpful with patients living far from the centers and/or in area where rehabilitation therapy is not provided. Having well understood the diagnosis, the average treatment time (prognosis) and the honest success rate may give to both partners the sense of having found the right road to cure vulvar pain and get back to a happier intimate and general life.

Box 11.18: Key Issues of Partners of Women with Vulvar Pain

- *Sexual*
  - *Loss of men's sexual desire due to*:
    - Her chronic pain complaint
    - Fear of hurting a loved partner and causing more pain
    - Erectile deficit, with maintenance difficulties
    - Type, extension, and duration of treatment ("caregiver burnout"), when the neuropathic component and associated behavioral changes become very demanding
  - *Difficulty in penetration* because of pain, vaginal dryness, stenosis, retraction, and the feeling of vaginal shortness (particularly in iatrogenic vulvar pain after oncologic treatments)
  - *Loss of pleasure in oral sex* (for both he and she partner) because of:
    - Loss of the "scent of woman" due to changes in genital scent when vulvar pain is associated with VVA, caused by premature menopause, loss of estrogens and testosterone, and related changes in the vaginal ecosystem and smell of vaginal secretions. These changes are more frequent in VVA after the menopause, when menopausal hormone therapy is not feasible (because of hormone-dependent cancer) or not desired.
    - Changes in the taste of vulvar skin and vaginal secretions, due to on the one hand the loss of sexual hormones and on the other hand to the aversive taste of vaginal creams, lubricant, and suppositories.
  - *Her loss of interest in sex due to lowered androgens*, fatigue, iron deficiency anemia, loss of energy, depression, and pain
  - *Her orgasmic difficulties* because of loss of testosterone (after ovariectomy or CT or RT) and consequences of treatment, or because of clitoralgia or clitorodynia, or FGM/C
  - *Her fear about his ability to obtain or sustain an erection*:
    - Vaginal dryness itself can challenge the quality of the erection. It can be perceived by the man as a sign of refusal and/or an indication of her "unsensitivity" to his sexual request and approach.
- *Psychological*
  - Difficulties in communication for:
  - The taboo of discussing intimate sexual issues
  - The fear of hurting the woman
  - Reactive anxiety, depression, and uncertainty about the future
  - Fears and concerns related to additional roles, family responsibilities, and economic costs during diagnosis, treatment, and recovery
  - Feelings of guilt about wanting to increase sexual intimacy or having a new partner

Modified from Graziottin et al. (2016)

Conclusions

Vulvar pain is a diagnostic and therapeutic challenge in the lifespan. It is underreported, underdiagnosed, and undertreated. The "collusion of silence" is rooted on two factors: the intimate nature of the disorder, on women's side, and the substantial lack of adequate training in the diagnosis and treatment of vulvar pain, on the side of healthcare providers.

Therapy of acute vulvar pain, chronic vulvar pain, and neuropathic vulvar pain presents very different challenges. The focus of the treatment moves in parallel from a "vulva-centered" approach, in the acute and usually short-living inflammation, to a "systemic brain-centered" approach, in the chronic and neuropathic progression of vulvar inflammation.

Cornerstones of the treatment include substantial change/improvement of lifestyles, when inadequate, and improvement of vulvar care. Specific pharmacologic treatments are finalized to reducing *Candida* recurrences, the mast cell and glial hyperactivity, and the pelvic floor hyperactivity, either primary or secondary to chronic inflammation and pain, and optimizing the hormonal levels, when loss of sexual hormones is a contributing factor.

Specific antalgic treatments are to be considered in the neuropathic evolution:

1. With neuroactive drugs, such as amitriptyline, antiepileptics, serotonin selective reuptake inhibitors (SSRIs), and serotonin-norepinephrine reuptake inhibitors (SNRIs)
2. With supplements, such as palmithoylethanolamide (PEA) and alpha-lipoic acid (ALA), that are increasingly used as useful complements of the pharmacologic treatment.

Antalgic block, made by a very experienced anesthesiologist with a specific training, is to be reserved to cases refractory to pharmacologic treatments.

Surgery is the last resort and must be considered with extreme caution as the risk is to perform a short-living ablation of proliferated vestibular pain fibers. There is a high (and now increasingly recognized) risk of pain recurrence either because the other unaddressed contributors renovate the vestibular trauma, inflammation, and proliferation of pain fibers and/or because the phenomenon of the phantom vestibular syndrome may be present.

Partners need to be counselled to optimize the expectations and address problems and needs. They may turn into very supportive once they have been explained the real cause of her vulvar pain and how to treat it.

The current therapeutic challenges are threefold:

1. To increase an early diagnosis of vulvar pain to optimize a resolving therapeutic strategy
2. To improve the healthcare providers training to increase their competence and confidence in dealing with the objectively challenging vulvar pain and its associated pelvic, sexual, and systemic comorbidities
3. Design-controlled studies in homogeneous group of patients to better define the standard of effective care in different types of vulvar pain

References

Abraham L, Pinkerton JV, Messig M, Ryan KA, Komm BS, Mirkin s. Menopause-specific quality of life across varying menopausal populations with conjugated estrogens/ba edoxifene. Maturitas. 2014;78(3):212–8. doi:10.1016/j.maturitas.2014.04.008. Epub 2014 Apr 26.
Aranda J, Edwards L. Retrospective chart review of 28 women on pregabalin for Vulvodynia. Paper presented at: XIX World Congress of the International Society for the Study of Vulvovaginal Diseases Meeting, July 2007; Alaska.
Bachmann G, Bobula J, Mirkin s. Effects of bazedoxifene/conjugated estrogens on quality of life in postmenopausal women with symptoms of vulvar/vaginal atrophy. Climacteric. 2010;13(2):132–40.
Bergeron S, Likes WM, Steben M. Psychosexual aspects of vulvovaginal pain. Best Pract Res Clin Obstet Gynaecol. 2014;28(7):991–9. doi:10.1016/j.bpobgyn.2014.07.007. Epub 2014 Jul 17.
Bertolasi L, Frasson E, Cappelletti JY, Vicentini S, Bordignon M, Graziottin A. Botulinum neurotoxin type A injections for vaginismus secondary to vulvar vestibulitis syndrome. Obstet Gynecol. 2009;114(5):1008–16.
Bohm-Starke N, Rylander E. Surgery for localized, provoked vestibulodynia: a long-term follow-up study. J Reprod Med. 2008;53:83–9.
Booth FW, Roberts CK, Laye MJ. Lack of exercise is a major cause of chronic diseases. Compr Physiol. 2012;2(2):1143–211.
Borghi A, Corazza M, Minghetti S, Toni G, Virgili A. Continuous vs. tapering application of the potent topical corticosteroid mometasone furoate in the treatment of vulvar lichen sclerosus: results of a randomized trial. Br J Dermatol. 2015;173(6):1381–6.
Bouchard C, Labrie F, Derogatis L, Girard G, Ayotte N, Gallagher J, Cusan L, Archer DF, Portman D, Lavoie L, Beauregard A, Côté I, Martel C, Vaillancourt M, Balser J, Moyneur E, VVA Prasterone Group. Effect of intravaginal dehydroepiandrosterone (DHEA) on the female sexual function in postmenopausal women: ERC-230 open-label study. Horm Mol Biol Clin Investig. 2016;25(3):181–90. doi:10.1515/hmbci-2015-0044.
Bruyniks N, Nappi RE, Castelo-Branco C, de Villiers TJ, Simon J. Effect of ospemifene on moderate or severe symptoms of vulvar and vaginal atrophy. Climacteric. 2016;19(1):60–5. doi:10.3109/13697137.2015.1113517. Epub 2015 Nov 19.
Carroll D, Moore RA, McQuay HJ, Fairman F, Trame M, Leijon G. Transcutaneous electrical nerve stimulation (TENS) for chronic pain. Cochrane Database Syst Rev. 2012;14(3):CD006276.
Dahir MM, Travers-Gustafson D. Breast cancer, aromatase inhibitor therapy, and sexual functioning: a pilot study of the effects of vaginal testosterone therapy. Sex Med. 2014;2(1):8–15.
Davis VJ. What the paediatrician should know about paediatric and adolescent gynecology: The perspective of a gynecologist. Paediatr Child Health. 2003;8(8):491–5.
Davis SR, Worsley R, Miller KK, Parish SJ, Santoro N. Androgens and female sexual function and dysfunction – findings from the fourth international consultation of sexual medicine. J Sex Med. 2016;13(2):168–78.
Derry HM, Padin AG, Kuo JL, Hughes S, Kiecolt-Glaser JK. Sex differences in depression: does inflammation play a role? Curr Psychiatry Rep. 2015;17(10):78.
Dionisi B, Senatori R. Effect of transcutaneous electrical nerve stimulation on the postpartum dyspareunia treatment. J Obstet Gynaecol Res. 2011;37:750–3.
Donders G, Bellen G, Byttebier G, et al. Individualized decreasing-dose maintenance fluconazole regimen for recurrent vulvovaginal candidiasis (ReCiDiF trial). Am J Obstet Gynecol. 2008;199:613.e1–9.
Eanes A, Bair E, Martin C, Iyer P, Zolnoun D. Psychosexual correlates of persistent postsurgical pain in patients with vulvodynia. Int J Gynaecol Obstet. 2011;113(3):225–8. doi:10.1016/j.ijgo.2010.12.018. Epub 2011 Apr 9.
Eva LJ, MacLean AB, Reid WM, Rolfe KJ, Perrett CW. Estrogen receptor expression in vulvar vestibulitis syndrome. Am J Obstet Gynecol. 2003;189(2):458–61.
Faraut B, Léger D, Medkour T, Dubois A, Bayon V, Chennaoui M, Perrot S. Napping reverses increased pain sensitivity due to sleep restriction. PLoS One. 2015;10(2), e0117425. doi:10.1371/journal.pone.0117425. eCollection 2015.

Finan PH, Goodin BR, Smith MT. The association of sleep and pain: an update and a path forward. J Pain. 2013;14(12):1539–52.

Fistarol SK, Itin PH. Diagnosis and treatment of lichen sclerosus: an update. Am J Clin Dermatol. 2013;14:27–47.

Foster DC, Kotok MB, Huang LS, et al. Oral desipramine and topical lidocaine for vulvodynia: a randomized controlled trial. Obstet Gynecol. 2010;116(3):583e93.

Gambacciani M, Torelli MG, Martella L, Bracco GL, Casagrande AG, Albertin E, Tabanelli S, Viglietta M, D'Ambrogio G, Garone G, Cervigni M. Rationale and design for the Vaginal Erbium Laser Academy Study (VELAS): an international multicenter observational study on genitourinary syndrome of menopause and stress urinary incontinence. Climacteric. 2015;18 Suppl 1:43–8.

Goldstein A, Pukall C, Goldstein I. Female sexual pain disorders: evaluation and management. Wiley-Blackwell: Oxford; 2009.

Graziottin A. Sexual pain disorders: dyspareunia and vaginismus. In: Porst H, Buvat J, ISSM (International Society of Sexual Medicine) Standard Committee Book, editors. Standard practice in sexual medicine. Oxford: Blackwell; 2006. p. 342–50.

Graziottin A. Mast cells and their role in sexual pain disorders. In: Goldstein A, Pukall C, Goldstein I, editors. Female sexual pain disorders: evaluation and management. Chichester/Hoboken: Blackwell Publishing; 2009. p. 176–9.

Graziottin A. Recurrent cystitis after intercourse: why the gynaecologist has a say. In: Studd J, Seang LT, Chervenak FA, editors. Current progress in obstetrics and gynaecology, vol. 2. Mumbai: Suketu P. Kothari/TreeLife Media; 2014. p. 319–36.

Graziottin A. Vaginal biological and sexual health – the unmet needs. Climacteric. 2015;18 Suppl 1:9–12.

Graziottin A. Unmet needs in vulvovaginal atrophy (VVA). Abstract book, 10th Congress of the European Menopause Society on "Promoting translation of science into clinical practice in midlife health and beyond", Madrid, Spain, 20–22 May 2015b, Maturitas 82 (3): 320–321, Nov 2015.

Graziottin A, Gambini D. Female sexual dysfunction: treatment. In: Bø K, Berghmans B, Mørkved S, Van Kampen M, editors. Evidence-based physical therapy for the pelvic floor – bridging science and clinical practice. 2nd ed. Oxford: Elsevier; 2015a. p. 258–70.

Graziottin A, Gambini D. Anatomy and physiology of genital organs – Women. In: Vodusek D, Boller F, editors. Neurology of sexual and bladder disorders (Handbook of clinical neurology, Volume 130, 3rd Series). Elsevier; 2015b. p. 39–60

Graziottin A, Gambini D. Evaluation of genito-pelvic pain penetration disorder. In: Waguih WI, editor. The textbook of sexual medicine. Springer Verlag; 2016

Graziottin A, Lukasiewicz M. Female sexual dysfunction and premature menopause. In: Lipshultz L, Pastuszak A, Perelman M, Giraldi AM, Buster J, editors. Sexual health in the couple: management of sexual dysfunction in men and women. New York: Springer; 2016.

Graziottin A, Murina F. Clinical management of vulvodynia. Milano: Springer Verlag Italia; 2011.

Graziottin A, Gambini D, Bertolasi L. Genital and sexual pain in women. In: Vodusek D, Boller F, editors. Neurology of sexual and bladder disorders (Handbook of clinical neurology, Vol. 130, 3rd Series), Elsevier; 2015, p. 395–412.

Graziottin A, Lukasiewicz M, Serafini A. Sexual rehabilitation after gynecologic cancers. In: Gianotten W, Reisman Y, editors. Sexual rehabilitation. Springer Verlag;2016.

Graziottin A, Skaper S, Fusco M. Inflammation and chronic pelvic pain: a biological trigger for depression in women? J Depress Anxiety. 2013;3:142–50.

Graziottin A, Skaper S, Fusco M. Mast cells in chronic inflammation, pelvic pain and depression in women. Gynecol Endocrinol. 2014a;30(7):472–7.

Graziottin A, Zanello PP. Pathogenic biofilms as triggers of recurrent vaginitis and cystitis. Proceedings of the 20th World Congress on Controversies in Obstetrics, Gynecology & Infertility (COGI), Paris, France, 4–7 Dec 2014, Monduzzi Editore, 2015.

Gurney EP, Nachtigall MJ, Nachtigall LE, Naftolin F. The women's health initiative trial and related studies: 10 years later: a clinician's view. J Steroid Biochem Mol Biol. 2014;142:4–11.

Hartmann EH, Nelson C. The perceived effectiveness of physical therapy treatment on women complaining of vulvar pain and diagnosed with either vulvar vestibulitis syndrome or dysesthetic vulvodynia. J Sect Women's Health. 2001;25:13–8.

Hartmann D, Sarton J. Chronic pelvic floor dysfunction. Best Pract Res Clin Obstet Gynaecol. 2014;28(7):977–90.

Impellizzeri D, Bruschetta G, Cordaro M, Crupi R, Siracusa R, Esposito E, Cuzzocrea S. Micronized/ultramicronized palmitoylethanolamide displays superior oral efficacy compared to nonmicronized palmitoylethanolamide in a rat model of inflammatory pain. J Neuroinflammation. 2014;11:136–41.

Kagan R, Williams RS, Pan K, Mirkin S, Pickar JH. A randomized, placebo- and active-controlled trial of bazedoxifene/conjugated estrogens for treatment of moderate to severe vulvar/vaginal atrophy in postmenopausal women. Menopause. 2010;17(2):281–9.

Kirtschig G, Becker K, Günthert A, Jasaitiene D, Cooper S, Chi CC, Kreuter A, Rall KK, Aberer W, Riechardt S, Casabona F, Powell J, Brackenbury F, Erdmann R, Lazzeri M, Barbagli G, Wojnarowska F. Evidence-based (S3) guideline on (anogenital) Lichen sclerosus. J Eur Acad Dermatol Venereol. 2015;29(10):e1–43. doi:10.1111/jdv.13136.

Labrie F, Archer DF, Koltun W, Vachon A, Young D, Frenette L, Portman D, Montesino M, Côté I, Parent J, Lavoie L, Beauregard A, Martel C, Vaillancourt M, Balser J, Moyneur E, VVA PrasteroneResearch Group. Efficacy of intravaginal dehydroepiandrosterone (DHEA) on moderate to severe dyspareunia and vaginal dryness, symptoms of vulvovaginal atrophy, and of the genitourinary syndrome of menopause. Menopause. 2016;23(3):243–56. doi:10.1097/GME.0000000000000571.

Lee CH, Sugiyama T, Kataoka A, Kudo A, Fujino F, Chen YW, Mitsuyama Y, Nomura S, Yoshioka T. Analysis for distinctive activation patterns of pain and itchy in the human brain cortex measured using near infrared spectroscopy (NIRS). PLoS One. 2013;8(10), e75360. doi:10.1371/journal.pone.0075360. eCollection 2013.

Leo RJ, Dewani S. A systematic review of the utility of antidepressant pharmacotherapy in the treatment of vulvodynia pain. J Sex Med. 2013;10(10):2497–505.

Lukasiewicz ME, Graziottin A. Women' sexuality after gynecologic cancers. In: Studd J, Seang LT, Chervenak FA, editors. Current progress in obstetrics and gynaecology, vol. 3. 2nd ed. Mumbai: Kothari Medical; 2015. p. 95–116.

Meury SN, Erb T, Schaad UB, et al. Randomized, comparative efficacy trial of oral penicillin versus cefuroxime for perianal streptococcal dermatitis in children. J Pediatr. 2008;153(6):799e802.

Moore RA, Wiffen PJ, Derry S, McQuay HJ. Gabapentin for chronic neuropathic pain and fibromyalgia in adults. Cochrane Database Syst Rev. 2011;16(3):CD007938. doi: 10.1002/14651858.CD007938.pub2.

Murina F, Bianco V, Radici G, Felice R, Di Martino M, Nicolini U. Transcutaneous electrical nerve stimulation to treat vestibulodynia: a randomised controlled trial. BJOG. 2008;115:1165–70.

Murina F, Graziottin A, Felice R, Radici GL, Di Francesco S. The recurrent vulvovaginal candidiasis: proposal of a personalized therapeutic protocol. ISRN Obstet Gynecol. 2011;2011:806065.

Murina F, Graziottin A, Felice R, Radici G, Tognocchi C. Vestibulodynia: synergy between palmitoylethanolamide + transpolydatin and transcutaneous electrical nerve stimulation. J Low Genit Tract Dis. 2013;17:111–6.

Murina F, Graziottin A, Vicariotto F, De Seta F. Can Lactobacillus fermentum LF10 and Lactobacillus acidophilus LA02 in a slow-release vaginal product be useful for prevention of recurrent vulvovaginal candidiasis? J Clin Gastroenterol. 2014;48:S102–5.

Murina F, Rehman S, Di Francesco S, Mantegazza V, Felice R, Bianco V. Vulvar lichen sclerosus: a comparison of the short-term topical application of clobetasol dipropionate 0.05% versus mometasone furoate 0.1%. J Lower Gen Tract Dis. 2015;19(2):149–51.

Murina F, Graziottin A, Raffaele F, Di Francesco S. Coital pain in the elderly: could a low dose estriol gel thrill the vulvar vestibule? Eur J Obstet Gynecol Reprod Biol. 2016a;207:121–4.

Murina F, Graziottin A, Felice R, Gambini D. Alpha lipoic acid plus omega-3 fatty acids for vestibulodynia associated with painful bladder syndrome. 2017b (in press).

Murina F, Graziottin A, Felice R, Gambini D. Alpha lipoic acid plus omega-3 fatty acids for vestibulodynia associated with painful bladder syndrome. 2016b. in press.

Nascimento OJ, Pessoa BL, Orsini M, Ribeiro P, Davidovich E, Pupe C, Filho PM, Dornas RM, Masiero L, Bittencourt J, Bastos VH. Neuropathic pain treatment: still a challenge. Neurol Int. 2016;8(2):6322. doi:10.4081/ni.2016.6322. eCollection 2016.

National Institute for Health and Clinical Excellence (NICE). Neuropathic pain – Pharmacological management CG96. 2010. http://guidance.nice.org.uk/CG96.

Pedersen BK. The diseasome of physical inactivity – and the role of myokines in muscle – fat cross talk. J Physiol. 2009;587(Pt 23):5559–68. doi:10.1113/jphysiol.2009.179515. Epub 2009 Sep 14. Review.

Pelletier F, Parratte B, Penz S, Moreno JP, Aubin F, Humbert P. Efficacy of high doses of botulinum toxin A for treating provoked vestibulodynia. Br J Dermatol. 2011;164:617Y22.

Pieralli A, Fallani MG, Becorpi A, Bianchi C, Corioni S, Longinotti M, Tredici Z, Guaschino S. Fractional CO2 laser for vulvovaginal atrophy (VVA) dyspareunia relief in breast cancer survivors. Arch Gynecol Obstet. 2016;294:841–6 [Epub ahead of print].

Podorozhansky YM, Podorozhansky Y, Hoffstetter S, Gavard JA. Role of vulvar care guidelines in the initial management of vulvar complaints. J Low Genit Tract Dis. 2012;16(2):88–91.

Rahn DD, Carberry C, Sanses TV, Mamik MM, Ward RM, Meriwether KV, Olivera CK, Abed H, Balk EM, Murphy M, Society of Gynecologic Surgeons Systematic Review Group. Vaginal estrogen for genitourinary syndrome of menopause: a systematic review. Obstet Gynecol. 2014;124(6):1147–56. doi:10.1097/AOG.0000000000000526.

Romero R, Nygaard I. CDC updates guidelines for treating sexually transmitted diseases. Am J Obstet Gynecol. 2015;213:117–8.

Salonia A, Clementi MC, Graziottin A, Nappi RE, Castiglione F, Ferrari M, Capitanio U, Damiano R, Montorsi F. Secondary provoked vestibulodynia in sexually-active women with recurrent uncomplicated urinary tract infections. J Sex Med. 2013;10(9):2265–73.

Shay KP, Moreau RF, Smith EJ, Smith AR, Hagen TM. Alpha-lipoic acid as a dietary supplement: molecular mechanisms and therapeutic potential. Biochim Biophys Acta. 2009;1790(10):1149–60. doi:10.1016/j.bbagen.2009.07.026. Epub 2009 Aug 4. Review.

Simonetta C, Burns EK, Guo MA. Vulvar dermatoses: a review and update. Mo Med. 2015;112(4):301–7.

Simpson RC, Murphy R. Paediatric vulvar disease. Best Pract Res Clin Obstet Gynaecol. 2014;28(7):1028–41. doi:10.1016/j.bpobgyn.2014.07.004. Epub 2014 Jul 17. Review.

Skaper SD, Facci L, Barbierato M, Zusso M, Bruschetta G, Impellizzeri D, Cuzzocrea S, Giusti P. N-Palmitoylethanolamine and Neuroinflammation: a Novel Therapeutic Strategy of Resolution. Mol Neurobiol. 2015;52(2):1034–42.

Slavich GM, Irwin MR. From stress to inflammation and major depressive disorder: a social signal transduction theory of depression. Psychol Bull. 2014;140(3):774–815. doi:10.1037/a0035302. Epub 2014 Jan 13.

Sobel JD. Recurrent vulvovaginal candidiasis. Am J Obstet Gynecol. 2016;214(1):15–21.

Sobel JD, Wiesenfeld HC, Martens M. Maintenance fluconazole therapy for recurrent vulvovaginal candidiasis. N Engl J Med. 2004;351:876–83.

Spoelstra S, Borg C, Weijmar Schiltz WW. Anticonvulsant pharmacotherapy for generalized and localized vulvodynia: a critical review of the literature. J Psychosom Obstet Gynecol. 2013;34(3):133–8.

Stockdale CK, Lawson HW. 2013 vulvodynia guideline update. J Low Genit Tract Dis. 2014;18(2):93–100.

Tommola P, Unkila-Kallio L, Paavonen J. Long-term follow up of posterior vestibulectomy for treating vulvar vestibulitis. Acta Obstet Gynecol Scand. 2011;90:1225Y31.

Vandenkerkhof EG, Macdonald HM, Jones GT, Power C, Macfarlane GJ. Diet, lifestyle and chronic widespread pain: results from the 1958 British Birth Cohort Study. Pain Res Manag. 2011;16(2):87–92.

Vincenti E. Chronic non-malignant pelvic-perineal pain: management by anesthetic blocks. From theory to practice. I: philosophic and pathophysiologic approach. Pelviperineology. 2014;33:103–9.

Vincenti E, Graziottin A. Sexual pain disorders: management by anesthetic blocks. In: Goldstein I, Meston C, Davis S, Traish A, editors. Women's sexual function and dysfunction: study, diagnosis and treatment. London: Taylor and Francis; 2006. p. 524–8.

Virgili A, Borghi A, Minghetti S, Corazza M. Mometasone fuoroate 0.1% ointment in the treatment of vulvar lichen sclerosus: a study of efficacy and safety on a large cohort of patients. J Eur Acad Dermatol Venereol. 2014;28:943–8.

Walker AK, Kavelaars A, Heijnen CJ, Dantzer R. Neuroinflammation and comorbidity of pain and depression. Pharmacol Rev. 2013;66(1):80–101.

Watson JC, Dyck PJ. Peripheral neuropathy: a practical approach to diagnosis and symptom management. Mayo Clin Proc. 2015;90(7):940–51.

Witherby S, Johnson J, Demers L, Mount S, Littenberg B, Maclean CD, Wood M, Muss H. Topical testosterone for breast cancer patients with vaginal atrophy related to aromatase inhibitors: a phase I/II study. Oncologist. 2011;16(4):424–31. doi:10.1634/theoncologist.2010-0435. Epub 2011 Mar 8.

Xanthos DN, Gaderer S, Drdla R, Nuro E, Abramova A, Ellmeier W, Sandkühler J. Central nervous system mast cells in peripheral inflammatory nociception. Mol Pain. 2011;7:42. doi:10.1186/1744-8069-7-42.

Zendell K. Genital lichen planus: update on diagnosis and treatment. Semin Cutan Med Surg. 2015;34(4):182–6.

Ziegler D, Low PA, Litchy WJ, Boulton AJ, Vinik AI, Freeman R, Samigullin R, Tritschler H, Munzel U, Maus J, Schütte K, Dyck PJ. Efficacy and safety of antioxidant treatment with α-Lipoic acid over 4 years in diabetic polyneuropathy: the NATHAN 1 trial. Diabetes Care. 2011;34(9):2054–60.

Zolnoun DA, Hartmann KE, Steege JF. Overnight 5% lidocaine ointment for treatment of vulvar vestibulitis. Obstet Gynecol. 2003;102(1):84e7.46.

Clinical Cases 12

Case histories may help students and learning physicians to focus on the real complaint of *vulvar pain* and associated comorbidities, sexual and urogenital, with their impact on the real life of patients. They will illustrate how sexual pain can affect a woman's life and how an early diagnosis can definitely change the woman's and couple's sexual experience for the better while curing a disturbing vulvar pain and associated symptoms. All names in the following case stories have been changed. Readers should focus on what should be listened to and selected as critical info from the narrative of the problem. Symptoms should be evaluated with a pathophysiologic reading of predisposing, precipitating, and perpetuating factors, to get the proper diagnosis and a well-tailored effective treatment (Graziottin and Murina 2011; Graziottin and Gambini 2016).

Case 1

I've always been shy and reserved, so different from my schoolmates. I had pain from the very first intercourse. Sex has always caused problems to me. I hoped it would have gone better over time. I tried many times, but pain became more and more excruciating. I had tears every time we tried. When I tried to make love, I felt that my vagina was tight and dry. I tried but my body did not respond. Sometimes I also had a sense of burning pain at the entrance of the vagina. He immediately stopped making love for fear of hurting me. No, I do not think we ever had a complete intercourse. Maybe I'm still virgin, I do not know. Now I cannot get aroused any more, not even a little bit, because I'm afraid of pain. Even my sexual desire has gone away. My family physician prescribed the contraceptive pill for me, suggesting that perhaps I was afraid of getting pregnant and did not relax. The pain didn't change. It's 3 years now that we do nothing. We have lost any type of intimacy, for fear that he gets aroused and we try again to have sex. We are very close, and he is so patient with me! I feel guilty for disappointing him and being unable to do what is so easy and funny for the majority of women. Now I'm here because we would love to have a child....

Alicia, 33 years of age

A. Graziottin, F. Murina, *Vulvar Pain*, DOI 10.1007/978-3-319-42677-8_12

12.1 Clinical Evaluation

Alicia's wording suggests a lifelong vaginismus with an unconsummated marriage, acquired loss of desire, arousal difficulties, and significant distress. The burning pain suggests comorbidity with lifelong vulvar vestibulitis/provoked vestibulodynia (VVS/PVD).

When asked, Alicia reports that:

(a) Since her first period, she could not use tampons during menstruation, because she could not insert them: "I felt I had a wall there."
(b) Since she was a girl, she was afraid of feeling pain at intercourse, in spite of longing for a closer intimacy with her boyfriend. Probably something she heard about "how painful is to stay with a man," in a conversation between her mother and her aunt, could have increased her fears. Interestingly, the mother said she had the same problem, when Laura dares to ask her about "problems with dad" after the first therapeutic sessions.
(c) She was not abused or harassed.
(d) She received a strict catholic education, where sex was not considered appropriate for a girl until marriage.

These observations suggest that she could have lifelong vaginismus, severe enough to prevent intercourse, leading to the non-consummation of her marriage and a hyperactive pelvic floor. Attempts of penetration may have caused microabrasions of the mucosa at the entrance of the vagina leading to VVS/PVD, sufficient to worsen the vaginismic attitude and further predispose her to lifelong introital dyspareunia, so frightening that she gave up any intimacy (Graziottin 2006; Graziottin and Murina 2011; Graziottin and Gambini 2016).

12.2 Clinical Examination

Her body language indicated a systemic anxiety and fear of being examined. She could not relax in spite of her physician's reassuring manner. A third-degree vaginismus (according to John Lamont classification) was diagnosed. Exquisite pain was elicited at 5 and 7 o'clock (when viewing the vaginal opening as a clock face with the anus at 6 o'clock), between the hymen remnants and the introitus vaginae (the opening of the vagina), when using gently a swab to design the "pain map" in the vestibular area. With the gentle examining gloved hand, tender points were elicited where the muscle levator ani inserts at the spine on both sides, with more intense pain on the left side. This "asymmetry" is frequent (72 % in the personal series – unpublished data). It may reflect postural problems and be worsened by the habit of keeping the legs tightly crossed most of the time. Postural issues and correct position of legs in the seated position should be addressed in the therapeutic plan.

12.3 Diagnosis

Lifelong vaginismus and dyspareunia, with unconsummated marriage, comorbid with vulvar vestibulitis/provoked vestibulodynia and a tightened, myalgic pelvic floor (Graziottin 2006; Graziottin and Murina 2011). Lifelong vaginismus could be the predisposing factor to dyspareunia. Both vaginismus and VVS/PVD have been discussed in the chapter on the pathophysiology of vulvar pain. Acquired genital arousal disorder and acquired loss of sexual desire were the comorbid female sexual disorders (FSD). According to the DSM V, currently the diagnosis would be genito-pelvic pain penetration disorder (GPPPD), comorbid with other FSD (Graziottin and Gambini 2016).

12.4 Comment

Comorbidity between different FSDs and between FSD and medical conditions is frequent in women. A careful clinical history is essential to identify predisposing, precipitating, and maintaining/perpetuating factors, which may be biological, psychosexual, and/or relational. In this case, the natural history of the current complaint had vaginismus as a likely predisposing factor, while intercourse was the precipitating one. Maintaining factors were biological (vulvar vestibulitis/provoked vestibulodynia), psychosexual (systemic fear and anxiety about pain), and relational: a shared fear of the natural "aggressiveness" intrinsic to penetration (Graziottin 2006; Graziottin and Murina 2011; Graziottin and Gambini 2016). Acquired desire and arousal disorders increased the vulnerability of the introital mucosa to the mechanical trauma, due to the lack of lubrication in response to sexual stimulation. The partner respectful attitude was positive in maintaining the emotional intimacy between the partners. However, this a bit "passive" behavior contributed to the acceptance of a nonsexual relationship for years, until the desire of children becomes prominent.

Case 2

The first problem was a cystitis, with blood in the urine, 4 years ago, after my first intercourse at 19. I was treated with antibiotics. Things seemed to go better but then I had new cystitis, three-four times a year, always 1 or 2 days after the intercourse, and recurrent Candida vaginitis. Now I have continuous pain in the bladder, that gets worse after intercourse, and burning pain at the entrance of the vagina. Urine exams showed *Escherichia coli* in the first episodes. Now most of the time the urine exam is negative and I still have bladder symptoms! I consulted seven physicians: urologists keep on prescribing antibiotics, gynaecologists give me vaginal creams and antimycotic, but none seems to understand what's going wrong… I feel helpless.

Paula, 23 years of age

12.5 Clinical Evaluation

Paula's history is typical: her symptoms started with recurrent cystitis, with antibiotics triggering *Candida* infections, leading to inflammation of the vestibular region, consequent introital dyspareunia, and symptoms of urinary urgency/frequency, pelvic pain, and nocturia, currently in the absence of bacterial infection or any other identifiable pathology.

12.6 Clinical Examination

Relevant examination findings are tenderness of the urethra and bladder base and tenderness to pressure with a cotton swab at the vestibule. Hypertonic/hyperactive pelvic floor dysfunction with muscle tenderness, myofascial pain, and tender points is also present.

12.7 Diagnosis

Painful bladder syndrome, with a history of recurrent (postcoital) cystitis, comorbid with vestibulodynia and recurrent *Candida* vaginitis, introital dyspareunia, and hyperactive myalgic pelvic floor.

12.8 Comment

Interstitial cystitis/painful bladder syndrome (IC/PBS) is a chronic bladder disorder characterized by *inflammation* of the bladder wall, pelvic pain, and irritative voiding symptoms. The symptoms of IC/PBS can overlap with such conditions as vestibulodynia, recurrent urinary tract infection, and chronic pelvic pain. IC/BPS and vulvodynia are frequently seen as comorbid to each other (in about 25 % of patients according to Reed et al. 2012 up to 60 % according to Salonia et al. 2013). Hypertonic/hyperactive pelvic floor dysfunction (HTPFD) is commonly seen in both conditions. It is still unclear if HTPFD results from chronic pain of IC/BPS and vulvodynia or if it is a precipitating factor or both.

An interesting survey on women affected with IC/PBS and controls (Peters et al. 2007) well indicates that affected women are significantly more likely to have suffered from lifelong vaginismus, lifelong fear of pain at intercourse, and lifelong introital dyspareunia than controls. This supports the hypothesis that a lifelong hyperactive pelvic floor, associated with vaginismus and/or lifelong dyspareunia, can be a "biomechanical" predisposing factor to recurrent postcoital cystitis (which are complained of 24–72 h after intercourse). When unaddressed, the persistent bladder inflammation caused by the intercourse and associated pathogenic biofilms of *Escherichia coli* (or other pathogens) contributes to PBS (Graziottin and Zanello 2015). If unaddressed, it can become as well a perpetuating factor for both the bladder and vestibular symptoms. This contributes to maintain the pelvic chronic inflammations while increasing the neuroinflammation and the shifting of pain from nociceptive to neuropathic, a real disease per se.

Neuropathic vestibular pain can include peripheral and central nervous system components. In the vestibulum, noxious insults trigger inflammatory mediators, neurotransmitters, and nerve growth factor activity, which can result in nociceptor sensitization or ectopic excitability of afferent neurons. This results in innocuous stimuli at the site of inflammation, such as light touch, warm, or cool temperatures, being perceived as painful (*allodynia*), and stimuli that usually are felt as uncomfortable or slightly painful, such as a pinprick, becoming extremely painful (*hyperalgesia*) central neurons.

Peripheral vestibular sensitization characteristically occurs after peripheral inflammation and comprises a reduction in threshold and an increase in the excitability of the peripheral terminals of nociceptors in response to sensitizing inflammatory mediators.

Nerve grow factor (NGF) appears to be a key molecule in the orchestration (also) of vestibular/vulvar peripheral inflammation. Inflammation-driven release of cytokines from immune cells provokes hyperalgesia through stimulation and production of other proinflammatory agents (Schaible 2015). Peripheral mast cell activation at vestibular level is generally considered proinflammatory and pro-nociceptive.

Physical, chemical, and mechanical stimuli activate local mast cells, causing degranulation and secretion of mediators that have been found to sensitize and induce the proliferation of C-afferent nerve fibers. These nerve fibers release inflammatory mediators, including NGF, which increase the proliferation and degranulation of mast cells, causing hyperesthesia, and enhance the inflammatory response. Mast cells show particular complexity in relation to the inflammatory response, and their density in inflamed tissue changes over time. In tissue where there is an acute inflammatory response, the concentration of mast cells is high (Graziottin 2009; Graziottin et al. 2013, 2014; Chatterjea and Martinov 2015). As the inflammation becomes more chronic, the number of mast cells decreases, and there is a parallel increase in neuronal proliferation. At this stage of the inflammatory process, neuropathic symptoms became prominent, but mast cell reactivation can occur at any time, with an exacerbation of symptoms or acceleration of neurogenic inflammatory processes (Xanthos et al. 2011).

HTPFD can exacerbate symptoms and can itself worsen in response to IC/BPS or vulvodynia flares. A multidisciplinary approach, including referrals to a well-trained physiotherapist or midwife to retraining the pelvic floor, is essential (Graziottin and Gambini 2016). A well-tuned teamwork is vital to address the biological, sexual, and psychosocial factors that contribute to the persistence of vulvar and bladder inflammation that keep on worsening pain in vulvodynia and PBS/IC.

Key Points

Every healthcare provider involved in the diagnosis and cure of vulvar pain in the lifespan should be familiar with the concepts that:

1. Acute vulvar pain can evolve to chronic and neuropathic if etiological factors are not *timely* addressed, particularly in the subset of women with immune-allergic inadequacies/vulnerabilities.
2. Chronic tissue inflammation mediated by the hyperactivated mast cells and other inflammatory cells is the first etiologic factor in vulvar pain.

3. It triggers neuroinflammation with progressive central sensitization and neurogenic neuroinflammation.
4. This changes over time the characteristics of pain perception and reporting by women complaining of vestibular/vulvar pain; of associated introital dyspareunia, either acquired or lifelong; and of medical and sexual comorbidities.
5. Attention to the hyperactivity of the pelvic floor, so frequently associated with vulvar pain, is a mandatory part of the clinical examination and treatment plan.

Cases 3 and 4

I loved making love. I had a satisfying sexual life since my first intercourse, at age 16. I do not want to catch diseases, so I had always used condoms as a protection against sexually transmitted infections (STI) and as contraceptive. I never had STI. My last gynaecological examination was performed 3 years ago, with a normal record and normal pap-smear. Everything was perfect. Then, 2 years ago something started to change. Sometimes I had pain in some positions when penetration was deeper. So I avoided them. Pain got really worse in the last year. Now I have a worsening acute pain during intercourse at deep penetration in every position. Sometimes it is like a stabbing pain. I have to stop in tears. It's a nightmare! Yes, periods were progressively more painful since my adolescence. They are now so debilitating, that I have to take 2 days off work to stay home because of my 'cramping' periods. And my boy-friend cannot understand why I turned to be 'sex-avoidant,' whilst I was so fond of making love with him before!.

Diana, 26 years of age

I detest having periods! They are a curse! Every months I have 2 days of pain, I cannot go to school, meet my friends, do anything. I'm just lying in the bed ingurgitating pain killers until pain goes down a bit. Last year I had my first intercourse. At that time I had little pain at the entrance of the vagina and an horrible pain deep in the vagina. Now I have pain everywhere: at the entrance and deep! My gynaecologist says that I have both vulvodynia and endometriosis, located in the vaginal wall between the vagina and the rectum. He showed me the picture on the atlas and showed that endometriosis invades the "utero-sacral" ligaments that connect the uterus to the sacrum. This is why intercourse is so painful. He says I should do a complex treatment for vulvodynia and be operated for the endometriosis, but I'm very afraid… Why am I so unfortunate?!.

Claudia, 21 years of age

12.9 Clinical Evaluation

Diana's and Claudia's wording suggests endometriosis. Two leading suggestive symptoms are the invalidating and worsening pain during periods and coital pain deep in the vagina, suggesting endometriosis of the uterosacral ligaments and/or in the Douglas pouch, in the posterior fornix, or in the rectovaginal septum. Claudia developed vestibulodynia as well: the comorbidity between the two pathologies induces clinicians to talk about "the evil twins."

12.10 Clinical Examination

At examination, Diana has a specific tenderness at the location of the uterosacral ligaments, with acutely elicited pain when these ligaments are palpated. An ovarian cyst of apricot size is objectively present on the right side. Claudia reports an acute pain and a stabbing pain, at the gynecological examination, when the uterosacral ligament is investigated. She says she has the very same pain when she has intercourse and when she underwent vaginal ecographic evaluation.

Key Practical Point

To explore well the pelvic area, the gynecologist should put the examining index finger between the cervix and the posterior vaginal wall, in the vaginal posterior fornix, to "put in tension" the uterosacral ligaments. If deep endometriosis is present, this maneuver elicits acute pain, exactly the same the woman experiences during intercourse. Every clinician should gently perform this maneuver when patients complain of deep dyspareunia. This provoked pain can be *the first sign of a deep endometriosis* – when the islands of ectopic endometrium are still too little (<2 mm of diameter) to be "seen" with ultrasound, MRI, or even laparoscopy. Yet they contain already some 10–20.000 cells which undergo the typical changes across the menstrual cycle and bleed within the tissue during periods, thus causing a very intense tissue inflammatory response and pain (Graziottin and Gambini 2016).

Therefore, women complaining of severe dysmenorrhea and deep dyspareunia should not be told "you have nothing" when exams are not informative, but "the endometriotic spots that cause your pain are *still too little* to be seen with the current instrumental methods. Yet they are active enough to cause deep inflammation of your pelvic tissues, causing the severe pain you are complaining of. I trust your pain and I'll do my best to relieve it!". This is *an example of a good and respectful communication* aiming at creating a solid trust between the patient and her physician. Then an appropriate medical treatment should be started immediately after the diagnosis: either with a continuous pill (Graziottin 2015a) or a progestogen.

Every specialist in vulvar pain clinics should be aware of the frequent comorbidity between endometriosis, leading to deep dyspareunia, and vulvodynia, causing introital dyspareunia. He/she should look carefully for both conditions as they contribute to increase the "river of inflammation" and the probability of a progressive neuroinflammation (Graziottin et al. 2013, 2014). The brain involvement then translates into a progressive shift to neuropathic pain, sickness behavior, depression, and progressive neurogenic neuroinflammation that can further potentiate the neuropathic pain associated with both conditions (Graziottin et al. 2014).

12.11 Exams

In Diana, the blood sample of the specific marker CA-125 is elevated (56 mU/ml). The ultrasound confirms an ovarian cyst of 5.2 cm in diameter, on the right, suggestive of endometriosis. RM confirms these findings and tiny endometriotic spots deep at the level of the uterosacral ligament. In Claudia, exams are not yet informative.

Key Point

The different exam findings in spite of similar symptoms point out to the need of looking at the "narrative" of a disease, say, its evolution over time that can be different in different people. The moment of the diagnosis is just a photogram in the movie of that disease. This stresses as well the importance of listening carefully to the symptoms' wording (severe dysmenorrhea and deep dyspareunia), as they are very informative about endometriosis as a leading etiological factor. With a rule of thumb, *between symptoms and exams, always trust symptoms first*. And try to give a clinical "meaning" to them with a solid pathophysiologic reading of symptoms and comorbidities.

12.12 Diagnosis

Acquired deep dyspareunia, due to pelvic endometriosis. Diana describes an increasing comorbidity with an avoidant attitude (sexual avoidance), self-protective, to avoid further excruciating pain. Claudia presents with introital dyspareunia, comorbid with VVS/PVD, and deep dyspareunia, comorbid with endometriosis (the "evil twins"). The cases well indicate that comorbidity – sexual and nonsexual – is very frequent and must be diagnosed in her complexity. Attention to the pathophysiologic relationship between different somatic and sexual symptoms should be accurate and comprehensive.

12.13 Comment

The incapacitating dysmenorrhea is a key symptom of endometriosis. Unfortunately it is often neglected or ignored for years until more serious conditions develop, such as ovarian endometrioma, deep dyspareunia, chronic pelvic pain, and/or infertility. Besides endometriosis, which is the most frequent etiology of deep dyspareunia, pelvic inflammatory disease (PID) should be considered as the second leading cause of deep dyspareunia, particularly in promiscuous women who do not use condom consistently. Chronic pelvic pain is the third leading contributor of deep dyspareunia. It can be comorbid with either endometriosis or pelvic inflammatory disease. Irritable bowel syndrome (IBS) is another contributor to abdominal and pelvic pain that should be considered in the clinical evaluation.

Case 5

I never had a problem. I was happy and healthy. I had my first intercourse when I was 17. Little pain the first time, then sex was fun and love. Last year, at 29, I had recurrent bronchitis and had two strong antibiotic treatments. Two weeks later I had a very painful vaginitis from Candida, that never went away completely. Sex became more and more painful at the entrance of the vagina. Even worse, this burning pain may last up to 2–3 days or more. Yes, since that antibiotic treatment, even my bowel habits have changed. I have alternating days of diarrhoea and constipation. Could this contribute to my symptoms? I read that I should eliminate sugars and yeast containing foods from my diet, is that correct?.

Michelle, 30 years of age

12.14 Clinical Evaluation

Michelle' wording suggests that *Candida* vaginitis has been triggered by two strong antibiotic courses, with major consequences on the intestinal and vaginal microbiota (Jayaram et al. 2014; Graziottin and Zanello 2015). Recurrent vaginal *Candida* is the precipitating cause of acquired vulvar vestibulitis/provoked vestibulodynia and acquired introital dyspareunia. Up to 70 % of women complaining of VVS/PVD have comorbidity with recurrent *Candida* vaginitis (see chapter on vulvar pain in adolescents). Irritable bowel syndrome (IBS) is often comorbid after repeated antibiotic courses. Mast cell-driven inflammation, typical of IBS, affects the colonic wall, increasing the vulnerability to allergies and food intolerance. Mast cells are leading as well the inflammatory immunoallergic response to *Candida* infections, contributing to VVS/PVD (see chapter on vulvar pain in adolescents) (Graziottin 2009; Graziottin et al. 2014; Chatterjea and Martinov 2015).

12.15 Clinical Examination

At inspection, the genital region appears inflamed (Fig. 12.1). The vulva is red, with white dense "cottage-cheese-like" leakage suggesting a *Candida* vaginitis; the centrum tendineum of the perineum is retracted and the pelvic floor is tightened. When the woman is requested to breath in with abdominal breathing and then push, she pulls instead. This suggests an "inverted command" of the pelvic floor, and it is an indication to electromyographic biofeedback to help the woman improve her awareness about the pelvic floor muscle relaxation while having an analgesic effect too on the introital pain.

The swab test elicits an acute burning pain at five and seven, when looking at the vaginal entrance as a clockface. At the insertion of the levator ani at the ischiatic spine, mid vagina left and right, tender points are appreciated suggesting levator ani myalgia and the need of biofeedback relaxation training. The remaining gynecological examination is within the normal range. The colon appears tense ("corda colica") and inflamed, suggesting a likely comorbidity with irritable bowel syndrome (IBS), with diarrhea alternated to constipation, often comorbid with VVS/VP, more frequent after antibiotic courses (Graziottin and Gambini 2016).

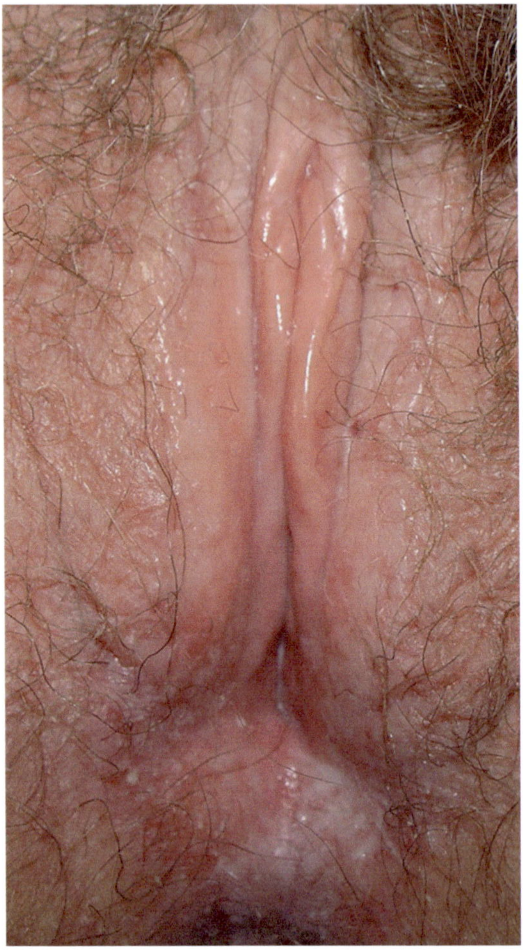

Fig. 12.1 Vulvovaginal candidiasis

12.16 Diagnosis

Candida vulvovaginitis, acquired vulvar vestibulitis/provoked vestibulodynia, acquired introital dyspareunia, and levator ani myalgia, comorbid with IBS.

12.17 Comment

In rats, three episodes of vaginal *Candida* are sufficient to trigger acquired vulvar vestibulitis/PV (Farmer et al. 2011).

Polymorphism in the gene coding for mannose-binding lectin, an innate immune antimicrobial protein that inhibits *Candida* proliferation, and polymorphisms in the genes coding for inflammasomes (macromolecules that regulate the release of interleukin IL-1ß) reduce the production of active IL-1ß necessary for recruitment of immune cells that inactivate yeast. This polymorphism and its associated immune incompetence are more common in vestibulodynia patients with recurrent VVC (Babula et al. 2008).

When a biopsy of the vestibular area is performed, the immunostaining indicates a significant increase of mast cells, on degranulated mast cells and mast cells close to pain fibers. This triad strongly supports the inflammatory nature of the pathophysiological process involving the vestibulum. In the first *Candida* attack, pain is "nociceptive," i.e., a friend signal that indicated the need to withdraw from and/or cure the agent causing pain. When pain becomes chronic, because the etiologic agent has not been recognized and cured, the inflammatory process involves neighbor organs leading to pelvic comorbidities. If still neglected, the inflammatory molecules produced by the mast cells literally "flood" the brain (Graziottin 2009; Graziottin et al. 2013, 2014). A progressive neuroinflammation leads to a maladaptive sickness with malaise, low mood, sleep disorders, impaired cognition, and memory in the most severe cases. Flares of pain may be triggered during periods by the fall of estrogens and progesterone, further stimulating the degranulation of mast cells in the inflamed organs (including the brain). When neuroinflammation persists, the brain takes the lead in the inflammatory process (Skaper et al. 2014; Walker et al. 2013):

- A *neuroinflammation-driven depression* complicates the clinical picture (Graziottin et al. 2013, 2014).
- A *neurogenic peripheral inflammation* contributes to maintain pain in the affected peripheral organ, including the vulva in this case, even when the peripheral etiological factors have been removed.
- A *neurogenic neuroinflammation* maintains active the inflammatory process within the brain. Pain, including vulvar pain, shifts from nociceptive to neuropathic, a real disease per se: the "dynia" phase of vulvar pain (vestibulodynia, vulvodynia, clitorodynia) becomes then the protagonist of the clinical picture.

Moreover, the vagina itself is relatively insensitive to pain, while the vulva and particularly the vulvar vestibule have a high level of free nerve endings (Schober et al. 2015). The levator ani hyperactivity can be provoked or worsened by the increasing inflammation and pain. IBS can be comorbid with VVS/PV in 30–50 % of cases: "the evil twins." Treatment should consider normalizing the bowel inflammation as well, in synergy with a competent gastroenterologist.

A diet with reduced yeast-containing processed food and sugars, with preference for fresh food, vegetables, fish, rice, cereals, and probiotics may improve the intestinal microbiota and contribute to reduce the bowel inflammation. This may positively modulate the "gut-brain" *axis* connection which otherwise may further contribute to the *river of inflammation and pain*.

Case 6

Nobody told me that having a baby could have been such a disaster for a woman. For her health. Her sexual life. Her marriage, too. I'm on the edge of a nervous breakdown! Sex was good until I got pregnant. Then I started to fear that having intercourse would have damaged the child or the pregnancy course. I avoided any more penetration. The delivery has been a nightmare. There were complications. The physician made me a big cut on the genitals (episiotomy) and then jumped on my belly to push the child out (Kristeller's maneuver). I had a terrible pain: I felt I was broken into pieces. The cutting was low to heal, very painful. When we tried to have intercourse after 3 months, pain was horrible, like having a knife pushing inside. I shouted so loud that he lost his erection. I cried all my tears. I have no more desire as I'm so afraid of pain. Yes, I'm still without periods as I'm breastfeeding. My husband is very nervous and aggressive now. He was supportive at the beginning, but now he says that after 2 years without sex he cannot think of spending his whole life in such a way. He says that if I do not find a solution he will get divorce.

Matilda, 35 years of age

12.18 Clinical Evaluation

Matilda's wording suggests postpartum dyspareunia, comorbid with acquired low desire (hypoactive sexual desire disorder, HSDD) and genital arousal difficulties. She looks depressed, and this aspect should be carefully evaluated and treated as well. A severe crisis of the marital relationship is in play.

12.19 Clinical Examination

Her episiotomy scar was tense, retracted, and painful. The vaginal pH was 6, suggesting vaginal dryness caused by the lack of estrogens, due to the continued breastfeeding, and a substantial change of the vaginal microbiota (Graziottin and Zanello 2015). This could be a concomitant etiological factor. Depression substantially contributes to the persistent loss of desire. The aggressive attitude of her husband further complicates the emotional and clinical scenario.

12.20 Diagnosis

Persisting vulvar pain after episiotomy and vaginal dryness concomitant with breastfeeding. Acquired dyspareunia, acquired genital arousal disorder, and acquired loss of sexual desire, causing severe distress and interpersonal difficulties. Comorbidity with depression.

12.21 Comment

The postpartum period is a difficult transitional phase for the woman and the couple ("transition to parenthood"). Besides making the adjustment to meeting their infant's needs, the parent/couple has to face a major reassessment of the erotic intimacy. The most frequent complaint is the vaginal dryness, which correlates with a genital arousal disorder. Comorbidity with low desire is common, more so when a postpartum iron deficiency anemia (IDA) is not adequately cured with iron supplementation, folic acid, vitamin B12, vitamin C, and lactoferrin. Introital dyspareunia is more frequent when episiotomy/episiorrhaphy has been performed with a poor scarring outcome (Barrett et al. 2000; Smith et al. 2013; Graziottin and Gambini 2016).

"Iatrogenic vulvar pain" is the precipitating cause of postpartum vulvar pain (see chapter on vulvar pain in pregnancy and after delivery). It can be further worsened by a dramatic worldwide perpetuating factor: "lack of professional recognition," i.e., medical neglect of sexual pain after delivery, as Glazener stigmatized in her paper about genital sexual pain/dyspareunia in 1997. This neglect about women's and couples' sex life after delivery is still the leading cause of persisting pain even 18 month after delivery in 23 % of women (McDonald et al. 2015). Factor contributing to vulvar pain includes operative deliveries, macrosomic baby, poor surgical outcomes, persisting breastfeeding with vaginal dryness, and lack of genital arousal.

Psychological morbidity is significantly higher in women with vestibulodynia/vulvodynia compared with asymptomatic women. Many studies demonstrate high degrees of anxiety, depressive symptoms, somatization disorders, and hypochondriacal symptoms in vulvodynia patients (Bergeron et al. 2014). Psychological factor activates the corticotrophin-releasing pathway, which increases the vulnerability to pain. However, neuroinflammation is a major biological contributor to depression, sickness behavior, and behavioral correlates (changes in sleep pattern, energy, cognition, memory, coping abilities) in patient affected with chronic inflammation and pain, including those affected by vulvar vestibulitis/provoked vestibulodynia. Neuroinflammation-based depression becomes progressively prominent with the evolution of pain to neuropathic. Restrictive episiotomy with a carefully individualized selection of women seems to be the best choice to reduce the negative impact of episiotomy on women's general and sexual health after delivery (Carroli and Mignini 2009).

Key Point

The "psychogenic" reading of vulvar pain as an "invention" of a woman's mind should therefore be deleted from physicians' diagnostic and curing attitude. The concept of neuroinflammation and associated behavioral changes, including mood swings, must be familiar to every HCP dealing with vulvar pain (and, indeed, with all types of chronic and/or neuropathic pain!).

Case 7

Carol is a 46 nice looking smart lady. Married, no children. She was diagnosed breast cancer at 40, underwent mastectomy of the left breast and immediate breast reconstruction, that looked fairly nice. She had chemotherapy, with anticipated menopause, and then adjuvant treatment with aromatase inhibitors for 5 year. She completed her treatment last year. She is complaining of severe vaginal dryness and introital dyspareunia. Her husband and herself do not like lubricants: 'a fiction of arousal,' as her husband describes it. They are emotionally very close; he has been very supportive with her. She tells the doctor she is very grateful to him because she has seen so many women with breast cancer divorcing because of sexual problems.

He is such a nice guy, doctor! I'm very fortunate to have him in my life. Facing breast cancer with a loving companion is a completely different story than being alone and desperate! That's why I absolutely want to improve my sex life, doctor: for him, for me, for us).

So she was very happy when she read about ospemifene marketed also for women who had completed all the adjuvant treatments after breast cancer. She immediately asked the consulted gynecologist to prescribe it. He confirmed that she had a severe vulvovaginal atrophy. She expected a marvelous change. To her disappointment nothing magic did happen. After more than 1 month the vaginal dryness and introital dyspareunia were almost unchanged. She asked for a second opinion to understand why the drug did not work with her. 'When do you take the drug?', the new gynecologist asked her. 'Well – she said –after breakfast.' 'And what do you usually eat at breakfast?'. 'Just a tea and a skimmed yoghurt.' 'Which is your more important meal?'. 'The dinner, because I enjoy sharing a nice meal with my husband, with a little sweets in the end.' 'Well, my first recommendation is that you take ospemifene after dinner: a higher content in fat in your meal can double and even triple the absorption of the drug. If the drug is not adequately absorbed it cannot work and help you! And by the way, I also recommend that you take it possibly at the same hour of the day, to guarantee the constancy of the blood level. Another help for a better result.' 'If you have severe pain at intercourse it is very likely that vaginal dryness is not the only critical factor. I'm sure that other causes are in play….'

Her clinical examination proved to be extremely useful in understanding why the drug 'did not work (yet).' The vestibular area was very sensitive to pain at 5 and 7 'o clock, when explored with the swab test and the gloved finger. A very tightened hyperactive pelvic floor was as well diagnosed. 'Ospemifene cannot work if we do not first cure the vulvar vestibulitis/provoked vestibulodynia that is clearly causing the pain you have at the beginning of the penetration and if we do nor relax your pelvic floor. It is so tightened!'.

The new gynecologist recommended rehabilitation of the pelvic floor with physiotherapy, hands-on massage and stretching of the posterior part of the levator ani and moulds while curing the VVs/PVD. 'I'm so happy you explain all these reasons to me doctor. I'll do everything you recommend because I really want to get out of this problem!'.

After 4 months, twelve session of physiotherapy and the pharmacologic treatment for VVS/PVD Carol came back with a great smile: 'You were right doctor. The drug I was prescribed was correct but there were some info and work missing. The physiotherapist you suggested is just great. She did a marvelous work on my pelvic floor. I feel a different woman altogether. And now ospemifene works very well! It's like a dream coming true after so many years of pain. My husband sends his grateful greetings as well!'.

Carol, 46 years old

12.22 Clinical Evaluation

Carol presents with the typical severe VVA of women who had menopause and underwent aromatase inhibitor adjuvant treatment. However, the evaluation must not be minimalistic. When severe acquired introital dyspareunia is complained of, other factors can contribute. A hyperactive pelvic floor is to be carefully considered as a key contributor of introital pain, independently from VVA, particularly in women who are nulliparous or who had cesarean section, because their pubococcygeus muscle has never been dilated by delivery. A tightened pelvic floor is even more likely to be diagnosed in nulliparous women after the menopause, when muscle fibers tend to be substituted by collagen. Vulvar vestibulitis/vestibular vulvodynia is another cause of acquired introital pain to be considered *also* after the menopause.

12.23 Clinical Examination

At first visual inspection, a hyperactive pelvic floor is clearly in play. The centrum tendineum of the perineum is very retracted; a sentinel hemorrhoid at twelve suggests an "inverted command" of the pelvic floor. This means that the woman pulls the pelvic floor when she intends to push: this is per se a clear indication to physiotherapy and electromyographic feedback to learn how to properly command the relaxation of the pelvic floor when she pushes. With the examining swab, pain is exquisitely elicited at 5 and 7 of the vestibulum, suggesting VVS/PVD. At physical evaluation, tender points are elicited at the insertion of the levator ani at the ischiatic spine bilaterally. A myalgic levator ani is appreciated along the palpation of the pubococcygeus muscle bilaterally. Both the hyperactive myalgic pelvic floor and VVS/PVD must be adequately treated before the SERM ospemifene can express its full therapeutic potential. The vaginal pH is 7, as expected, coherently with a prolonged lack of estrogens and severe VVA.

12.24 Diagnosis

Severe VVA, VVS/PVD, hyperactive myalgic pelvic floor with inverted command, acquired introital dyspareunia in a breast cancer patient with anticipated iatrogenic menopause who has completed the adjuvant treatments. She is candidate to ospemifene therapy once VVS/PVD and the hyperactive myalgic pelvic floor have been treated.

12.25 Comment

Carol's clinical history clearly stresses the absolute need of a careful detailed comprehensive diagnosis of the likely multifactorial etiology of acquired introital dyspareunia, more so after breast cancer.

A multifactorial therapy is to be planned to allow ospemifene to specifically improve the VVA-related contribution of vaginal dryness and introital dyspareunia.

Case 8

Elisabeth is a 63-year-old woman. She has been happily married for almost 40 years. She enjoys four children and five grandchildren. She had no specific symptoms at menopause, besides moderate hot flashes, so she decided not to use hormone therapy. She has developed progressive vaginal dryness. In the last year intercourse has become frankly painful.

I love my husband and I do not want to make him feel rejected. He feels that if I'm dry I have no more desire for him. Well, yes, I do not have the drive I was used to, but I still enjoy our intimacy were it not for that pain that is becoming worse and worse. Yes, I often suffer from vaginitis and cystitis caused by the same germ, *Escherichia coli*… I feel dry in my vagina [she indicates the vulva!]. Is there an effective treatment for me? In the last year my body caused me so much pain and symptoms that I suddenly felt I'm getting old….

Elizabeth, 63 years of age

12.26 Clinical Evaluation

Elizabeth's wording suggests specific menopause-triggered biological problems: vulvovaginal atrophy (VVA) and vaginal dryness, predisposing to introital dyspareunia, and recurrent vaginitis and cystitis from *Escherichia coli*, a saprophytic germ of colonic origin, in the context of a good couple relationship and a serene family life. Interestingly, she calls "vagina" the vulva, i.e., the external genitalia, as many women do (Graziottin, 2015b).

As a practical note, physicians should always clarify with their patients where exactly symptoms are perceived/referred to: the vulva, the vagina, or both, as it is the case in the postmenopausal vulvovaginal atrophy (VVA, a subset of the genitourinary syndrome of menopause, GSM) (see chapter on vulvar pain after the menopause).

12.27 Clinical Examination

External genitalia present with vulvar dystrophy, dry skin, involution of the labia, and white hair. The vagina looks atrophic as well, with a subtle, pale rose mucosa. The vaginal pH is 7.0, which suggests vaginal atrophy because of the persistent lack of estrogens.

12.28 Diagnosis

Vulvovaginal atrophy (VVA). Acquired genital arousal disorder with acquired dyspareunia and personal distress. Comorbidity with recurrent vaginitis and cystitis from saprophytic pathogens (*Escherichia coli*).

12.29 Comment

Vaginal dryness is the second most frequent sexual complaint during the postmenopausal years, after loss of desire. Comorbidity with recurrent vaginitis and cystitis is frequent. Comorbidity between genital arousal disorder and acquired introital dyspareunia is also frequent, when the atrophic vaginitis is complicated by vulvar dystrophy, which contributes to introital dyspareunia.

Unfortunately, vaginal dryness is underreported, underdiagnosed, and undertreated in the majority of postmenopausal women (see chapter on vulvar pain after the menopause). An easy to be treated problem may therefore turn into a major cause of loss of sexual intimacy and sexual avoidance even between loving partners.

These cases well illustrate that vulvar pain and pain during intercourse can present in many different ways, depending on where in her reproductive cycle the woman is, besides other factors.

Case 9

I had my menopause at 52, I did not do any hormonal treatment because I was afraid of breast cancer. Now, at 56, sex is impossible because of pain. I'm so narrow that nothing gets in. The young doctor who tried to do the pap-smears could not insert the speculum. She said I had a disease of the vulva ('lichen sclerosus') that has almost closed the entrance of the vagina. And that it can turn into a cancer! Is there any treatment to avoid the cancer and open the vagina? I have a new partner….

Sophia, 56 years of age

12.30 Clinical Evaluation

Night itch is Sophia's main symptom, with some daily flares of itch as well. She complains also of painful intercourse (acquired introital dyspareunia) and vulvar/vestibular pain as a consequence of erosions, fissures, and introital narrowing.

12.31 Clinical Examination

Typical lesions like porcelain-white papules and plaques are visible, often associated with areas of ecchymosis and scratching lesions. Architectural modifications, also designated as "scarring," resulting from adhesions (synechiae) between two contiguous surfaces involved by the disease, are other relevant findings.

12.32 Diagnosis

Severe vulvar lichen sclerosus, with labial conglutination and stenosis of the vaginal introitus. Acquired introital dyspareunia (Fig. 12.2).

12.33 Comments

Lichen sclerosus is a chronic inflammatory – and probably autoimmune – disorder which commonly affects the ano-genital-vulvar skin. The most common symptoms are *pruritus/itching*, mostly perceived at night, and pain with frequent relapses and remissions. The lifetime risk of squamous cell carcinoma of the vulva is low but not negligible, in the order of 5 %.

Adhesions of the clitoral hood can result in the formation of a retention pseudocyst, and narrowing of the introitus can make intercourse and/or micturition difficult or impossible to treat from the medical (i.e., with drugs) point of view.

Conventionally, ultrapotent topical corticosteroid cream or ointment is the recommended treatment of choice: high response rates have been reported from large case series of women diagnosed with lichen sclerosus, with either complete or partial resolution of symptoms in 54–96 % of women (Simonetta et al. 2015). Topical estriol on the vestibule and the vagina, and testosterone cream (prepared by the

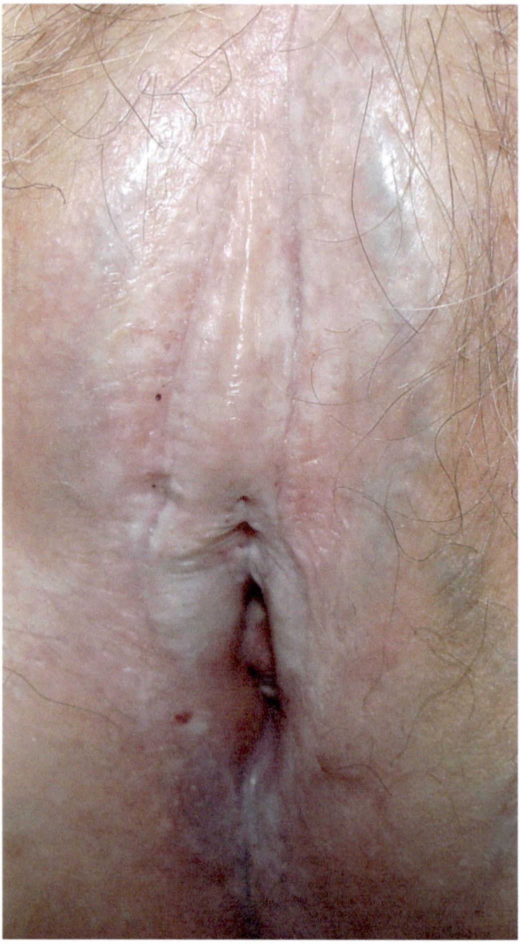

Fig. 12.2 Lichen sclerosus

pharmacist), should be applied on the vulva and in the vagina, with a careful application of the anterior vaginal wall, to improve the urethral symptoms as well. This combined treatment definitely improves the vaginal stenosis.

Progressive massage and stretching of the vaginal introitus and rehabilitation of the pelvic floor (when hyperactivity of the elevator ani is in place) address the "biomechanical" component of the introital coital pain in patients with lichen sclerosus and vulvar pain. The physical therapy should be combined with topical creams/gels.

The clitoral adhesions can be divided surgically. Surgery for vulvar lichen sclerosus should be considered to counteract the effects of the scarring produced by the disease with different goals according to the individual problem: dissection of a buried clitoris, division of fused labia or clitoral hood, or release of introital fusion or stenosis (Gurumurthy et al. 2012).

Conclusions

Clinical cases have been selected, illustrated, and commented with a few specific goals:

- Highlight the fact that *vulvar pain exists* and is complained of in the lifespan.
- Stress the importance of a careful:
  - Listening of the *woman's wording*, of the narrative of *pain experience* with special attention to the *predisposing*, *precipitating*, and *perpetuating factors* (including a persistent diagnostic omission of the biological truth of vulvar pain).
  - Reporting in the medical record the first symptoms and affected organ (not necessarily the vulva) and then the progression of symptoms and associated comorbidities, both pelvic and systemic, including depression.
  - *Physical examination* that is essential to diagnose the etiology of vulvar pain: no exam can surrogate a very accurate inspection and palpation of the vulva, elevator ani, internal genitals, and deep pelvic structures.
- Stimulate colleagues to update their knowledge in anatomy, endocrinology, pathophysiology, and semeiology of the vulvar organ and to improve their ability to "read" with a clinically competent sight what they see.

The perception of an increased motivation and skill in diagnosing and treating vulvar pain in the daily office activity would be the most rewarding feedback from our readers. Please let us know.

References

Babula O, Linhares IM, Bongiovanni AM, Ledger WJ, Witkin SS. Association between primary vulvar vestibulitis syndrome, defective induction of tumor necrosis factor-alpha, and carriage of the mannose-binding lectin codon 54 gene polymorphism. Am J Obstet Gynecol. 2008; 198:101.e1–4.

Barrett G, Pendry E, Peacock J, Victor C, Thakar R, Manyonda I. Women's sexual health after childbirth. BJOG. 2000;107:186–95.

Bergeron S, Likes WM, Steben M. Psychosexual aspects of vulvovaginal pain. Best Pract Res Clin Obstet Gynaecol. 2014;28:991–9.

Carroli G, Mignini L. Episiotomy for vaginal birth. Cochrane Database Syste Rev. 2009;(1):CD000081. doi:10.1002/14651858.CD000081. pub2. (Meta-Analysis).

Chatterjea D, Martinov T. Mast cells: versatile gatekeepers of pain. Mol Immunol. 2015;63(1):38–44.

Farmer MA, Taylor AM, Bailey AL, Tuttle AH, MacIntyre LC, Milagrosa ZE. Repeated vulvovaginal fungal infections cause persistent pain in a mouse model of vulvodynia. Sci Transl Med. 2011;3:101ra91.

Glazener CM. Sexual function after childbirth: women's experiences, persistent morbidity and lack of professional recognition. Br J Obstet Gynaecol. 1997;104(3):330–5.

Graziottin A. Sexual pain disorders: dyspareunia and vaginismus. In: Porst H, Buvat J, editors. ISSM (International Society of Sexual Medicine) Standard Committee Book, Standard practice in Sexual Medicine. Oxford: Blackwell; 2006. p. 342–50.

Graziottin A. Mast cells and their role in sexual pain disorders. In: Goldstein A, Pukall C, Goldstein I, editors. Female sexual pain disorders: evaluation and management. Chichester: Blackwell Publishing; 2009. p. 176–9.

Graziottin A. "The shorter, the better": a review of the evidence for a shorter contraception hormone-free interval. Eur J Contrac Repro Health Care. 2015a;20:1–13. [Epub ahead of print].

Graziottin A. Vaginal biological and sexual health: the unmet needs. Climacteric. 2015b;18 Suppl 1:9–12. doi:10.3109/13697137.2015.1079408.

Graziottin A, Gambini D. Evaluation of genito-pelvic pain penetration disorder. In: Waguih WI, editor. The textbook of sexual medicine. Boston: Springer; 2016.

Graziottin A, Murina F. Clinical management of vulvodynia. Milan: Springer; 2011.

Graziottin A, Skaper S, Fusco M. Inflammation and chronic pelvic pain: a biological trigger for depression in women? J Depress Anxiety. 2013;3:142–50.

Graziottin A, Skaper S, Fusco M. Mast cells in chronic inflammation, pelvic pain and depression in women. Gynecol Endocrinol. 2014;30(7):472–7.

Graziottin A, Zanello PP. Pathogenic biofilms: their role in recurrent cystitis and vaginitis (with focus on D-mannose as a new prophylactic strategy). In: Studd J, Seang LT, Chervenak FA, editors. Current progress in obstetrics and gynaecology, vol. 3. 2nd ed. Mumbai: Kothari Medical; 2015. p. 218–38.

Gurumurthy M, Morah N, Gioffre G, Cruickshank ME. The surgical management of complications of vulval lichen sclerosus. Eur J Obstet Gynecol Reprod Biol. 2012;162(1):79–82.

Jayaram A, Witkin SS, Zhou X, Brown CJ, Rey GE, Linhares IM, Ledger WJ, Forney LJ. The bacterial microbiome in paired vaginal and vestibular samples from women with vulvarvestibulitis syndrome. Pathog Dis. 2014;72(3):161–6.

McDonald EA, Gartland D, Small R, Brown SJ. Dyspareunia and childbirth: a prospective cohort study. BJOG. 2015;122(5):672–9. doi:10.1111/1471-0528.13263. Epub 2015 Jan 21.

Peters KM, Killinger KA, Carrico DJ, Ibrahim IA, Diokno AC, Graziottin A. Sexual function and sexual distress in women with interstitial cystitis: a case control study. Urology. 2007;70(3):543–7.

Reed BD, Harlow SD, Sen A, Edwards RM, Chen D, Haefner HK. Relationship between vulvodynia and chronic comorbid pain conditions. Obstet Gynecol. 2012;120:145–51.

Salonia A, Clementi MC, Graziottin A, Nappi RE, Castiglione F, Ferrari M, Capitanio U, Damiano R, Montorsi F. Secondary provoked vestibulodynia in sexually-active women with recurrent uncomplicated urinary tract infections. J Sex Med. 2013;10(9):2265–73.

Schaible HG. Emerging concepts of pain therapy based on neuronal mechanisms. Handb Exp Pharmacol. 2015;227:1–14.

Schober J, Aardsma N, Mayoglou L, Pfaff D, Martín-Alguacil N. Terminal innervation of female genitalia, cutaneous sensory receptors of the epithelium of the labia minora. Clin Anat. 2015;28(3):392–8.

Simonetta C, Burns EK, Guo MA. Vulvar dermatoses: a review and update. Mo Med. 2015;112(4):301–7.

Skaper SD, Facci L, Giusti P. Mastcells, glia and neuroinflammation: partners in crime? Immunology. 2014;141(3):314–27. doi:10.1111/imm.12170.

Smith LA, Price N, Simonite V, Burns EE. Incidence of and risk factors for perineal trauma: a prospective observational study. BMC Pregnancy Childbirth. 2013;13:59.

Walker AK, Kavelaars A, Heijnen CJ, Dantzer R. Neuroinflammation and comorbidity of pain and depression. Pharmacol Rev. 2013;66(1):80–101.

Xanthos DN, Gaderer S, Drdla R, Nuro E, Abramova A, Ellmeier W, Sandkühler J. Central nervous system mast cells in peripheral inflammatory nociception. Mol Pain. 2011;7:42. doi:10.1186/1744-8069-7-42.

MIX
Papier aus verantwortungsvollen Quellen
Paper from responsible sources
FSC® C105338

If you have any concerns about our products,
you can contact us on
ProductSafety@springernature.com

In case Publisher is established outside the EU,
the EU authorized representative is:
Springer Nature Customer Service Center GmbH
Europaplatz 3, 69115 Heidelberg, Germany

Printed by Libri Plureos GmbH
in Hamburg, Germany